SURGERY FOR NURSES

KU-600-645

THE AUTHOR

# JAMES MORONEY

M.B., Ch.B., F.R.C.S.(Eng.), L.R.C.P.(Lond.)

Consultant Surgeon, Broadgreen Hospital, Liverpool
Clinical Lecturer in Surgery, University of Liverpool
Examiner in Surgery to the
General Nursing Council for England and Wales
Formerly Hunterian Professor,
Royal College of Surgeons of England

# SURGERY FOR NURSES

JAMES MORONEY

THIRTEENTH EDITION

CHURCHILL LIVINGSTONE
EDINBURGH LONDON AND NEW YORK 1975

Churchill Livingstone

Medical Division of Longman Group Limited

Distributed in the United States of America by Longman Inc., New York and by associated companies, branches and representatives throughout the world.

© LONGMAN GROUP LIMITED, 1975

*All rights reserved. No part of this publication may be reproduced, stored in a retrieval system, or transmitted in any form or by any means, electronic, mechanical, photo-copying, recording or otherwise, without the prior permis-sion of the publishers (Churchill Livingstone, 23 Ravelston Terrace, Edinburgh)*

| | |
|---|---|
| First Edition | 1950 |
| Second Edition | 1952 |
| Reprinted | 1954 |
| Third Edition | 1955 |
| Fourth Edition | 1956 |
| Fifth Edition | 1958 |
| Sixth Edition | 1959 |
| Seventh Edition | 1961 |
| Eighth Edition | 1962 |
| Ninth Edition | 1964 |
| Tenth Edition | 1966 |
| Eleventh Edition | 1967 |
| Eleventh Edition Reprinted | 1969 |
| Twelfth Edition | 1971 |
| Twelfth Edition Reprinted | 1972 |
| E.L.B.S. Edition first published | 1971 |
| E.L.B.S. Edition Reprinted | 1972 |
| Thirteenth Edition | 1975 |
| E.L.B.S. Edition of Thirteenth Edition | 1975 |

ISBN 0 443 01186 9

**Library of Congress Cataloging in Publication Data**
Moroney, James.
  Surgery for nurses.
  Bibliography: p.
  Includes index.
  1. Surgical Nursing. 2. Operations, Surgical.
I. Title [DNLM: 1. Surgery, Operative–Nursing texts.
2. Surgical nursing. WY161 M868s].
RD99.M73     1975     610.73'677     74-81756

Printed in Great Britain
by R. & R. Clark Ltd, Edinburgh

# Preface to the Thirteenth Edition

THE decision to print this edition by a new process has presented me with a splendid opportunity to re-write the whole book as well as to remake every illustration.

There are new chapters on Pain, The Nature of Disease, and Iatrogenic Disorders. More than thirty nursing procedures have been described in considerable detail and this fulfils more completely the ambition expressed in the second paragraph of the Preface to the First Edition more than a quarter of a century ago. The aim of the book to provide a simple, well-illustrated up-to-date text for the student nurse remains unchanged.

*1975*                                                   James Moroney

# Extract from the Preface to the First Edition

IN writing this book for nurses I have had constantly in mind the difficulties and anxieties which confront the student nurse preparing for the Final State Examination and at the same time undertaking an increasing amount of responsible work in the wards.

The subject matter is based on the syllabus of the General Nursing Council, and in each section I have endeavoured to include an account of the nursing care which is so inseparable a part of the treatment of every surgical condition.

Without unduly sacrificing the space devoted to general surgery, sections on the more specialised branches of surgery have been included.

While it is written primarily for the student I hope that the trained nurse may find it a useful book of reference.

1949                                                     James Moroney

# Acknowledgements

The author gratefully acknowledges his indebtedness to many who have helped in the preparation of this book:

*Special Contributions*

    H. M. Alty (Dental and facio-maxillary surgery)
    D. M. J. Burns (Ophthalmology)
    John Campbell (Haematology)
    R. B. Crosbie (Neonatal surgery)
    F. Ronald Edwards (Cardiothoracic and oesophageal surgery)
    Mark Moroney (Biographical notes)
    J. C. Richardson (Resuscitation in all its aspects)
    P. M. Stell (Ear, nose and throat surgery)
    Charles West (Neurosurgery)

*Preparation of the Manuscript*

| | |
|---|---|
| Joan Bowstead | Margaret Lane |
| M. R. Colmer | J. N. Rimmer |
| M. E. Jackson | V. E. Wigley |

*Preparation of Illustrations*

| | |
|---|---|
| C. J. Fitz-Simons | E. Oliver |
| E. Wilkinson | |

*Proof-reading and Index*

| | |
|---|---|
| Paul Aukland | E. E. Fenn |

*Overall Editing and Collation*

    Mark Moroney

*Nursing Procedures*

    Broadgreen Hospital School of Nursing

*Clinical Photographs*

    Mr A. B. Wallace and the *Lancet*
    Mr P. P. Rickham and *Pediatric Clinics of North America*
    Mr P. P. Rickham
    Surgeons of Alder Hey Hospital, Liverpool
    (Neonatal and Paediatric conditions)

*Illustrations*

    *British Medical Journal* and Dr Howes and Osborn

# Contents

CHAPTER                                                                          PAGE
1 Surgery, the Nurse, and the Patient . . . . 1
2 Surgical Diagnosis and the Nurse . . . . 7
3 Identification of the Patient . . . . . 14
4 The Preoperative and Postoperative Care of the
   Patient . . . . . . . . 18
5 Pain . . . . . . . . . 35
6 Infection and Immunity . . . . . 40
7 Microbiology . . . . . . . 48
8 Inflammation . . . . . . . 63
9 The Specific Surgical Infections . . . . 70
10 Sterilisation . . . . . . . . 80
11 Asepsis and Theatre Technique . . . . 86
12 Surgical Ward Dressings . . . . . 101
13 Haemorrhage . . . . . . . 108
14 Thrombosis and Embolism . .. . . 127
15 Acute Circulatory Failure . . . . . 135
16 Fluid and Electrolyte Balance . . . . 146
17 Fluid Administration . . . . . . 153
18 Respiratory Failure . . . . . . 162
19 Burns and Scalds . . . . . . . 181
20 Trauma . . . . . . . . 190
21 Diseases of the Skin, Muscle and Tendon . . 198
22 New Growths . . . . . . . 210
23 Diseases of the Peripheral Arteries and Gangrene . 225
24 Varicose Veins . . . . . . . 237
25 The Nature of Disease . . . . . . 240
26 The Lymphatic System and the Spleen . . . 248
27 Organ and Tissue Transplantation . . . . 252
28 The Mouth, the Face, and the Tongue . . . 257
29 The Endocrine Glands . . . . . . 275
30 Diseases of the Breast . . . . . . 287

31  Diseases of the Lungs and Thorax . . . . 303
32  Surgery of the Heart . . . . . . 318
33  Diseases of the Oesophagus . . . . . 326
34  The Acute Abdomen . . . . . . 333
35  Stomach and Duodenum . . . . . 359
36  Diseases of the Liver, the Gall-bladder and the
      Pancreas . . . . . . . . 384
37  Diseases of the Small Intestine . . . . 402
38  Diseases of the Caecum and the Colon . . . 408
39  Diseases of the Rectum and the Anus . . . 423
40  Hernia . . . . . . . . 437
41  Diseases of the Kidney and Ureter . . . . 441
42  Diseases of the Bladder, the Prostate, and the
      Male Genital Organs . . . . . . 466
43  Neonatal Surgery (The Surgery of the Newborn) . 492
44  Surgical Aspects of Tropical Diseases . . . 502
45  Injuries and Diseases of the Central Nervous System 505
46  The Peripheral Nerves . . . . . . 531
47  Fractures . . . . . . . . 539
48  Diseases of Bone . . . . . . . 557
49  Diseases of the Joints . . . . . . 562
50  Diseases of the Ear, the Nose, and the Throat . . 572
51  Diseases of the Eye . . . . . . 586
52  Gynaecology . . . . . . . 603
53  Iatrogenic Disorders . . . . . . 629
54  Some Biographical Notes . . . . . 636
    Table of Approximate Normal Values . . . 645
    Index . . . . . . . . . 646

# CHAPTER 1
# Surgery, the Nurse, and the Patient

Surgery is one of the most ancient arts in the world. Its oldest branch, obstetric surgery, is almost as old as the world itself. The daring and manual dexterity of the barber-surgeon were surpassed only by the courage and forbearance of his conscious patient. Survival of such an ordeal was followed by many months in bed, during which time 'laudable' pus drained from the wound. Much less than a century ago the surgeon of that day operated without even washing his hands, and was clad in a top hat and a frock coat well stained with blood and pus. For convenience, he carried his ligature and suture materials in the buttonhole of his lapel!

The discovery of anaesthetics and the appreciation of the importance of eliminating infection in the patient's wound have transformed the surgical art. Each year adds much to the vast store of knowledge, even to the knowledge of such fundamentals as the sciences of anaesthetics and asepsis. The comparatively recent advances of blood transfusion and chemotherapy are examples of some of the outstanding achievements of contemporary scientists.

A century ago there were no skilled nurses as we know them today. The nurse's predecessor was often an illiterate, rough, dirty handywoman, and in many institutions a patient was in great measure dependent on what help he could secure from the patient in the adjoining bed.

Surgery, surgeons, and nurses have changed considerably in a century, but the plea for relief from suffering has remained essentially the same. Every patient is a man, woman, or child living and working in different surroundings and in different spheres of activity. They are all different—different in outlook, different in character, different in their reaction to the same disease. Appreciation of the importance of this individual variation is a fundamental principle of good nursing.

Surgical treatment is usually undertaken away from the patient's own home. The advantages are overwhelming, for many procedures would be impossible even in the home of a millionaire. There is one serious disadvantage, however, in that hospital staffs have few opportunities of visiting ill patients in their own homes. It is surprising at times to see what 'home' means, and the advice given to a patient on leaving hospital must be considered against this background. The current trend of nursing education aims at a 'wider basic training' with secondment of the student to the community nurse.

The patient's mental outlook, his fears, his hopes, and his will, may play a part equal in importance to the purely physical treatment of his disease. To ignore, to be unaware of, or to neglect these factors may make a patient prefer death to a struggle, and then no amount of effort may be able to regain the valuable ground which has been lost or opportunities which have been cast away.

The nurse can do much to allay and alleviate the inevitable anxieties of the surgical patient, on arrival, and throughout his stay in the ward. Success, or failure, will be determined by:

## THE APPLICATION OF PROFESSIONAL KNOWLEDGE

There can be no substitute for knowledge gained by study and experience. Since its projection is ultimately on human beings, its first impact is on the patient's mind.

It is obvious that the patient's confidence will be gained and maintained only by a combination of knowledge and understanding.

## HER APPRECIATION OF THE AIMS OF MODERN SURGICAL TREATMENT

Without a high order of technical competence and anatomical knowledge, in surgeon and nurse alike, no operation could be a success. The operation, however, is only a part, albeit an important part, of treatment. To the patient it is dominant and likely to be most feared. While a scar may be the only visible anatomical distortion, physiological and psychological changes may be profound and with the passage of time may cause increasing disability. To diminish or alleviate these disabilities requires the exercise of sympathy and judgment at least equal to the operative skill.

An operation is not an inevitable sequel of admission to a surgical ward, because many conditions subside without operative treatment. An operation may be:

1. An emergency. This is performed only when there is an immediate threat to life from haemorrhage, respiratory or intestinal obstruction, or a spreading infection not likely to be controlled by conservative measures alone.
2. Planned (elective). Strategically this is the most desirable, because it can be undertaken when the patient's general and local conditions are controlled to the maximal degree.
3. Multistaged. This may be necessary because:
    (a) The patient's condition is not good enough to do all that is necessary at once, or

(b) The first operation may be designed to rest or drain an organ or cavity, so that subsequent curative measures can be safely undertaken.

(c) Reoperation. This may be necessary for a complication and is particularly distressing to the patient and disappointing to the surgeon and nurse.

The aim of surgery is to assist and not to usurp the place of natural healing. For this reason timing may be as important as the nature and extent of the operation.

*Human sympathy and understanding*

It is a fair presumption that one becomes a nurse because one is activated by a desire to help others in distress. In addition, one must have an imaginative mind and considerable tact and patience. Only by imagining oneself in the patient's position can it be realised how he is feeling and how one can help. The background of professional knowledge and detailed care is discussed in Chapter 4. The following aspects of some of these subjects are discussed from the point of view of the nurse–patient relationship.

RECEPTION

The relationship must be established at once—it is that of the good hostess and the welcome guest—natural, kind, and cheerful. Questions should be answered simply and there is no place for dramatisation. Many questions can be answered only by the sister of the ward who will refer all questions on diagnosis and prognosis to the medical staff. Arrangements should be made for the patient to see his relatives, the medical social worker, and a minister of religion if he so desires— all of whom have a part to play in assisting him to settle down peacefully and quietly.

PREPARATION OF THE PATIENT

The patient may be admitted for an emergency operation, or for one where time is a less urgent factor. Where there are several days in hand, the nurse can get to know the patient as an individual and consider how he will react to the various preparations, and how they are best undertaken. It is now customary to admit a patient the evening before or even on the day of operation. Many preliminary preparations are undertaken as an outpatient.

1. *Consent form.* This has to be signed by the patient before any operative procedure can be undertaken. It is a medical responsibility to see that this is done (p. 89).

2. *Collection of specimens.* Blood may have to be taken by the doctor or by the phlebotomist for examination or for cross-matching. This is the first experience of a hospital procedure.

The reason given for the procedure, and how it is performed, may well determine the patient's future attitude. An efficient vein tourniquet and really sharp needles, with an adequate choice to ensure that the smallest possible needle is used, are important in fulfilling the promise that it is really 'only a little prick'. Urine is tested without the patient's knowledge, but it is usually better that he should be told about it.

3. *Dental hygiene* may have been poor and require correction.

4. *Physiotherapy* may be necessary to improve pulmonary function.

5. *Skin preparation.* This is discussed fully on page 29. Plenty of soap should be used. Disposable razors are cheap and hygienic. A quiet unhurried preparation with the patient engaged in conversation may well increase his confidence.

6. *Bowel.* In the few cases where an enema or washout is necessary the patient will require reassurance, and a simple explanation makes the nurse's task easier.

SPECIAL POINTS TO BEAR IN MIND IN THE POSTOPERATIVE PERIOD

The nurse must always look beyond the operation to the postoperative period and anticipate how her own difficulties may be diminished by a judicious word beforehand. The patient is made to feel that everything will be done to minimise the discomfort.

*Pain and sleep.* The patient quite rightly desires reassurance that he will not be kept awake by pain.

*Diet.* While everyone may appear very satisfied with the patient, he may be wondering how he will recover on a diet of fluids alone. A simple reassurance of the importance of a fluid diet at this stage can often allay these fears.

*Blood transfusion.* If a postoperative blood transfusion is likely to be running, it is as well to say beforehand that this is usual. The patient will feel that he is being well cared for and not that some unexpected complication has arisen.

*Oxygen therapy* may be particularly alarming, as many patients consider it to be a last desperate measure. If it is to be used postoperatively he should be accustomed to it before operation.

*Breathing exercises* are important but may be painful, and special care must be taken if the best result is to be achieved. Arrangements may be made for him to see the physiotherapist preoperatively.

*Fear of bursting a wound.* This is a point on which all patients desire reassurance, because this is exactly the sensation that arises from distension of viscera beneath an abdominal wound. Unless they are reassured, they will not move about freely in bed.

*Drainage tubes.* Their removal causes some discomfort, and an analgesic such as aspirin 600 mg one or two hours beforehand may be given but is not usually necessary.

*Care of wound.* A clean wound is kept covered, and no special treatment is necessary unless there is reason to suspect that it has become infected. Drainage tubes are usually sited away from the main wound. Daily dressing of the drainage tube site and cleansing should be performed. Not unnaturally, the patient, who is encouraged to move his legs and his chest, may think that his wound has been forgotten and a word of explanation is necessary to ease what may be a suppressed anxiety on this account.

*Removal of the stitches.* Anticipation always worries the patient. It can be quietly explained that it is only the stitch that is cut.

*Any other postoperative procedure* which may worry the patient should be anticipated in advance, for example, the cuff of the sphygmomanometer can be put on the patient's arm preoperatively if frequent postoperative blood-pressure estimations are required. In some units these readings may be monitored.

The patient in whom a gross mutilation has to be undertaken requires more than ordinary care, as well as special sympathy, and the nurse cannot know too much about the various devices and treatment to help these patients. The patient, when he leaves hospital, should feel that, in his misfortune, be it minor or serious, everything possible was done to rehabilitate him. At least he should have no reason to feel that they —'they' in this case being the hospital staff—never realised what they had done to him.

### RELATIONSHIP OF DISEASE TO EMOTION AND OF EMOTION TO DISEASE

With experience, these relationships become well known to the nurse, but there is always the proviso that if they are taken too much for granted as a routine the patient's complaint may be neglected.

Certain lesions, such as thyrotoxicosis, peptic ulcer, and ulcerative colitis, are conditions where stress seems to play a part in their aetiology or their aggravation. All patients suffering from these conditions are anxious but, of course, there are other causes of anxiety.

The overanxious patient is liable to a higher incidence of complications which a more phlegmatic character may avoid. They include:

1. *Retention of urine.* In many cases, where there is no mechanical obstruction, retention may be purely nervous in

origin, particularly following operations on the perineum and anus or on any occasion when the recumbent position has to be assumed postoperatively.

2. *Air swallowing.* Air swallowing (aerophagy) sometimes results in dilatation of the stomach and again is a nervous reaction.

3. *Thrombosis.* This is more liable to occur in the patient who lies stiff and immobile in bed and movement must be encouraged.

4. *Tachycardia.* Many patients develop postoperative tachycardia in the absence of haemorrhage or toxaemia, and it can in itself be very wearisome. Sedation is usually indicated.

5. *General exhaustion* from:
   (a) Lack of rest and inadequate sleep;
   (b) Failure to take adequate nourishment because of nervous upset of digestion;
   (c) Persistent hiccough which is particularly difficult to control.

The mind and body are an integrated whole, and any attempt to manage them in isolation from one another is doomed to failure. The patient may be shy, reserved, taciturn and resent loss of dignity—he may be worried about his job or his family.

In addition to some of the detailed points which have been discussed above, the following are of considerable importance to the patients:

*The pattern of his day.* The more normal this can be the more normally we can expect the patient to react. Most patients are not accustomed to being awakened in the early hours of the morning, and if this can be avoided it is a great advantage.

*The elimination of noise.* It is unfortunately true that the hospital environment is often noisy and disturbed rather than quiet and peaceful.

*Explanation.* A simple explanation of what is happening is too often avoided.

# CHAPTER 2

# Surgical Diagnosis and the Nurse

Accurate diagnosis is the corner-stone of treatment. It is the doctor who makes the diagnosis after he has elucidated all the facts. The nurse's observation may be most important, particularly over a period when the patient's condition is changing.

## HISTORY

A careful history is the most important single part of diagnosis. What the patient has observed is nearly always significant. He should have the opportunity of giving his account unhurriedly and without interruption in a room or examination bay. His family history, previous medical history, occupation, and the like are sometimes valuable. For example, a 'cellulitis of the arm' may be a case of anthrax if the patient works in a tannery or handles hides as a transport worker. An obscure rash on a patient in a general hospital may be smallpox in a traveller. A fistula-in-ano may be the first sign of pulmonary tuberculosis, and further inquiry may reveal that someone in the patient's home is a known sufferer from tuberculosis. Another example of the importance of the history is the tendency for some diseases to have a hereditary incidence—carcinoma of the colon is a very striking instance in families suffering from familial polyposis, and haemophilia in males is a well-known example. It is not the nurse's duty to obtain a detailed history as a routine, but patients will often mention to a nurse some fact of great importance which they thought was too trivial to mention to the surgeon. When the nurse is attending to the patient, however, she should always obtain a clear history if the patient complains of a new symptom; the exact complaint, if it is pain, its nature, site, radiation, aggravating and relieving factors, should be obtained at once. Sometimes before the doctor arrives the patient's condition may become such that he is unable to give as clear an account, and in rare cases he may be unconscious. The patient's complaints are known as symptoms, for example pain–what is elicited on examination, such as tenderness or a swelling, is known as a sign.

7

## CLINICAL EXAMINATION

Facts discovered by examination are known as 'signs', and for their orderly elucidation the following plan is always advisable.

*Inspection* reveals that which can be observed by looking. It is surprising how much can be missed by impatience or too cursory a glance. For example, in a patient's face may be seen:

  Anxiety or distress
  Fright
  Depression
  Indifference
  Stupor
  A flush
  Pallor
  Cyanosis
  Jaundice
  Oedema
  Partial paralysis
  A swelling
  A rash
  Exophthalmos
  Sweat

Any of these observations may be informative. The pallor and sweat may be the result of haemorrhage, and cyanosis may signify increasing respiratory obstruction. Jaundice may be due to obstruction of the bile duct or haemolysis from a recent blood transfusion. Facial paralysis may be caused by a draught from lack of care in the ward, an extending intracranial condition, or the spread of middle-ear disease to the brain or mastoid antrum.

Elsewhere similar observations should be made, and in all sites previous scars, dilated veins, or the presence of a swelling are important. Anything abnormal should be reported by the nurse, however trivial it may appear.

*Palpation* or examination by feeling with the hands is next performed. To be of value the palpation must always be gentle and the hands must be warm. Tenderness, guarding (stiffness or spasm of the underlying muscles), or a swelling may be discovered. It is well to remember that patients who are in hospital for some other condition are not immune from acute abdominal conditions. Hernias still strangulate and peptic ulcers may still perforate. It has been said with no little truth that the most dangerous place for a patient suffering from a peptic ulcer to perforate is in a hospital!

*Percussion* consists of setting up artificial vibrations in the tissues by means of a sharp tap, usually with the fingers. Considerable experience is required in its interpretation. It is a sign by which a distended bladder gives rise to a dull note on percussion, thus differentiating it from a distended intestine which on percussion is described as being tympanitic (resonant).

*Auscultation* is particularly valuable to the nurse in the diagnosis and control of atrial fibrillation. It is impossible to control digitalis therapy unless the heart apex rate as well as the pulse rate are counted and charted separately.

The presence of the increased peristaltic sounds of intestinal obstruction may be heard with the stethoscope, but of greater interest is the reappearance of normal peristaltic sounds in the recovery from paralytic ileus, in which condition they disappear completely.

## SPECIAL INVESTIGATIONS

Special tests may be necessary to confirm or aid diagnosis, and in carrying out investigations it is important that the regime of preparation is carefully followed.

Radiological diagnosis is based on contrast of shadows, and radio-opacity is proportional to atomic weight. The bones of the skeleton are readily visualised by 'straight' X-rays, and X-ray diagnosis can be almost completely accurate. Soft tissues may be examined by a modification of the type of ray: soft X-rays are used extensively in the diagnosis of chest disease. In general, however, the soft tissues are examined by outlining their cavities by filling them with opaque media. The barium meal, the barium enema, the bronchogram, and the retrograde injection of radio-opaque media into the kidneys are all examples of direct outlining of the interior of organs or tracts. Cholecystography for gall-bladder disease and the intravenous pyelogram are indirect methods of outlining organs, and also of testing their function. The examination of the blood vessels and the areas they supply or drain necessitate direct injection of a contrast medium into the vessel. Cine radiography will record the progress of opaque media and allow study at leisure—an image intensifier gives a television account of the conditions in the part X-rayed.

All these examinations depend on the careful co-operation of the nurse. For example, a patient should not take food or drink six hours before a barium meal examination. If a patient vomits the 'dye' taken for a cholecystogram, or diarrhoea follows ingestion of the 'dye', a radiologist should be informed. Contrast media contain iodide materials to which the patient may be sensitive, so antihistamines, adrenaline and hydrocortisone, diuretics and intravenous equipment should be readily available in case the patient collapses.

Radioactive isotopes are now used to determine the function or the absence of function in many glands and organs. Deep-seated areas of the body may be outlined by such techniques and direct writing by a Geiger counter on a machine produces what is known as a Scanogram. Radioactive isotopes are discussed in some detail on page 220.

Good organisation should reduce to a minimum the necessity to repeat radiological examinations. Diagnostic radiology adds to the hazards from radiation to the individual and the community at large. Amongst the most notable are the genetic effects and the possibility of development of leukaemia.

*Radiological examination of women of reproductive age*

It has become vitally necessary, in the light of present knowledge, to reduce the possibility of performing a radiological examination on any female patient between the ages of 15 and 50 who might be pregnant. It is, therefore, necessary to restrict certain X-rays in these patients to a time when it should not be possible for them to be pregnant, i.e. in that period of the menstrual cycle prior to ovulation. Therefore it is necessary to enter the date of the last menstrual period on all X-ray request forms in patients of this age and it may also be necessary to indicate, for the benefit of a clerk, that the examination should be carried out only between certain dates. These would normally be the ten days commencing with the first day of the period or the first day of the next expected period.

The examinations in question are:

   Straight abdomen
   Intravenous and retrograde pyelogram, and cystogram
   Cholecystogram
   Barium meal and enema
   Lumbar spine, sacroiliac joints, sacrum and pelvis
   Hips
   Myelogram
   Hysterosalpingogram
   Lymphangiogram

It may be justifiable to ignore the above rule (known as the 'ten-day rule'). The grounds for ignoring it are: (1) medical urgency; (2) the patient is taking effective contraceptive precautions and the possibility of pregnancy can be reasonably ignored. If either is applicable it should be indicated on the X-ray request form.

Only by fulfilling the above recommendations can the Code of Practice for those exposed to ionising radiations be observed.

Many laboratory findings are invalidated because the specimens collected are not accurately labelled by the nurse or there has been undue delay in sending them to the laboratory.

Ultrasonic devices, by recording sound waves, give valuable clinical information. The presence of a thrombus in a vein (p.130) as well as early pregnancy, may be detected by this means. It can also be used to monitor the sounds of the foetal heart.

Visual inspection of the interior of many organs is possible either directly or by indirect means, and these procedures are known as endoscopic inspections. They include cystoscopy, laryngoscopy, bronchoscopy, oesophagoscopy, sigmoidoscopy, gastroscopy, and peritoneoscopy. With all these procedures a biopsy may be taken.

## THE NURSE'S SPECIAL CONTRIBUTION TO DIAGNOSIS

Careful observation, accurately recorded, is of great value. The patient in hospital, particularly in a surgical ward, is in highly artificial surroundings. This is greatly exaggerated as treatment progress, whether by the administration of drugs, artificial feeding, or operation. The patient's physical condition, too, is often quite unstable during the 21 days following an uneventful operation, even though he may have resumed work, and he is more liable to sudden complications—for example, pulmonary embolism. The following examples serve as general illustrations of the care which is necessary:

1. **Haemorrhage.** An increasing pulse rate, a falling blood pressure and a subnormal temperature are characteristic of haemorrhage. For this reason alone it is important to chart a slight fall of temperature below the normal. Increasing pallor is characteristic, but in jaundiced patients it is unobservable, so particular attention to the pulse is essential.

After many operations—for example, mastectomy or cholecystectomy—a drainage tube is inserted. There is always some bloodstained discharge, but repacking of the outer dressings once or even twice is quite safe, provided the pulse rate is not rapid and the patient's colour is good.

Following prostatectomy, if the drainage is light pink in colour haemorrhage is not excessive.

2. **Abnormal discharges.** The presence of bile from a gallbladder wound when the common bile duct has not been opened, or of a faecal discharge from an abdominal wound, should be reported at once.

3. **Continuous suction and irrigation apparatus.** These treatments can be very treacherous if the nurse is unaware of cer-

tain dangers. There is a danger of any suction apparatus becoming blocked and the nurse thinking the cavity is dry while, in fact, fluid is welling up and distending the cavity of an organ, such as increasing haemorrhage, causing paralysis of the muscular walls. For this reason intermittent suction of the stomach is usually preferable.

Continuous irrigation is sometimes used after bladder operations and a complete suppression of urine may pass unobserved for days unless a strict check of the volume of fluid run in and the volume recovered has been kept.

4. **Analgesics and other measures of symptomatic relief.** The patient in severe pain or vomiting is naturally interested only in securing immediate relief. Analgesics and sedatives should never be ordered until a diagnosis is made. They give temporary relief but do not arrest a progressive disease and do, in fact, make its diagnosis more difficult by masking symptoms and signs. Pain is essentially a protective mechanism.

For the relief of vomiting, aspiration of the stomach by a nasogastric tube is excellent, but it must not be used until a diagnosis has been made because, again, dangerous obstructive symptoms may be masked.

5. **Patients admitted in coma.** These patients present special difficulties because a clear history is not always available, but in all cases the nurse should be alert to the possibility of the presence of associated injuries. Fractures without deformity can easily pass unnoticed in the comatose patient and delayed signs of internal injuries may appear some hours or days after admission. The level of consciousness is noted and assessed regularly.

The size of the pupils, whether they are equal or not, whether they are contracted or dilated, and their reaction to light, are essential observations, and any changes which occur should be written down.

The onset of a fit, its type, spread, duration and other features are frequently seen only by the nurse, and her report of the fit may be decisive in some cases. The appearance of slight weakness (paresis) in any muscles, as well as complete paralysis, is important. If this is done by means of a simple diagram, the right and left side should be clearly labelled.

6. **Enemas.** Enemas may be prescribed for diagnostic purposes, and the deciding factor as to whether an intestinal obstruction is complete and requires operation, or is incomplete, may be the report of the nurse that no flatus has been passed after an enema.

The passage of flatus by a rectal tube when the patient is suffering from peritonitis or paralytic ileus is a sign that the condition is responding to treatment.

7. **General observation when the patient is washed** may be very important. A swelling, an ulcer, a rash, oedema, or fullness may be noticed when a patient is being washed, and such an observation may be the final clue to the solution of the pathology in an otherwise obscure case.

8. **Changes in personality and behaviour** should be watched very carefully. The effect of the mind on a patient's bodily ills can be profound, and in a surgical ward it is no less disastrous than elsewhere. Patients with a poor psychological background may break down completely before or, what is worse, after an operation. Chronic alcoholics are bad operative subjects and require special care. Not all mental manifestations have their origin in diseases of the mind and the following are examples of gross organic disease which may be present or appearing:

(a) *Slight confusion* is common preceding cerebral thrombosis.

(b) *Confusion, drowsiness and incoherent speech* may indicate the presence of a cerebral tumour which may be primary or secondary. A considerable amount of major surgery is 'cancer' surgery, and secondary deposits are characteristic of a cancer. The brain is one of the sites where a secondary deposit may lodge, and early recognition is important so that the attempt to remove the primary growth is abandoned, as it would now prove fruitless.

(c) *Polydipsia.* Excessive thirst and polyuria (excessive urinary output) are characteristic of diabetes insipidus. This condition is due to disease or injury of the pituitary body situated in the sella turcica in the middle fossa of the skull. Occasionally the condition is caused by a fracture in this area, with consequent damage to the pituitary gland.

9. **Pulmonary embolism.** Pulmonary embolism (p. 131) is a condition of which every nurse in every surgical ward in every hospital must be aware. It is the one condition which will kill a fit patient with dramatic suddenness.

Careful observation will always be necessary. The evaluation of findings and history is already in a small way being computerised. In the future the use of computers will be an added aid in the management of a patient.

# CHAPTER 3

# Identification of the Patient

The complexity of modern medical practice arises partly from the rapid increase in scientific knowledge and partly from the fact that the application of this knowledge for the patient's benefit demands that a greater and greater number of people are directly or indirectly concerned in his treatment. The amount of scientific equipment and the range of chemical re-agents used in the treatment of a single patient can hardly be realised. Well-equipped operating theatres, laboratories and other departments of investigation and treatment are expensive to build and to staff. For this reason alone, the type of work which the acute general hospital undertakes becomes even more complex.

The result is that the treatment of a particular patient has become and will become more specific. That is to say that the treatment will be so well designed for him and his condition that the first essential is that he must be identifiable with certainty. There is greater liability to mistake or to human error today than ever before, and the consequences are liable to be more crippling and more lethal because many drugs and fluids have narrower margins of safety and are more potent in their effects than similar drugs in the past.

For this reason, the nurse must always ask herself two questions:

1. Is this patient William Smith (or whatever his name may be)?
2. Is this the correct injection, tablet or blood for William Smith?

She must also be able to ask herself these questions in reverse, namely:

1. Is the next patient for the removal of his appendix William Smith?
2. Is this William Smith now being lifted on to the trolley whom I am taking to the theatre for the removal of his appendix?

Certain well-known facts emerge about patients' behaviour in the stress and strain of going to the operating theatre, receiving injections or even in going from the waiting room to the consulting room of a clinic. For example, a patient sometimes thinks that he has been called when in fact another patient's name has been called. Some patients, hard of hearing, do not like to admit it and even though addressed by another patient's name, keep on saying 'yes' to everything!

This is now the paradoxical situation, that as care and treatment become more specific, more effective and more carefully planned (more personal, in fact), the risk that the plan may misfire through misidentification is greater and more serious.

Many patients have similar names and their place in the ward may be changed, so that identification such as 'third bed from the end on the left' is quite unreliable. A bed card on the wall or locker is certainly useful, but the patient may be moved in the ward and his bed card left, so that this method is not entirely foolproof. The patient's case sheet and records are not suitably kept at the end of the bed so they are not a method of identification. The only safe method is to have a separate identification marked on the bed; either on the bed or on a piece of strapping attached to the crossbar. More recently addressing machines have been used which produce a sheet of labels stating the patient's name, address, date of birth, sex, ward and unit number. Seriously ill patients and all patients going to the theatre should have their name on their wrist. Ident-A-Band, which is a plastic bracelet, can be used and cannot be removed by the patient. The importance of identification of the patient is even greater when he is unconscious and may require an injection such as insulin, or a transfusion of blood.

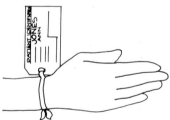

Fig. 3.1    Label attached to patient's wrist for identification.

## IDENTIFICATION OF THE PATIENT'S SPECIMENS

It is vitally important that every specimen for examination taken from a patient either in the ward or operating theatre should be carefully labelled. In the ward there are certain cardinal points to avoid mishap:

1. Everything necessary to collect the specimen should be taken to the bedside.

2. The label should be written out and attached by the person taking the specimen in the presence of the patient and at the bedside.
3. Specimens should never be collected from two patients and then two labels written out together.

Blood specimens from patients suspected of suffering from serum viral hepatitis should carry a warning label (p. 386).

In the theatre, specimens removed at operations are labelled and sealed after each operation.

## THERAPEUTIC FLUIDS, TABLETS, AND OTHER AGENTS

Of all the therapeutic fluids, the one most liable to cause sudden and irreparable damage is incompatible blood. This will be stressed again in the chapter on blood transfusion. The following elementary precautions are essential:

1. The patient must be identified with certainty.
2. The label indicating the cross-match against the patient's blood must be checked against the patient and the bottle of blood and also the blood group.

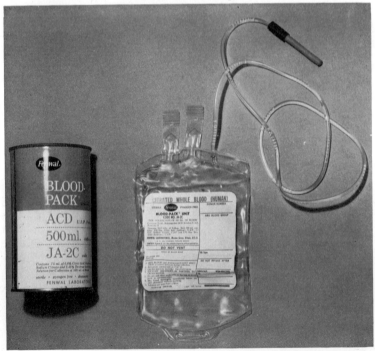

FIG. 3.2   Plastic blood pack unit (Fenwal bag). It is removed sterile from the sealed metal container before use.

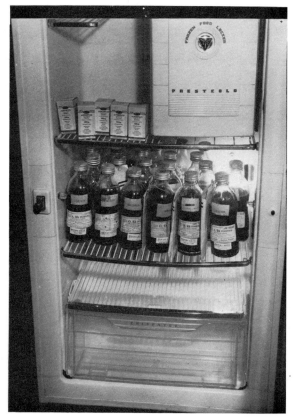

Fig. 3.3   Special care must be taken to remove the correct bottle from the refrigerator.

The maze inside a blood refrigerator (Fig. 3.3) illustrates how easy it is to pick up the wrong bottle.

Other substances particularly liable to cause harm are the anticoagulants, insulin, radium and sedatives. The tragedy of a mistake in the identification of a patient requires no emphasis and in the rush of a busy day it is more likely to occur. Even the coincidence of an identical name, occupation, and disease may play a part, so that the sole identifiable mark may be the patient's home address and his date of birth. If a nurse is in doubt she should never hesitate to share her doubt at once with a more senior member of the staff.

Finally it is essential for the nurse to be able to identify the contents of a medical gas cylinder by its colour. Gas cylinders are now pin indexed—that is, the attachment is so contrived that coupling can be effected only to the correct point on a machine for that particular gas.

# CHAPTER 4

# The Preoperative and Postoperative Care of the Patient

The preoperative preparation and the after-care of the patient is a subject to which an increasing amount of attention has been devoted in recent years. Complications once believed to be unavoidable have been reduced to very small proportions, and the convalescence of a larger number of patients has been more comfortable. The final result of an operation is much more likely to be entirely satisfactory in the absence of complications.

The great variation which appears to exist among the methods favoured by different surgeons is undoubtedly a cause of considerable bewilderment and confusion to the junior nurse. However, it must be realised that the differences are not differences of principle but of method.

The principles of preoperative and postoperative care can be readily understood by a moment's reflection on what an operation really means to a patient. In his mind arise thoughts of a wound, loss of blood, an anaesthetic, a period of incapacity in bed, weakness when he gets up, pain and fear of the end result—perhaps of death, perhaps of some incapacity which may prevent him from carrying on his normal life.

Before all operations, but particularly in an emergency, a nurse must inquire if the patient is taking any drugs. (The term drugs covers all medicines including those which are self-prescribed.) Many of these influence the preoperative preparation. Obvious examples are the steroids, which must always be increased; insulin or other antidiabetic drugs, and anticoagulants (p. 130). Oestrogens (which are contained in some contraceptive pills) increase the risk of thrombosis. Cytotoxic drugs, or any drug liable to damage the white blood corpuscles, delay healing. Diuretics may lower the blood potassium and prolong the action of muscle relaxants after anaesthesia. Antihypertensive drugs may cause an undesirable fall in blood pressure. Monoamine oxidase inhibitors react with anaesthetic agents.

All drug therapy, quite apart from those listed above, should be considered with special reference to its effect on anaesthesia, haemorrhage and all the factors possibly arising in the patient's convalescence.

THE PRINCIPLES OF TREATMENT, THEREFORE, ARE:

1. To render safe the administration of an anaesthetic and to ensure that the patient recovers consciousness without mishap.
2. To prevent or treat circulatory failure.
3. To achieve healing of the wound as rapidly as possible.
4. To prevent or treat complications which may arise as a result of recumbency in bed.
5. To restore rapidly the function in all the organs of the body as well as in the mind.

The operation should be undertaken when the patient is in the best possible condition and for this reason the planned operation, where the patient can be assessed several days before admission, is preferable to the emergency operation. The chest is X-rayed, a blood haemoglobin is performed and an estimation of the blood urea and electrolytes is undertaken if there is reason to suspect they may be altered. If necessary, pulmonary function tests are performed.

It is necessary to have the signed permission of the patient before performing an operation, or, if the patient is under 16 years of age, in Great Britain, that of his parent or guardian. Before taking the patient to the theatre the nurse should check that she has the correct patient, his notes and X-ray films. Rings, earrings and hearing aids should be removed or covered with Sellotape so that there can be no contact between metal on the patient's body and diathermy current. The stomach should always be empty before the patient is anaesthetised. Usually this means prohibiting food for six hours previously and fluid for about three/four hours. If a fit patient must have an anaesthetic immediately, such as a sudden labour in a multiparous woman, a stomach tube must be passed without delay. The stomach of patients suffering from intestinal obstruction must be emptied by aspiration—not only must a tube be passed but it must be aspirated continuously until the anaesthetist has induced the anaesthetic and has passed and inflated the cuff of an endotracheal tube. The reason is that stomach contents may be aspirated into the bronchial tube.

THE OPERATION BED. The bed is made with clean linen, usually while the patient is having a bath. While the patient is in theatre, the bed is remade. The top bed clothes are double-rolled and then made into a pack. According to the patient's needs, other articles are prepared, e.g.

Post-anaesthetic tray
Oxygen
Charts

Because the preparation for operation, the care of the patient in the theatre and the immediate postoperative treatment are continuous in time they are considered together in this chapter.

## THE CARE OF THE PATIENT UNDER ANAESTHESIA

Before the administration of an anaesthetic the patient's heart and lungs are examined and a specimen of urine is tested for the presence of sugar and albumin. The finding of an abnormal constituent in the urine is reported at once. Further preparation of the patient may be necessary and the choice of anaesthetic may be influenced.

Freedom from colds and respiratory infections is desirable, and if the patient suffers from chronic bronchitis the operation should be deferred, if possible, until the warm summer months. He should be persuaded to stop smoking. If a cough is present a corset dressing on the abdominal wound may prevent postoperative complications. Preoperative breathing exercises may also be prescribed with advantage and smoking reduced. He must be warmly clad and covered in transit to and from the theatre.

### Premedication

This formerly took the form of morphia (10 to 15 mg), pethidine (50 to 100 mg) or omnopon (20 mg) provided that the

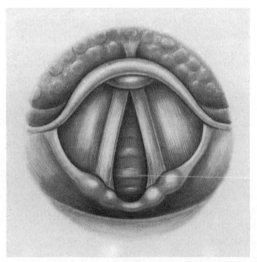

FIG. 4.1   Laryngoscopic view of vocal folds. The root of the tongue is shown above the V-shaped opening formed by the vocal folds between which the rings of the trachea are visible.

patient was not taking monoamine oxidase inhibitor drugs. Modern practice tends towards the administration of pure anxietolytic drugs such as Librium 10 mg, Droperidol 10 mg or Valium 10 mg. This helps to avoid the vomiting and nausea which must be attributed to the use of morphia. If a general anaesthetic is to be administered, atropine (0·6 mg) may be prescribed to prevent excessive secretion of mucus in the respiratory tract. With the increasing use of non-irritant anaesthetic techniques it has become quite common to omit the routine administration of atropine before operation. Instead, the drug may be given by the anaesthetist at the same time as anaesthesia is induced. This avoids the unpleasant dry mouth, tachycardia, and blurred vision caused by atropine. It may also avoid rises in temperature, particularly in children, due to the inhibition of sweating.

## ANAESTHESIA

This is a condition in which the patient loses consciousness and is insensible to the proceedings. It can be produced by various routes:

1. **Inhalation.** Known agents for this purpose are ether, ethyl chloride, chloroform, trilene, nitrous oxide, halothane (Fluothane), cyclopropane. Inhalation may be from:

(a) An open mask, for example, dripping ether on to a gauze pad.
(b) A semiclosed circuit—a large flow of gas from an anaesthetic machine is delivered to the patient's airway. With expiration the gases, including $CO_2$ from the lungs, escape from the apparatus by a one-way valve.
(c) A closed circuit. A small flow of gas is used. The expired gases are passed through soda lime to absorb $CO_2$ and the gas is then recirculated.

2. **Intravenously.** Thiopentone (Pentothal) and methohexitone (Brietal) are well-known examples.

## ANALGESIA

Analgesia is the loss of sensation to pain with or without loss of consciousness. It can be:

1. **General.** Examples are nitrous oxide or trilene in small dosage. This method is used extensively in dentistry and midwifery.

2. **Local.** Local may be—
(a) *Regional*, produced by blocking the nerves at a site proximal to the proposed region of operation.

(b) *Infiltration*, produced by blocking the nerve at the actual site of the operation.

(c) *Topical*, produced by blocking the nerve endings by the application of an analgesic agent to the surface.

**Epidural analgesia.** Epidural analgesia is induced by the introduction of local anaesthetic into the epidural space.

### MUSCLE RELAXANTS

Muscle relaxation is necessary for many operations, especially upper abdominal procedures, and this can be produced by injecting intravenously certain agents such as D-tubocurarine chloride, Pavulon (pencuronium bromide), Scoline or succinylcholine, which paralyse the voluntary muscles, including the diaphragm and intercostal muscles. If these drugs are used a perfect airway has to be maintained and the lungs must be artificially ventilated. At the end of the operation the effect of the muscle-relaxant drug has not completely worn off, and the anaesthetist gives the patient a counteracting drug (prostigmin). This is accompanied by an injection of atropine which prevents the undesirable effects of prostigmin, such as cardiac arrest. Even so a certain amount of weakness may remain in the vital respiratory muscles, so great vigilance is required. There is no antidote to Scoline, but the period of efficacy is short (minutes).

**Hypothermia.** Hypothermia is now only used to render controlled hypotension safer and is confined to the surgery of intracranial aneurysms.

Anaesthesia is induced in the usual way. Various drugs are given to diminish metabolism and lower the temperature, and in addition all warm bedclothing is removed and ice-bags placed all over the patient. When a satisfactory fall in temperature to about 32·2°C (90°F) is obtained the operation is performed. The patient's temperature is brought up very slowly postoperatively.

**The induction of anaesthesia.** General anaesthesia is usually induced by the intravenous injection of one of the barbiturate drugs such as Pentothal (thiopentone).

A peaceful atmosphere in the anaesthetic room comforts the patient and makes the induction of the anaesthetic easier.

If a local or epidural analgesic is used, ear plugs render the patient's ordeal in the theatre less distressing. The patient's eyes should be covered to prevent him from following the course of events by watching the reflection in the lamp. His attention should also be diverted from time to time by engaging him in conversation while the operation is proceeding.

*Maintenance of a free airway*

The maintenance of a free airway is essential. The clothing should not include any constricting bands around the waist or neck, and if the patient wears dentures they should be removed in the ward and kept in a place of safety.

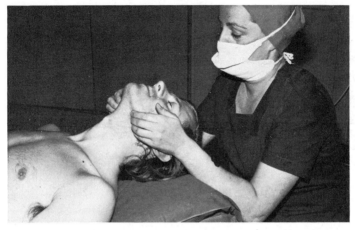

FIG. 4.2   The jaw of the unconscious patient is held forward to prevent his tongue falling back into the air passages and a rubber airway is left in until it is coughed out.

After operations on the mouth the following complications are particularly liable to occur:

1. Asphyxia due to:
   (a) Blood and mucus running down the trachea.
   (b) Haemorrhage blocking the naso- and oropharynx.
   (c) The tongue falling back.
2. Inhalation pneumonia from the aspiration of pus or other material.

After induction of the anaesthetic a cuffed endotracheal tube is passed. The patient's throat is packed with a continuing length of gauze. Afterwards he is nursed on his side. The pack must be removed and the nurse must note that this has been done. All swabs and packs used by the anaesthetist are coloured so that they cannot be confused with those used by the surgeon. Exudates of mucus and blood are aspirated and an airway is usually inserted before the patient leaves the theatre.

The jaw of an unconscious patient should always be held well forward; if this is done the tongue cannot slip back. An artificial pharyngeal airway must also be kept on the theatre trolley, and if this instrument is introduced it should not be removed by a nurse until the patient resents its presence.

No patient should be taken from the theatre back to the ward until the anaesthetist has given permission to move him.

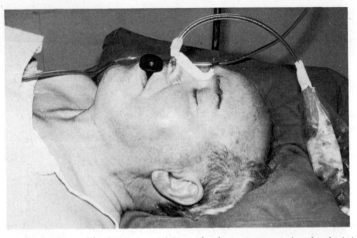

FIG. 4.3    Patient with airway in position. Also has a nasogastric tube draining into a plastic bag.

### Care of the limbs

While unconscious the patient's legs and arms should be kept in the correct position, and at all times special care should be taken to avoid pressure on the nerves, otherwise paralysis is liable to occur. There is particular danger of radial paralysis if the patient's arm is allowed to hang over the edge of the table. Arms should not be extended over boards whilst the patient is in the head-down position with shoulder supports because of the risk of damage to the brachial plexus.

### Care of the bladder

For almost all operations the bladder should be empty. The important exceptions are cystoscopic examinations and operations on the bladder.

### On return to bed

During transit from the theatre the patient must be warmly clad and, if bald, the head should be covered with a shawl or small blanket. On return to the ward the patient is laid on his side and propped over on his shoulder. Turning the head to one side is not advised as this makes it almost impossible for the patient to vomit (if necessary) and breathing with the twisted neck is very difficult. He should not be left unattended before he is able to speak. When consciousness has returned, the position varies considerably with the nature of the operation which has been peformed, but in most cases it is a good rule to allow the patient to assume the position he finds most comfortable. The area of the wound is inspected for bleeding.

It may be noticed that on return to the ward, although the airway is clear, his respiration is unsatisfactory and he is becoming cyanosed. This is particularly liable to occur after the use of the relaxant drugs, where full respiratory function has not been recovered. Oxygen should be given and the anaesthetist summoned at once—further assisted respiration with the anaesthetic machine may be advised. If the pulse is good, the patient sweating and of good colour, respiration may still be unsatisfactory. This failure is due to excessive retention of carbon dioxide in the blood and it is necessary to remove the excess by a carbon-dioxide absorber, using assisted respiration. It is essential to differentiate between respiratory obstruction in which the patient is struggling to breathe and respiratory depression which is caused by relaxant drugs or circulatory failure.

However, the anaesthetist will give precise instructions on the management of the patient before the patient leaves the theatre.

Visiting in open wards on operation days is undesirable and patients recovering from anaesthesia behind screens are in a position of great peril. A better alternative if visiting is allowed is a recovery area in the ward where constant observation is possible.

**The aspiration of gastric contents.** Patients who vomit during anaesthesia are liable to inhale gastric contents which are highly acidic.

If this occurs the patient may develop Mendelsohn's syndrome, giving rise to serious pulmonary complications. Such patients are treated by bronchial toilet and the administration of large doses of corticosteroids and antibiotics.

*Postoperative vomiting.* Postoperative vomiting, if excessive, leads to rapid salt and water depletion. In most cases the vomiting ceases very quickly; if it does not, Maxolon 10 mg or chlorpromazine (Largactil) 25 mg is usually effective. If the vomiting persists, however, the stomach is aspirated with a nasogastric tube. The patient is given only fluid at first until the bowel sounds have returned, after which a normal diet is resumed.

Persistent hiccough is sometimes a very distressing complication of an operation. The best treatment is to administer $CO_2$ (carbon dioxide) 5 per cent; if there is no response, 10 per cent $CO_2$ may be given. Largactil 25 mg is sometimes of value. In intractable cases the administration of hyoscine (0·4 mg) or 'blocking' of the left phrenic nerve may be advisable.

### The care of the mouth

After gastric operations fluids by mouth are usually forbidden for 24 hours, and after that the quantity is restricted for a further 24 hours.

When a patient who is confined to bed can clean his own teeth, he is given a beaker of water or mouth wash, and a bowl in which to spit.

When a patient is unable to use his hands but is otherwise well, the nurse can clean his teeth for him, using the patient's own toothbrush, and toothpaste, and allow him to rinse his own mouth, spitting into a bowl held by the nurse.

When the patient cannot co-operate in caring for his mouth, a special technique is required along the following lines.

The nurse washes and dries her hands. If possible an explanation is given to the patient. Privacy is ensured. A hand towel

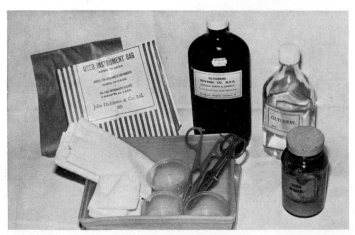

FIG. 4.4   Oral hygiene.

*Contents of disposable pack*
　Lotions—
　　Aqueous sol. sod. bicarbonate 1 : 160
　　Glycerin of thymol compound, B.P.C.
　　Glycerin
　3 gallipots
　Gauze swabs
　Disposable forceps

is placed over the patient's chest for protection. Using the fingers, a cotton wool swab or a lint square is firmly fixed into the teeth of a pair of forceps which clip, e.g. artery forceps. The swab is dipped into a solution of sodium bicarbonate in water, strength of 1 in 160.

The mouth is opened and is cleaned in a systematic order, e.g. lips, cheeks, gums, teeth, palate, tongue. If necessary the tongue can be depressed using a tongue depressor. Each swab is used only once. It is removed from the forceps using a pair of dissecting forceps, and is discarded into the soiled dressing bag.

When the mouth has been cleaned, it can be freshened using a swab dipped into glycothymoline.

The lips can be kept moist by a thin film of vaseline or glycerine and borax.

The face is dried, the towel removed and the patient made comfortable. The equipment is removed and discarded.

The nurse washes and dries her hands.

Any unusual condition of the mouth is reported to the Sister or Charge Nurse, who will order any special treatment.

CARE OF DENTURES

When a patient can clean his own dentures, he is given a bowl of tepid water in which to do so, and also a beaker of water or mouthwash with which to rinse his mouth.

When it is necessary for a nurse to clean the patient's dentures, they are removed and placed into a denture container. Taking the dentures and the patient's toothbrush to the bathroom, she cleans the dentures over a sink of tepid water, brushing the dentures under a running tap. They are returned to the patient, who is allowed to rinse his mouth before replacing them.

When a patient does not wish to retain his dentures, or in the case of a very weak or unconscious patient, the dentures are first cleaned and then placed in a denture container labelled with the patient's name, and stored in his locker. Before replacing the dentures which have been stored, they should be rinsed in cold water.

*Maintenance of nutrition*

If the operation is a short one, such as uncomplicated appendicectomy, no special difficulty arises in feeding. The patient takes fluids shortly after recovering consciousness and soon resumes a normal diet. Following a long period of anaesthesia, the maintenance of nutrition is essential, and of all the constituents of diet, fluid is the most important. Until the patient is able to drink, the fluid balance is maintained by the administration of fluid by other routes (Chapter 17).

*Deep-breathing exercises*

Deep-breathing exercises, particularly in the 48 hours following the operation, do much to eliminate pulmonary complications. These should be taught by the physiotherapist in the pre-operative waiting period if possible.

# THE WOUND

### THE DIMINUTION OR ELIMINATION OF INFECTION AT THE SITE OF THE DISEASE

A wound will heal rapidly only if it is non-infected. The wound includes not only the incision in the skin, fascia and muscles, but in all the deeper organs which have been opened. If infection is present in the organ to be operated on it should, if possible, be controlled before the operation takes place. Not only is the operation easier and safer, but the patient's convalescence is smoother.

In some cases several weeks' preparation may be necessary before the operation is undertaken. To illustrate this principle, operations at the following sites may be taken as examples:

1. **The lungs.** In Chapter 31 this problem is considered in detail. In the condition known as bronchiectasis, for which a lobe of the lung is removed, every effort is made to empty the cavities of pus and render their walls as clean as possible. Expectorant mixtures, antibiotics, postural drainage, breathing exercises, and physiotherapy are all prescribed for this purpose.

2. **The stomach and duodenum.** Operation is commonly undertaken for chronic gastric and duodenal ulceration which has failed to respond to medical treatment, or because the ulcer has produced an obstruction to the outlet of the stomach (pyloric stenosis). If the emptying of the stomach is defective, gross infection results in the stagnant food. The stomach must be washed out repeatedly.

A chronic gastric or duodenal ulcer becomes larger and deeper, and when it is active the patient is unable to work. Strict medical treatment, although it may have failed to heal the ulcer sufficiently to allow the patient to work, will always produce considerable shrinkage in the size of the ulcer, and when the effect is maximal the operation can be undertaken with greater ease.

3. **The intestine.** It is almost impossible to sterilise the intestinal contents, but the degree of infectivity can be reduced considerably. The incision and suture of a septic swollen intestine are fraught with considerable danger. The stitches may cut out, resulting in leakage of the intestinal contents. Before an

operation on the intestine, the diet should consist of food which leaves no residue, so that faecal accumulation is diminished. Sulphonamide drugs which are not absorbed, such as sulfasuxidine, or antibiotics such as neomycin are administered to reduce infectivity. Colonic lavage clears the bowel of faecal material, but it is necessary only for operations on the large bowel.

4. **The urinary tract.** A wound communicating with the urinary tract will be very slow to heal in the presence of grossly infected urine. The consumption of about 3000 ml of fluid daily is adequate to ensure elimination of waste products and not too excessive to dilute the concentration of antibacterial drugs in the kidneys.

The same principle applies to all sites where an operation may be performed, whether it be the mouth, the eye, the ear, or the joints. The methods of controlling infection will be discussed in detail (p. 45). Some surgeons like to operate under an 'antibiotic umbrella' if there is a risk of infection, but experience has shown that this is not as effective as one may think (p. 53).

THE PREPARATION OF THE SKIN

The preparation of the skin is a procedure common to almost all operations. The skin should be shaved, and if the patient is fit a bath or better a shower is given to remove loose hairs. The skin is then washed with Derl soap (2 per cent hexachlorophane) and water and dried on a clean towel. After this preparation the patient is put into a theatre gown and goes to bed in freshly laundered sheets. No antiseptic, towelling or dressings are applied in the ward.

The skin of the thighs of a patient who is incontinent of faeces requires special preparation if anaerobic infections are to be avoided after operations such as amputation or nailing operations for fracture of the femoral neck.

THE IMPORTANCE OF ADEQUATE VITAMIN C IN THE BODY

If vitamin C is deficient the healing of the wound may be delayed or fail to occur, but in the United Kingdom vitamin C deficiency is now uncommon except in the elderly who live alone.

THE CARE OF THE WOUND

This is considered in detail in Chapter 12.

**PREVENTION AND TREATMENT OF CIRCULATORY FAILURE (SHOCK)**

This subject is considered in detail in Chapter 15.

Usually until four hours before the operation the patient may drink freely. If drinking is difficult or the patient is vomiting, fluids must be administered by the intravenous route. In pyloric stenosis, or intestinal obstruction as fluid cannot leave the stomach, fluid by mouth is prohibited for hours or even days preoperatively. A patient depleted of salt and water becomes collapsed very rapidly. Severe purgation, once thought to be a good preoperative measure, is now known to be harmful since it produces severe dehydration and loss of electrolytes. In most cases a reduction of diet is all that is necessary.

An anaemic patient collapses very easily, and slight haemorrhage increases this tendency (p. 135). A preliminary blood transfusion is given and may be continued during the operation. Fear predisposes to circulatory failure and sedatives and hypnotics may be useful. The relief of pain and the promotion of sleep are important. Analgesic and hypnotic drugs are administered, but an uncomfortable bandage or an awkward position in bed should be corrected. The patient must be returned to a warm bed, but further treatment by heat only increases the degree of circulatory failure.

After operation the nurse should note carefully the patient's colour and the state of his skin, any increase in the rate of the pulse, its quality, and any irregularity, and a strict check on the blood pressure is also indicated. In more serious cases a half-hourly check is recorded or the heart rate is monitored. Basically the treatment is relief of pain, elevation of the foot of the bed, blood transfusion and, if necessary, packing of the wound.

### THE PREVENTION AND TREATMENT OF COMPLICATIONS WHICH ARISE AS A RESULT OF RECUMBENCY IN BED

With very few exceptions no patient should be confined to bed before operation. The principal exception is a patient suffering from thyrotoxicosis and even in this condition confinement to bed to secure complete rest to the heart is now rarely necessary as modern antithyroid drugs control the toxicity so effectively.

The complications which may arise are:

1. **Difficulty with micturition.** Many patients find it difficult to pass urine while lying flat in bed and the difficulty is increased if there is an abdominal wound. The patient may sit or stand up or use a commode. Relaxation is necessary and the relief of pain essential. The treatment of this condition is discussed in Chapter 42. Catheterisation is not resorted to until all other measures have failed. A patient suffering from a minor degree of prostatic obstruction should have a catheter

passed in the theatre after any operation which may precipi-
tate retention. It can be removed in a day or two when he is
up and about and pain has diminished.

2. **Difficulty with defaecation.** Difficulty in defaecation
arises from conditions similar to those which interfere with
micturition. The main factor in this condition, however, is intestinal distension with gas causing pain, and in all cases it
should be relieved at regular intervals by the passage of a flatus tube—otherwise the heart and lungs may be embarrassed
and the onset of the condition known as paralytic ileus may be
encouraged.

Distension may be induced by an unsuitable diet during the
two days before operation. Foods likely to cause residue and
flatulence, such as vegetables, pastries, and large quantities of
milk, should be avoided. The immediate preoperative care
of the bowel has been discussed on page 29, but if the bowel
is the site of the operation, as in removal of a portion of the
colon, extra precautions are necessary (p. 415).

3. **Respiratory complications.** Respiratory complications
are very common. Many anaesthetic mixtures are irritant and
produce excessive secretion. This may result in bronchitis or
massive lobar collapse of the lungs. Pneumonia is an occasional complication. Many patients are afraid to take deep
breaths because of fear of damage to their wounds, and lack of
movement and shallow breathing increase the liability to pulmonary complications. They need help and supervision. The
patient is encouraged to use his hands to support the abdominal wound.

Inhalations, of which steam is the most important, are sometimes of value. Alternatively an ultrasonic nebuliser producing
'cold steam' or an electric nebuliser may be used. Nebulisers
may be fitted to the oxygen supply. The moisture produced
by either method reaches the smaller bronchioles and liquefies
the mucus.

Pulmonary complications following operation are much
commoner after interference in the upper abdomen and in all
operations are more closely related to pre-existing bronchitis
rather than the type of anaesthetic. Preoperative assessment
and treatment with antibiotics, bronchial dilators, breathing
exercises and, if necessary steroids, diminish the risk. In addition of course the patient should stop smoking. Good postoperative physiotherapy is essential.

4. **Thrombosis.** Inactivity from rest in bed and an increase
in the number of platelets in the blood as the result of a
wound are conditions which favour the occurrence of a blood
clot (or thrombus) in the veins of the legs. Movement of the
clot into the general circulation (embolism) may give rise to

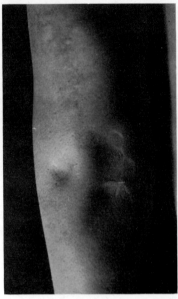

FIG. 4.5   Pitting oedema of the leg due to femoral thrombosis.

sudden death (p. 131). Measures to diminish thromboembolism are discussed on page 129. Preoperative oestrogens have already been mentioned as likely to increase thrombosis. Operating on the patient, with the legs slightly elevated off the table and continued slight bed elevation postoperatively, diminish the risk of thrombosis. In high-risk patients prophylactic heparin therapy may be prescribed (p.130).

5. **Bedsores.** Great care should be taken to prevent bedsores after operations and in any severe illness. Their treatment is described in Chapter 21.

6. **Muscular disuse and deformity.** Muscular disuse and deformity have to be carefully guarded against, especially in orthopaedic conditions where they are most likely to occur, but they are none the less important in all conditions where the patient has been confined to bed for a considerable period.

7. **Mental inactivity.** Many patients tend to deteriorate mentally during a long stay in bed, and occupational therapy has a useful part to play.

Postoperative mania may occur in unstable subjects after operation. Old people are liable to develop mental changes. This is also liable to occur in toxic conditions. Paraldehyde (7 to 10 ml) is usually prescribed if the patient is otherwise uncontrollable.

Delirium tremens may occur in chronic alcoholics.

8. **Diminution in circulating blood volume.** This occurs with bed rest and increases the risk of circulatory collapse (shock) during operation. It may be further aggravated by the vasodilatation produced by many anaesthetic agents in current use.

9. **Postoperative pyrexia.** Following operation many patients develop a rise in temperature which usually subsides after 24 hours. If it persists the following steps are advisable:

(a) The wound should be inspected for swelling or tenderness, which may be due to haematoma formation or infection.

(b) The urine is examined for pus and organisms.

(c) The legs are inspected for signs of thrombosis (p. 129).

(d) The chest is examined and a radiograph may show a segment of collapse.

(e) After an abdominal operation a residual abscess in the pelvis (detectable by rectal examination) or a subphrenic abscess (p. 345) should be suspected.

(f) A white blood count for leucocytosis.

## DAY SURGERY

The patient's general practitioner, together with the community nurse, will be able to continue treatment at home. In some cases where equipment or home help facilities are necessary the social services of the district authority may be used.

Day surgery requires the co-operation of the general practitioner, the community nurse and the hospital.

Preoperatively the suitability of the patient's home is assessed, a note is sent to the hospital of any drugs which the patient may be taking, X-rays, blood and urine examination are undertaken before the day of admission but urine must always be examined again on the day of operation. Before the patient is discharged following day surgery he should be—

(i) seen by the doctor at the hospital and kept in if there is any doubt;

(ii) given analgesics or a note of what is necessary;

(iii) warned about bleeding;

(iv) told to report back to the hospital if necessary.

### RESTORATION OF FUNCTION

The restoration of function in the organs of the body by rehabilitation, re-education, exercises, and an adequate convalescence are most important.

The advice given to a patient on leaving hospital on such

special points as diet, care of his wound, fitness for work, and other activities will do much to ensure a good result. Such advice must however be given against the knowledge of the patient's social background, his psychological attitude, education and personal character.

# CHAPTER 5

# Pain

Pain is one of the commonest presenting and continuing symptoms of organic and psychiatric disease. The mechanism of its production and perception are ill understood. It is rarely felt as an isolated sensation—a pin-prick is a mixture of touch and pain. The simple conception of pain receptors conveying impulses along a sensory nerve to a tract in the spinal cord and then to the cerebral cortex which localises the site of the pain is not confirmed by modern physiological research.

Pain arising in the skin can be localised accurately but pain of visceral origin is usually felt in the skin or muscular wall far distant from the organ involved. Conversely, it has been shown that vascular changes and alterations in the tone of a viscus can be produced by stimulating a localised area of skin. Such changes may provide a rational explanation for the use of counter-irritant measures and for acupuncture.

## GATE CONTROL THEORY OF PAIN

Melzack and Wall in 1965 postulated the theory of a gate control mechanism. The large 'A' fibres tend to close this gate and the small 'C' fibres tend to open it. If the large 'A' fibres are destroyed, as in herpes zoster, the smaller 'C' fibres have free play and the gate is opened giving rise to pain. Electrical stimulation of the larger nerve fibres in the posterior columns of the spinal cord is effective in the control of some types of pain. Work is at present proceeding to make this a practical possibility (p. 39).

Pain is protective. It is subjective and cannot be measured or monitored like the temperature or the pulse rate. A nurse will confirm from her own experience on the wards the apparently enormous variation in the degree of pain felt by two different patients from what appears to be an identical clinical lesion. In making this assessment the family doctor with intimate knowledge of a patient and his background has a great advantage over hospital staff. Anxiety and depression are important factors in the causation and escalation of pain. All pain is genuine and real to the patient and it may well be that pain of psychological origin is even more severe. To doubt this is to place oneself at a great disadvantage in the management of the patient. The only pain which is not genuine is one 'produced' for malingering or fraudulent purposes. Pain may be caused by tissue destruction with the release of chemical substances locally as well as by anoxia. The products of the inflammatory reaction are well recognised sources of the origin of pain although the exact nature of the substances and the mode of action are open to more doubt. That cancer produces so little pain in the earlier stages is an important cause of delay in diagnosis. Lack of oxygen is a well-recognised cause of myocardial pain as it is of intermittent claudicaton in peripheral arterial disease. Pressure on nerve roots is believed to be a cause of pain and in prolapsed intervertebral disc (p. 537) this is undoubtedly true because removal of the disc cures the pain. It is also believed that collapse of a vertebral body from secondary carcinoma causes pain by compressing the nerve root below, but the fact that removal of even one adrenal gland (p. 298) in a responsive case of breast cancer will relieve the pain immediately provides a nice enigma which baffles explanation on present knowledge. A single dose of oestrogens for a similar pain arising from cancer of the prostate may have the same dramatic effect.

The administration of steroids is effective in relieving susceptible pain but there is a danger that they may mask, exacerbate or reactivate a lesion which in their absence the body would overcome uneventfully. A healed peptic ulcer or a healed focus of pulmonary tuberculosis may become very active.

## CLINICAL MANAGEMENT

The significance of pain as a symptom of disease has to be evaluated by a full examination of the patient so that a diagnosis can be made. Analgesics are withheld in patients suffering from acute abdominal pain until a diagnosis is made (p. 333). Even in these conditions a sensible explanation will do much to relieve pain by allaying anxiety. In some acute situations an analgesic may have to be administered before transport of the patient to hospital, but the amount should be kept to the minimum and a note of what has been administered. The dosage and the time of administration should accompany the patient. Obviously the sooner the diagnosis is established and a plan of treatment instituted the better.

The converse situation also holds great danger for the patient. The diagnosis has been clearly established—the patient either complains of repeated pain or the pain suddenly becomes more severe. The alert nurse should ask herself two questions before repeating analgesics—'Is this the same situation?' or 'Has a complication arisen?' Two examples are:

1. The patient under medical treatment for a peptic ulcer may have repeated pain—one danger is perforation, and it is a regrettable truth that the mortality is higher if the patient in hospital perforates than at home or even on the street! Only awareness of the hazard and re-examination of the patient complaining of repeated or severe pain will enable the diagnosis of perforation to be made when it occurs and prolonged delay avoided by giving analgesics.
2. Most patients with gall stone colic are treated expectantly. Occasionally a gall stone will obstruct the small intestine—a condition which requires an urgent operation for its relief.

The ultimate relief of pain in acute organic disease is cure of the disease. As this will usually be of short duration the problem of the relief of pain is not a difficult one. Appropriate algesics are prescribed and the danger of addiction is negligible. None the less, the drugs are chosen after assessment of the pain arising from the local condition, the degree of anxiety or fear and the stability or otherwise of the psychological background. Above all else it must never be suggested to a patient that he or she is too intolerant of pain—pain is never to be equated with an endurance test. In practice the total amount of analgesics can be considerably reduced if they are given in small frequent doses before the pain recurs rather than after the patient has been in pain for some time.

*Drugs*

There is an endless variety and combination of drugs but in practice an individual unit will usually use a small number which have been found to be adequate. Rapid and effective absorption is essential for their action. If the patient is unable to eat or drink a parenteral route is essential. The only parenteral route which is effective in the shocked patient is the intravenous one. Subcutaneous or intramuscular injections are not absorbed when the patient is shocked and an undesirable cumulative dosage may arise as recovery occurs.

Analgesic drugs may cause respiratory depression, nausea, constipation or hypotension.

NARCOTIC ANALGESICS

*Pethidine* (50–100 mg) is an effective analgesic but is less powerful than morphine. It is less likely to cause respiratory depression but lowers blood pressure.

*Morphine* (10–15 mg) is an excellent analgesic but decreases respiration and therefore dangerous in bronchitic or asthmatic patients. Many patients complain of nausea and it tends to cause constipation.

*Methadone* (Physeptone) (5–10 mg) has less psychic effects than morphine.

*Pentazocine* (Fortral) (30–60 mg) is an intermediate between morphine and codeine. It has a low risk of addiction but can cause hallucination.

*Dihydrocodeine* (DF118) (30–60 mg) is suitable for moderate pain.

### NON-NARCOTIC ANALGESICS

*Aspirin* is the most widely used analgesic. There is a risk of gastric haemorrhage (p. 370) and it may interfere with blood coagulation by increasing the prothrombin time.

*Distalgesic tablets* are a mixture of dextropropoxyphene hydrochloride (32·5 mg) and paracetamol (32·5 mg) and are used for mild pain. Paracetamol (500 mg) or Paracodal are also used.

## CHRONIC PERSISTENT OR RECURRENT PAIN

Acute pain is fairly easily relieved by analgesics while measures are taken to cure its cause. The pain is protective. In many cases of persistent or recurrent pain the pain is in itself the dominant feature. Such patients may be divided into two categories:

1. Those in whom the expectation of life is short, usually a patient with advanced malignant disease.
2. Sufferers who have a normal life expectancy but persistent pain is overwhelming. These include arthritics, post-herpetic neuralgia and many other conditions.

The patient with malignant disease can be treated with analgesics and anxiolytic drugs and in severe pain there are a variety of methods listed below which may be effective in a particular case. The patients in the second group present a much more difficult problem. In all it is essential to be certain that pain is the symptom complained of and not just itching or numbness. A careful clinical examination and investigation is essential to exclude any obvious remedial cause. For intractable pain there are special pain clinics but treatment is always difficult and uncertain.

### Methods of treatment

1. *Analgesics* similar to those administered for acute pain are used—the danger of addiction in non-malignant patients is an

overriding consideration and should intensify the efforts to use other methods of control.

2. *Anxiolytic drug therapy.* Diazepam (Valium) (5–30 mg daily) or chlorpromazine (Largactil) (75–800 mg daily) are widely used for mild anxiety or agitation in combination with analgesics.

3. *Local injection* of nerves or nerve plexes. Long-acting local anaesthetics are injected.

4. *Destruction* of nerve routes or tracts by:
   (a) Phenol or alcohol.
   (b) Surgical section.
   (c) Electric coagulation.

Despite such radical measures in time the pain recurs in many patients. Trigeminal neuralgia (p. 534) which does not respond to carbomazepine (Tegretol) is treated by injection of the ganglion or nerve section.

5. *Radiotherapy* is often effective for the relief of secondary malignant deposits in the spine.

6. *Hormonal methods* including oophorectomy, adrenalectomy or hypophysectomy (p. 298).

7. *Sympathecomy* is indicated for true causalgia—a burning pain which occurs after injury to a peripheral nerve.

8. *Posterior-column stimulation.* A special electrode is attached to the dura mater and connected by a subcutaneous lead to a button implanted under the skin. The patient controls the button which is attached to a small transmitter on the skin. The patient can press on the button to stimulate the posterior columns.

The control of intractable pain is far from easy and with further understanding of its physiology better methods of control will be discovered.

CHAPTER 6

# Infection and Immunity

Infection is the successful invasion and growth of micro-organisms in a body tissue. The severity or mildness of the resulting disease is dependent upon:

1. The resistance of the patient.
2. The dosage and virulence of the organisms.

THE RESISTANCE OF THE PATIENT TO INFECTION

The main forces of resistance to infection are the white corpuscles of the blood and the antibodies (immune bodies) which are present in the blood and the tissue fluids. An intact skin or mucous surface is one of the greatest natural forces in avoiding infection, because the organisms on the body surface known as contaminants are denied access to the tissues.

**The white blood corpuscles (or leucocytes).** Normally there are 5000 to 10,000 white corpuscles per ml of blood, and they are present in the following forms:

| | |
|---|---|
| Polymorphonuclear leucocytes | 55 to 65 per cent |
| Lymphocytes | 25 to 35 per cent |
| Eosinophils | 1 to 3 per cent |
| Mononuclears | 2 to 10 per cent |
| Basophils | 1 per cent |

The polymorph, the basophil, and the eosinophil together constitute granular cells or granulocytes.

As a result of an acute infection, the number of white corpuscles present in the blood increases rapidly and the polymorphonuclear leucocytes may even account for 90 to 95 per cent of the total white count. If, for any reason, this increase should fail to occur, the disease takes a more severe course than would otherwise have been expected. Excessive irradiation and the excessive dosage of certain drugs, such as the sulphonamide drugs, thiouracil, chloramphenicol, and cytotoxic drugs (used in treating malignant disease), depress the production of leucocytes. If the production of granulocytes is markedly depressed the patient is unable to combat even the mildest infection and death results. This condition is known as

40

agranulocytosis (no polymorphonuclear leucocytes), but is more usually a granulocytopenia (diminished number of white cells). Clinically the most obvious feature of agranulocytosis is a destructive condition in the tissues of the mouth and throat because the patient has no resistance to the vast number of organisms he normally inhales and ingests without ill effect each day. The most valuable drugs for this condition are antibiotics which help to combat infection. ACTH (adrenocorticotrophic hormone), 100 units daily, increases the production of granulocytes and is said to be of value in this condition.

Almost all acute infections result in an increase in the white corpuscles, but there are important exceptions, e.g. in typhoid fever, in which the white cell count is below normal, of the order of 2000 to 3000 per ml. The term 'leucopenia' is applied to those states in which the white corpuscles are fewer than normal.

TYPES OF IMMUNE RESPONSE

Immunity to a particular disease is due to the presence of specific antibodies. Antibodies arise in the body either as a response to the presence of an antigen or are inherited.

Immunity is a response to previous infection or is created artificially by the administration of dead or weakened organisms to which there is a response (active immunisation) or by the administration of gammaglobulin (passive immunity).

The antibodies are produced by certain lymphocytes in response to an antigen and form the group of substances known as the immunoglobulins. When stimulated to produce antibodies the lymphocytes change in appearance and are known as plasma cells.

There are also cellular immune reactions in which lymphocytes embryologically distinct from those which produce antibodies become sensitised to the patient's own tissue or to implanted tissue. This forms the basis of a marked inflammatory reaction such as occurs in autoimmune disease—the rejection of transplanted organs. It may be rapid, when it is known as anaphylaxis; or slower, when it is known as rejection.

THE DEGREE OF IMMUNITY

This varies from patient to patient and with different types of organisms.

The following factors may alter, usually unfavourably, the degree of immunity:

1. *Age.* In infancy antibody production has not developed because the infant has not had the chance of exposure to latent infection. In extreme old age it may be depressed like all the

other vital functions.

2. *Race*. The introduction of a new infection to a native race is usually catastrophic. The inhabitants have no natural immunity to a new disease. For instance, tuberculosis has almost wiped out the Red Indians.

3. The following conditions diminish resistance to infection with a resultant lowering of the degree of immunity:

(a) Metabolic diseases, e.g. diabetes mellitus.
(b) Severe anaemias, hypoproteinaemia and blood diseases.
(c) Uraemia.
(d) Cold, exposure, starvation, haemorrhage, and metallic poisoning.
(e) Radioactivity.
(f) A poor blood supply or a wound filled with serum or haematoma.

## THE DOSAGE AND VIRULENCE OF ORGANISMS

By dosage we mean number of organisms. Obviously a more severe infection is produced by 10,000,000 organisms than by 1,000,000 of the same strain.

Different strains of the same organism vary in their inherent power to attack the body, and this property is known as virulence; organisms of the same strain vary in virulence under different conditions. The virulence is sometimes a property of the body of the organism, and sometimes it is due to a toxin or poison which it produces. In clinical practice the sensitivity or response to antibacterial drugs may well be decisive in assessing the virulence of the clinical infection.

## SUSCEPTIBILITY TO SURGICAL INFECTION

The susceptibility of a patient to infection depends upon the freedom of access of organisms to his body and the degree of immunity which he possesses to the particular organism once it is implanted on his tissues.

*Access of organisms*. An intact healthy skin or mucosa is the greatest barrier against infection. Organisms may gain access from a wound, be inhaled or swallowed.

The whole complex organisation of surgical technique is designed with the sole object of preventing the access of organisms to wounds. This is known as asepsis—literally, no infection.

# CLINICAL APPLICATION OF IMMUNITY

## 1. *Diagnostic*

The estimation of the presence of immune bodies in the blood may be of value in diagnosis. The test is usually performed on the blood serum. The specimen of blood should be collected with no anticoagulant in the specimen tube, so that the serum can separate from the clot. The Widal test for the diagnosis of typhoid fever and the Wassermann reaction for the diagnosis of syphilis are examples of its use.

## 2. *Prophylactic and therapeutic*

Tetanus toxoid is administered if the patient has been recently exposed to tetanus. Human antitetanus immunoglobulin is used in treatment of the disease.

Active immunisation is effected to prevent several diseases, for example, tetanus, smallpox, diphtheria, poliomyelitis and tuberculosis.

Active immunisation is undertaken for tetanus, and anyone liable to be at risk, such as agricultural workers, children, and members of the services, are included. The following schedule of active immunisation is advised in children: At the end of the first two weeks of life BCG (Bacille Calmette-Guérin) for tuberculosis; at 12 weeks first injection of diphtheria, pertussis, and tetanus, triple antigen, 1 ml; at five months a second injection; and at 11 months a third injection. Poliomyelitis inoculation (Salk vaccine) is given at five and 11 months. After the first year the child is inoculated against measles. Smallpox vaccination is usually undertaken at the second year. A booster dose of diphtheria and tetanus antigen should be given when the child starts school and again at the age of 10 years.

Immunisation in older children or adults can, of course, be given by an injection of tetanus toxoid on its own. This is usually given as two injections at four-weekly intervals. For complete protection booster doses should be given each year. There is a tendency to forget or neglect the necessity for immunisation when the disease is rarely seen.

### Immunisation programme

| | | |
|---|---|---|
| 1st Inoculation | 12 weeks | Diphtheria |
| | Triple | ←Tetanus |
| | Polio | Whooping cough |
| 2nd Inoculation | 5 months | Triple |
| | | Polio |

3rd Inoculation          11 months $<$ Triple
                                     Polio

After 1st year—Measles not Smallpox

## SERUM REACTIONS

Serum reactions may be of two types:

1. **Anaphylaxis.** This is a state of sensitisation. It does not occur when an injection of serum (the antigen) is given for the first time, but is liable to occur from the second injection if given after 10 days of the first. For this reason careful inquiry should always be made to elicit whether the patient has had a previous injection of serum or is allergic to foreign protein. If there is any doubt, small doses should be given (desensitisation); that is, an intradermal injection of 0·2 ml and wait for 15 minutes. If there is no reaction the same dose is repeated. Then if, after a further 15 minutes, there is no reaction the remainder of the dose ordered is administered. If there is a reaction doses of 0·5 ml are given at 15-minute intervals until the total amount prescribed has been administered. Anaphylaxis is a frightening condition—the most severe cases collapse and die almost at once in a state of acute circulatory respiratory embarrassment. For this reason an ampoule of adrenalin (1 : 1000 1 ml) and an additional syringe should always be available when antitetanic serum is to be administered intramuscularly or subcutaneously.

Hydrocortisone, 100 mg, by intravenous injection may be given to supplement the action of adrenalin.

2. **Serum sickness.** An injection of a single dose of antitoxic serum given for the first time may occasionally produce a reaction from foreign protein which comes on seven to 10 days afterwards and is characterised by an urticarial rash, albuminuria, headache, nausea, vomiting, joint pains, and loss of appetite. Antihistamine drugs such as Piriton 4 mg are useful in treatment, and for the skin irritation calamine lotion is applied.

3. **Accelerated reaction.** This is really serum sickness in a severe form and after a much shorter interval, a few hours after the injection up to two or three days. It usually, but not invariably, occurs in patients who have had a previous serum injection. The patient is acutely ill with fever, bronchospasm, headache, joint pains, and a rash. He should be admitted for treatment which may include adrenalin, the antihistamines and, possibly, corticosteroids.

## THE PREVENTION AND CONTROL OF INFECTION

Infection is always inimical to the interest of the surgical patient. It adds to his suffering, delays his recovery, and may cause such destruction to his tissues that his last state is worse than his first. If it is severe enough it may cause death.

Many surgical conditions are primarily infective and the prevention of the spread of infecting organisms to other patients is a cause of constant anxiety. In subsequent chapters considerable attention is paid to the practical details of this problem, but certain general principles are worthy of special notice.

1. *General measures of hygiene* are of the first importance for the patient and nurse. Cleanliness of the ward, the handling of food, crockery, and personal cleanliness are of the greatest importance. An individual thermometer for each patient, kept in a solution of 0·5 per cent Savlon, is an example of the type of measure which it is necessary to take.

2. *Control of special local conditions* in a surgical wound. Injury or bruising of a wound increases the risk of infection. The patient is instructed not to touch dressings or his skin which may have been contaminated by pus. Hand washing should be frequent and Chlorhexidine soap is used. Masks should not be touched with the fingers, changed frequently and as soon as a dressing has been finished the mask is discarded so that the nurse is able to breathe freely and diminish the risk of infection into her own nose. Naseptin, a mixture of neomycin and hibitane cream, may be used in the nose and is particularly valuable in nasal carriers.

3. *Special methods of protection* such as immunisation and prophylaxis.

The more specific the action of the organism the more highly developed are the measures to counteract its activity. In hospital it is the common pyogenic organisms which are particularly troublesome, and notable amongst these is the antibiotic-resistant staphylococcus.

4. *Recognition.* Because some degree of infection is inevitable, it is easy to fail to recognise the outbreak until it has reached serious proportions. Routine recordings of the temperature and pulse rate are invaluable. A separate register of any infection which arises in a wound may be kept in each ward; or better, a control of infection sister appointed to the hospital.

5. *Prevention.* The following measures are important:

(a) BED SPACING should be as generous as possible. A minimum of 2·4 metres is essential.

(b) STAFF with minor septic lesions should not be on duty in a surgical ward.

(c) CONTAMINATED DRESSINGS AND INSTRUMENTS are treated as appropriate by disinfection or incineration.

(d) STERILISATION must be effective and recontamination prevented (Chapter 10).

(e) BLANKETS are a special source of danger, and woollen blankets should be substituted by those made of cotton material or cellulose laundered when each patient is discharged. Gentleness in handling bedclothes reduces the risk of dissemination of infection.

(f) ANTIBIOTICS should be used with care and not indiscriminately (Chapter 7).

(g) THE DRESSING OF SURGICAL WOUNDS requires special care and protection and dressing only when really necessary. The patient should be instructed not to interfere with the dressing and to report if he requires attention for oozing of serum, pus or blood (Chapter 12).

(h) EXTRAORDINARY MEASURES are necessary for cases of homotransplantation (Chapter 27).

(i) NOTHING THAT IS TO BE PUT INTO THE BED SHOULD BE PLACED ON THE FLOOR—back rests, bed cradles and bedpans.

(j) SCREEN COVERS AND CURTAINS around the bed require regular laundering.

(k) ISOLATION. Where facilities are available, patients with infections due to organisms known to give rise to epidemics, e.g. certain staphylococcal infections, are barrier nursed in an isolation ward.

6. *Control.* Patients with an infected wound should, if possible, be isolated. If this is impossible barrier nursing has to be instituted at once. Infection spreads on the hands of the staff, fomites or clothes and through the air or by droplets. Hands should be washed inside the cubicle and *dried outside* to obviate contamination from paper cloths or paper towels stored in the cubicle. Unless gowns are used intelligently they are better not used at all. A surgeon dons a sterile gown before beginning an operation and discards it at the end. Only the same practice must be adopted in barrier nursing—such a practice need not add unduly to the laundry problem since the used gown usually need be only autoclaved and not laundered.

It may be desirable to close the ward to further admissions if the sepsis rate is rising or to empty the ward for cleaning and disinfection if there is a severe outbreak of infection.

Investigations should include bacteriological examination of:

(a) The wound.
(b) The mouth, hands, throat and skin of the staff.
(c) Careful examination to discover any specific lesions in other patients.

The appropriate chemotherapy will be used.

# CHAPTER 7

# Microbiology

All infections are caused by micro-organisms and these are divided into bacteria, viruses, fungi and protozoa. Bacteria can be seen with the aid of a microscope but viruses are very much smaller and can only be seen with the aid of an electron microscope.

Organisms which cause disease are known as pathogens; those incapable of causing disease non-pathogens.

## BACTERIA

MORPHOLOGY (SHAPE)

Micro-organisms which include bacteria and fungi are described according to their shape, as seen under the microscope:

1. Bacilli are rod-shaped.
2. Cocci are rounded.
3. Spirochaetes are corkscrew-shaped in appearance.
4. Fungi are much larger in size and branched.

Because organisms are colourless, staining is necessary to make them visible under the microscope.

PHYSIOLOGY

*Effect of atmosphere.* (1) Aerobic bacteria are organisms which cannot survive without oxygen. (2) Anaerobic organisms can survive only when free oxygen is absent. In the body anaerobic conditions are in practice only created when the blood supply has been cut off so that no oxygen reaches the part, for example, in dead muscle.

*Artificial growth of organisms.* This is known as culturing. Various substances known as media are used to grow organisms artificially; that most commonly used is agar. Pus containing organisms, swabbed on to an agar plate and kept at body temperature (37°C) overnight, will produce a growth varying in appearance with the strain of the organism. Viewed with the naked eye the effect appears rather like sugar icing on a cake or discrete colonies of the organism may be visible.

*Effect of temperature.* Conditions favourable to a growth of micro-organisms are warmth, moisture and an adequate supply of nutrients. Cold inhibits the growth of bacteria. It interferes with their ability to divide and multiply, but it never kills them. Some organisms provide for their survival by the formation of spores. A spore is the bacterium in a modified form, modified to protect itself in unfavourable surroundings. As soon as the conditions are more favourable it develops into a normal organism. While moist heat at 100°C (212°F) kills all organisms, spores require a temperature of 116°C (240°F) to 127°C (260°F) for their destruction.

*Reaction to Gram's stain.* All organisms are divided into those which are Gram-positive or Gram-negative. Organisms which stain and hold the stain are known as Gram-positive. Those in which it disappears after washing with alcohol are known as Gram-negative and require to be counterstained. Since the introduction of the antibiotics this has extended its significance beyond laboratory identification. For example, most Gram-positive cocci are sensitive to penicillin and most Gram-negative bacilli are sensitive to streptomycin.

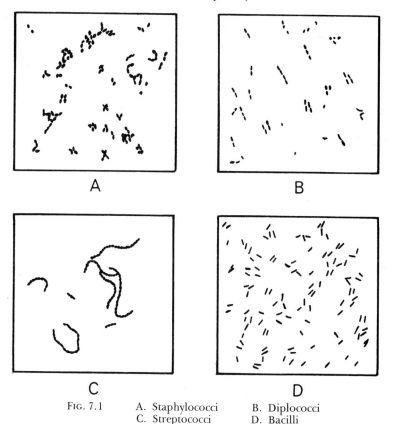

FIG. 7.1    A. Staphylococci    B. Diplococci
            C. Streptococci     D. Bacilli

As bacteria have acquired resistance to antibiotics, this pattern is tending to change, and it is customary to carry out in the laboratory sensitivity tests on the infective organisms prior to treatment. Where the patient's condition is such that there is no time for delay, substances such as gentamicin may be prescribed until the results of the sensitivity tests are available.

*Sensitivity to organisms.* This is determined by adding a particular antibiotic to the culture media and if growth is prevented the organism is described as sensitive.

### COMMON PYOGENIC ORGANISMS

The common pyogenic or pus-producing organisms include *staphylococci*, small rounded bacteria which, under the microscope, appear in clusters like bunches of grapes (Fig. 7.1).

The commonest group is the *Staphylococcus pyogenes*. Boils, carbuncles, and many abscesses in the skin and subcutaneous tissues are due to staphylococci. They are the most common cause of bone infection. Less frequently they cause infection elsewhere, for example, a perinephric abscess. Their tendency to acquire antibiotic resistance constitutes a major surgical problem. Sometimes they cause a fulminating enterocolitis which is a major threat to the patient's life.

*Streptococci*, viewed microscopically, appear in chains. Some strains haemolyse blood on a blood agar plate, and are then known as the haemolytic variety; the remainder as non-haemolytic. The haemolytic streptococci, which are much more virulent, are the causal organisms of many severe diseases such as septicaemia, bronchopneumonia, and empyema. A further danger is that they may be harboured in the throat of a healthy individual, causing no harm to the host, who spreads disease to others unknowingly. Such a person is known as a 'carrier'. Haemolytic streptococci are still usually sensitive to penicillin.

*Pneumococci* are always in pairs (diplococci). They are the usual cause of lobar pneumonia and occasionally are responsible for arthritis, empyema and meningitis. Very rarely they cause peritonitis in little girls. Pneumococci may be sensitive to penicillin and the sulphonamides.

*Escherichia coli* is a rod-shaped organism whose natural habitat is the intestine, where it is non-pathogenic. Like most Gram-negative organisms it produces a powerful endotoxin and may be a cause of bacteraemic shock. Perforation of the intestine enables the bacillus to gain access to the peritoneal cavity, where it is pathogenic (disease-causing). Hence it is a common cause of peritonitis secondary to appendicitis and diverticulitis. Urinary infections such as cystitis, and pyelonephritis are frequently due to the *E. coli*. It is penicillin-resistant, but is usually sensitive to the sulphonamide group of drugs, to streptomycin and chloramphenicol.

| Culture: *E. coli* | Penicillin | Streptomycin |
|---|---|---|
| | — | + |
| | Ampicillin | Tetracycline |
| | — | — |
| | Kanamycin | |
| | + | |

FIG. 7.2    Laboratory report stating the organism and the antibiotics to which it is sensitive and to which it is resistant.

The *Proteus group* of organisms of which the most common are *Proteus vulgaris* and *Proteus mirabilis* are well-recognised urinary tract pathogens where they cause pyelonephritis as well as lower urinary tract infections. They can also contaminate and infect wounds and burns.

*Pseudomonas aeruginosa* is a pathogenic organism which appears in wounds treated with antibiotics—it may cause persistent urinary infections as well as infection in machines used for assisted respiration. It is noted for the curious bluish-green of the pus. The most useful antibiotic is carbenicillin. It should be used not for the mere presence of the organism but when there is real danger from it. More recently the sulphamino penicillins have been tried. The great danger of *Pseudomonas* is that it develops in wounds when the competition from more sensitive bacteria has been removed. The young, the old, the burnt and patients receiving wide spectrum antibiotics or on steroid treatment are liable to develop this infection.

## VIRUSES

Virus diseases of special interest to the surgical nurse are poliomyelitis (infantile paralysis), viral hepatitis from blood products, and rubella (German measles) in the pregnant woman on account of the risk of congenital deformities to the foetus. The common cold and influenza are also due to viruses. Before it can cause disease a virus has to enter and multiply inside the body of the cell.

## FUNGI

*Monilia*, which is normally suppressed by harmless bacteria, may cause a virulent infection following broad-range antibiotics.

## THE PROTOZOA

Amoebic dysentery, malaria and hydatid disease are all caused by protozoa.

## ANTIBACTERIAL AGENTS

The antibiotics and chemotherapeutic agents are powerful antibacterial substances which have made surgical procedures safer and increased the scope of surgery. They have not however diminished the need for supportive measures such as good hygiene in the wards or the need for an incision to evacuate pus. Antibiotics are produced by moulds or by bacteria from which they are extracted, while chemotherapeutic agents are produced synthetically from chemical compounds. Some are bactericidal—that is they destroy the organism— others which prevent propagation are known as bacteriostatic.

Before discussing the more important agents briefly, some general principles should be considered:

1. **Choice of agent.** Modern chemotherapy has taught us to think not so much in terms of disease but in terms of sensitive organisms. If the organism is known and is sensitive to an antibiotic, cure is certain. This presupposes that the facilities for identification and tests for sensitivity are universally available. It also assumes that the organism can be readily isolated from the patient. Isolation, culture, assessment of sensitivity by the bacteriologist and the administration of the appropriate antibiotic is ideal. Unfortunately this is only possible in certain types of infection and in many cases it has to be assumed that the organism is the one commonly responsible for the condition and the antibiotic to which it is usually sensitive is chosen. The patient's response is used as an indication to sensitivity. If, after 72 hours, there is no response the antibiotic is changed or if, before this period has elapsed, the organism can be isolated and sensitivity tests show that a different antibiotic is indicated, therapy is changed.

When an antibiotic is prescribed it should be:

(a) Administered by the *correct route*. Penicillin, for example, is destroyed by gastric acid and has, therefore, to be given by intramuscular injection.

(b) Given at the stated intervals in the dose prescribed, so that its concentration in the bloodstream is maintained.

(c) Continued over a sufficient period of days to cure the infection.

A sufficient quantity of fluid has to be taken so that the antibiotic can be excreted by the kidney if this is its route of elimination, and if used for treatment of urinary infection the fluid intake should not be so great that the concentration of the antibiotic in the urine is so low as to be ineffective. An intake of 3 litres per day is probably the optimum.

It is inadvisable to prescribe antibacterial therapy for mild self-limiting infections. These substances are expensive, not without complications and may produce resistant organisms. It used to be thought that antibiotics given prophylactically would prevent postoperative infection, but experience has shown that this is not so and a careful aseptic technique is the best safeguard. There are, however, three conditions where they should be used before operation:

(i) Amputation for gangrene (p. 254).
(ii) Operations on patients with congenital or rheumatic heart disease.
(iii) Urethral dilatation.

A patient with a resistant organism sensitive to only one antibiotic should be nursed in isolation so that it is not propagated in the ward and may emerge resistant to every known antibiotic. Antibiotic therapy should cease when the period for which it has been prescribed has elapsed.

2. **Complications of antibiotic therapy.** (a) *Resistant organisms.* New antibiotics are being developed almost continuously. Penicillin and, in a lesser degree, streptomycin have a margin of safety not possessed by any other antibiotic. The need to use other antibiotics arises only when the organism is insensitive or resistant. One of the greatest current-day problems in hospital is the presence of resistant staphylococci. These arise in the following ways:

(i) Inadequate or too short a dosage of penicillin.
(ii) The difficulty of sterilising woollen blankets has been overcome by substituting cotton blankets.
(iii) Theatres attached to ward blocks are more liable to be infected with these resistant organisms than separate isolated theatre blocks. It is important to be certain that there are no defects in the air-conditioning plant. It is not unknown for defects to result in these organisms being sucked into the theatre from nearby wards and corridors. Even on the foggiest days in winter the atmosphere of an industrial town is reasonably sterile. The same cannot be said of the average hospital ward.
(iv) Patients for elective operations should be admitted into a clean unit.

(b) *Sensitisation* of the patient or staff may occur with any antibiotic. For this reason antibiotics are not prescribed for trivial infections. Sensitivity reactions take the form of a skin rash or even, in some cases, severe anaphylactic shock may result.

The following precautions are of value in protecting the nurse from sensitivity:

(i) The same needle can be put into the bottle of solution and also used for injection into the patient.

(ii) Air in the syringe should be expelled with the needle in the bottle. Spraying it into the atmosphere causes skin reaction on the face and arms.

(iii) The overall precaution, of course, is for the nurse to wear gloves.

(iv) Hermetically sealed or orally administered capsules of antibiotics prevent skin contact with the antibiotic. Disposable syringes and hand washing to remove any particles after handling antibiotics are probably as important in preventing reactions in the nurse.

3. **Toxic reactions.** Toxic reactions are almost unknown with penicillin, but damage to the 8th nerve may occur with the aminoglycoside antibiotics. Streptomycin and gentamicin affect particularly the vestibular branch while neomycin and kanamycin affect the auditory branch and both are more likely to occur in the presence of poor renal function. With local or topical use, neomycin, in addition to damage to the auditory division of the 8th nerve, is dangerous in the presence of hepatic failure as well as when renal function is impaired. It is recommended that inhalation of an aerosol of neomycin in bronchiectasis should be limited to 1 g daily. Similarly topical application to bedsores should not exceed 1 g daily.

Another well-known toxic reaction is the danger of aplastic anaemia from chloramphenicol. Many antibiotics of course are so toxic to the kidneys that they are unsuitable for use.

4. **Super infection.** Suppression of the normal flora by antibiotics may unleash the activities of organisms which are normally held in check. Examples are monilial infection and staphylococcal enterocolitis.

*Penicillin* was the first and is still the safest of the antibiotics. The original form sodium benzyl penicillin, known as crystalline penicillin, is effective against a large group of organisms of which the more important are:

Streptococcus
Gonococcus
Pneumococcus
Meningococcus
The gas gangrene bacillus, *Clostridium welchii*
Spirochaete of syphilis
*Cl. tetani*
*Bacillus anthracis*
*B. diphtheria*
Some staphylococci

It has no antibacterial action on:

*Escherichia coli*

*Salmonella typhosus*
*Mycobacterium tuberculosis*
*Pseudomonas aeruginosa*

## Administration and dosage

Penicillin may be administered:

### 1. SYSTEMICALLY

Intramuscular injection is the usual method of systemic administration, but with the present purified penicillin preparations the objection to the subcutaneous route because of painful reactions no longer holds, and this route may have some slight advantage in being followed by slower absorption. Penicillin dissolved in sterile distilled water or saline when injected is excreted by the kidneys in a few hours so that the concentration in the blood falls rapidly. This necessitates repeated injection every three hours. The dosage varies with the severity of the infection; 500,000 to 1 mega units six-hourly or twice daily is usually prescribed, and is continued for four to five days or longer. The dose is readily soluble in 1 ml of sterile water.

The absorption of penicillin may be delayed by dissolving the drug in procaine. The dose is 400,000 units once or twice daily. This preparation, while effective in most cases, is inadequate to maintain a high blood level of penicillin, and in severe infections or persistent infections due to a relatively resistant organism, sodium penicillin in water should be given.

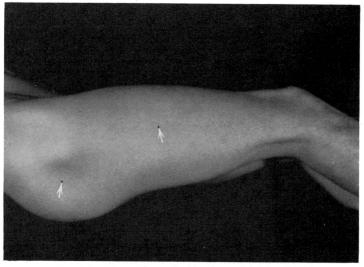

FIG. 7.3   The safe sites for intramuscular injection.

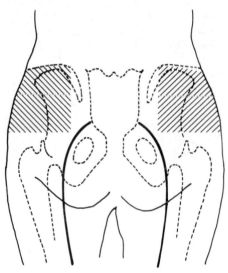

FIG. 7.4    If the buttock is used the upper and outer quadrant is the safe area.

*Intramuscular injection.* Requirements:
   Receiver
   5 or 10 ml syringe
   Needle—size 23G $1\frac{1}{4}$ (12) or 21G $1\frac{1}{2}$ (1)
   Needle—19G 2—for drawing up if required
   2 Mediswabs
   Prescription and recording sheet
   Disposable gloves should be worn when potentially sensitising drugs are to be injected.
   The injection is prepared in the treatment room. Using the aseptic technique the guarded needle and syringe are assembled and placed in the receiver. The drug is checked, the ampoule opened, or the cap of a multidose bottle wiped with a mediswab. The needle guard is removed. The drug is drawn up into the syringe, the amount being regulated according to the prescription. Air bubbles are expelled, the needle guard is secured, and the syringe and needle are replaced in the receiver together with a mediswab.
   The patient is advised of what is to happen. Privacy is ensured and the patient placed in a suitable position. The clothing is arranged so as to expose the site. The site chosen is the lateral aspect of the thigh. If this cannot be used, the ward sister or the unit officer is informed and they may give it into the buttock. The nurse and witness check with the prescription sheet. The nurse cleans the skin with the mediswab.
   The needle is inserted at an angle of 90°, care being taken to avoid touching the bone. The plunger is withdrawn slightly to

ensure a blood vessel has not been punctured. If blood is seen entering the syringe, the needle is withdrawn, and firm pressure applied to the puncture site for 10 seconds. An adjacent site is then chosen for the injection. If no blood is seen, the fluid is instilled gently. The mediswab is placed over the needle track and the needle withdrawn smoothly. The underlying tissues are massaged, and/or the patient is instructed to carry out 'quadriceps' exercises to aid absorption of the drug and to reduce discomfort. The patient is made comfortable and the recording sheet initialled by the nurse giving the injection. Used equipment is discarded, and the nurse washes and dries her hands.

*Subcutaneous or hypodermic injections.* Although not used for antibiotics they are necessary for the administration of many drugs.

*Requirements:*
>    Receiver
>    2 ml syringe
>    Needle—size 25G 1 (17)
>    Needle—21G 1½ (1)—for drawing up if required
>    2 Mediswabs
>    Prescription and recording sheet

The needle is inserted at an angle of 45°, care being taken not to insert it right up to the hub. The plunger is depressed

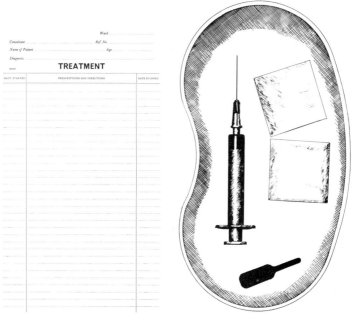

Fig. 7.5 Tray for intramuscular injection.

gently and the fluid instilled. The mediswab is placed over the needle track and the needle withdrawn smoothly. The skin is massaged gently to aid dispersion of the fluid.

The patient is made comfortable, and the recording sheet initialled by the nurse giving the injection. In the case of a DDA drug, the nurse and the witness sign the register. Used equipment is discarded, and the nurse washes and dries her hands.

## 2. LOCALLY.

Penicillin may be applied locally without the slightest harm to the tissues while killing or preventing the growth of susceptible organisms. It may be injected into the theca, joints, empyema or abscess cavities. However, local penicillin applications should be discouraged as sensitivity often develops.

Apart from a mild skin rash no toxic reactions from systemic penicillin have been reported, but as with any drug an acute sensitivity reaction may accrue. A few reports of fatal collapse following intrathecal penicillin have been reported. It is advisable to inquire if the patient is known to be sensitive to penicillin.

Penicillinase is an enzyme produced by bacteria which destroys benzyl penicillin and is responsible for the development of resistant organisms, particularly resistance of staphylococci.

The enzyme penicillinase is now procurable as 'Neutropen', and if given after a penicillin injection it destroys any drug left in the tissue and prevents sensitisation reactions.

*The later penicillins.* The basic nucleus of penicillin (6-aminopenicillanic acid) has been isolated, and from this any number of new penicillins can be made. This advance promises penicillins of wider antibacterial activity causing no reactions, together with a fresh approach to the problem of resistant organisms.

1. Phenoxyethyl penicillin (Broxil) has the advantage that it can be given by mouth.
2. Dimethoxyphenyl penicillin (Celbenin). This is invaluable in the treatment of penicillin resistant organisms, but it must be given by injection since, like penicillin, it is destroyed by the gastric acid.
3. Aminophenyl penicillin (Ampicillin, Penbritin) has a broader spectrum than any of the penicillins in use at present and active against Gram-negative bacilli. It has the advantage that it may be taken by mouth.
4. Phenoxypropyl penicillin (Ultrapen, Brocillin). This can also be given by mouth.
5. Cloxacillin (Orbenin) can be given by mouth in the treatment of resistant staphylococcal infection.

The development of penicillin will be taken further as time passes.

*Streptomycin* was the first product of intensive research following the demonstration of the powerful antibacterial properties of penicillin. By mouth its action is localised to the intestinal tract, from which it is not absorbed, so for systemic effect it has to be given by intramuscular injection. Its main disadvantages are the risk of damage to the eighth cranial nerve causing vertigo and deafness from prolonged administration, and the extraordinary rapidity with which resistance of bacteria to the drug can develop. For this reason it must be given in adequate doses at once if its use is advisable. It is the antibiotic of most value against the tubercle bacillus. It is important in cases of tuberculosis to combine its administration with PAS (para-aminosalicylic acid) or INAH (isonicotinic acid hydrazide) which delays the appearance of bacterial resistance. Used alone its most useful action in surgical practice is in the destruction of the *E. coli*.

DOSAGE. The usual dose is 1 g daily intramuscularly, but always combined with PAS or INAH by mouth in cases of tuberculosis. To diminish bacteria in the colon the usual dose is 1 g three times daily by mouth. It is excreted more slowly than penicillin by the kidneys and reaches a high concentration in the urine, where it is effective in destroying sensitive organisms. The urine must be alkaline for streptomycin to be effective in these infections. Streptomycin given systemically does not reach the cerebrospinal fluid and therefore must be injected intrathecally for meningeal infections.

*Chloramphenicol* (chloromycetin), which was the first antibiotic to be synthesised, is effective against a wider range of organisms than penicillin and streptomycin together. It is curative in typhoid fever, bacillary dysentery and acute brucellosis. It is effective against some virus diseases. It is administered by mouth or intravenously. The dosage is 250 to 500 mg six-hourly Vitamin B complex should be given as well. Nausea, vomiting and diarrhoea as well as agranulocytosis or aplastic anaemia may develop as toxic reactions so its administration should be limited to conditions where other antibiotics are inappropriate.

*The tetracyclines* include chlortetracycline (aureomycin), oxytetracycline (terramycin), tetracycline (achromycin), and dimethylchlortetracycline (ledermycin). They are all antibiotics of wide antibacterial activity and have the advantage that they are effective when taken by mouth but may also be administered intramuscularly or intravenously. Their great value is in conditions in which other antibiotics have failed to effect cure or resistance has developed.

DOSAGE. Average dosage is 250 mg six-hourly.

Like chloramphenicol, they may produce mild gastrointestinal disturbances and a raw tongue while, in addition, soreness of the buttocks and anus may occur. Vitamin B complex should be administered if treatment is prolonged. Tetracyclines given during pregnancy or in the first year of life cause permanent discoloration of developing teeth. If the prescribing of tretracyclines increases the future population will probably have teeth several shades deeper on average than hitherto. Oxytetracycline causes less discoloration.

*Other antibiotics* are bacitracin, polymyxin, and erythromycin. All are of value in appropriate cases. The main use of these antibiotics is when the organisms are resistant to penicillin or streptomycin.

*Erythromycin* has a similar range of activity to penicillin but its main disadvantage is that bacteria rapidly develop resistance. The dose is 250 to 500 mg six-hourly.

*Fucidin* is an antistaphylococcal antibiotic of the 'narrow spectrum' type. It is administered orally only in a dosage of 250 to 500 mg six-hourly.

*Lincomycin* (Lincocin) has recently been introduced as another antibiotic effective against staphylococcus as well as other organisms.

*Cephaloridine* (Ceporin) is an antibiotic effective against many other resistant Gram-negative organisms. It may be given in a dosage of 250 mg six-hourly intramuscularly. It may also be given by mouth.

*Trimethoprim* is an antibacterial substance similar in range to the sulphonamides. When combined with a sulphonamide, usually sulphamethoxazole, it has a greatly potentiated and very effective range of activity. Commercially it is supplied as Septrin or Bactrim.

Other antibiotics which are used occasionally are kanamycin, colomycin and gentamicin.

Bacitracin, polymyxin and neomycin are in the main used as local applications and are combined in a 'polybactrin spray'. Neomycin may be used for rapid sterilisation of the intestinal tract in preparation for surgery in a dose of 1 g every four to six hours for 24 hours. Nystatin is effective against monilial infections, for example, *Candida albicans*.

Griseofulvin in prolonged dosages of 1 g daily is effective in fungal infections of the skin, nails and the scalp.

## THE SULPHONAMIDE GROUP OF DRUGS

The sulphonamide group of drugs are, in general, effective against the same organisms as penicillin, with the important exception that *E. coli*, which is insensitive to penicillin, responds to the sulphonamides.

There are several separate sulphonamides which are divisible into two groups:

1. THOSE ABSORBABLE FROM THE INTESTINAL TRACT
   This group includes:

> Sulphathiazole and sulphadiazine
> Sulphadimidine, sulphamerazine and sulphafurazole (Gantrisin).

They are normally given by mouth. As they pass into the cerebrospinal fluid they are useful for prophylaxis following fractures of the skull. They are also very useful in the treatment of infections of the kidney. The usual dosage is 2 g initially, followed by 1 g four-hourly for four to five days or longer. A tablet containing a mixture of three sulphonamides—sulphatriad—was said to be less likely to cause toxic reactions, but investigation has shown that this is not true.

These preparations are insufficiently soluble for parenteral administration and must be given as their sodium salt in 1 ml of normal saline by the intravenous route.

A useful addition to the sulphonamide group of drugs is a long-acting sulphonamide which maintains a therapeutic blood level for at least 24 hours and a single daily dose of 0·5 g is sufficient. The untoward effects are, of course, also prolonged. There are three separate long-acting sulphonamides:

> Sulphamethoxypyridazine (marketed as Midicel and Lederkyn).
> Sulphaphenazole
> Sulphadimethozene 'Madribon'.

## Toxic reactions
*General:*
1. Nausea and vomiting.
2. Dizziness.
3. Cyanosis.

*Local:*
1. Damage to the active blood-forming tissue. This results in leucopenia (p. 40) and anaemia.
2. Skin rashes and drug fever.
3. Haematuria.
4. Crystallisation of the drug in the kidneys. This causes anuria (p. 444).

*Prevention*
1. The total dosage is normally limited to 30 g of short-acting sulphonamides in the adult.

2. A white blood count examination is undertaken in prolonged administration.

3. The fluid intake must be adequate, 3 litres daily to prevent crystallisation of the drug in the kidney. Because this is more likely to occur in acid urine, a mixture of potassium citrate is given to render the urine alkaline. A fluid balance chart should be kept.

4. A patient receiving sulphonamide therapy should be at rest and not ambulant.

LOCAL USE OF THE ABSORBABLE SULPHONAMIDES. As a powder or cream, sulphathiazole and sulphanilamide are used extensively to combat infection. Sulphacetamide is widely used as eye drops.

2. THOSE NON-ABSORBABLE FROM THE INTESTINAL TRACT

These preparations pass through the gastrointestinal tract almost unchanged, and are used in the treatment of infections such as dysentery. They are of great value in surgical practice in diminishing the infectivity of the bowel before and after operations, such as colectomy. Succinyl-sulphathiazole (sulfasuxidine) is the preparation in common use. Its administration, etc. is discussed under Diseases of the Colon.

Sulphasalazine (Salazopyrin) is taken up selectively by the connective tissue of the intestine; 1 g four or more times daily is the usual dosage. It is strictly speaking an absorbable sulphonamide but is later excreted into the intestinal tract.

### OTHER ANTIBACTERIAL CHEMOTHERAPEUTIC AGENTS

The nitrofurans are a distinct class of antimicrobial substances unrelated to the sulphonamides or the antibiotics. They produce their antibacterial activity by:

1. Inhibiting carbohydrate metabolism ⎫
2. Interfering with cellular respiration ⎭ of micro-organisms

Nitrofurantoin is administered orally for urinary infections. Furamide is used in bacillary dysentery, bacillary food-poisoning, and non-specific diarrhoea.

Nalidixic acid (Negram) is an antibacterial agent particularly active against Gram-negative organisms. A side-effect is photo-sensitivity of the skin producing a severe sunburn-like reaction on exposure to sunlight.

Noxyloilin (Noxyflex) is used in local treatment of wounds (aerosol spray) or in the bladder as an instillation.

# CHAPTER 8

# Inflammation

Inflammation is the response of the body to an irritant. The irritant may be a burn, a chemical, a wound, or a micro-organism. It is usually painful; pain warns the patient that the enemy has arrived and is an indication that his body has risen to the attack.

It is only the body tissues which can overcome the irritant. By treatment we can, at the best, only aid this struggle. If necessary, the body will sacrifice much loss of tissue to survive, and when its superiority has been established it will cleanse and repair its wound. The modern conception of inflammation recognises four stages as illustrated in wound healing. Wound healing always follows a regular pattern:

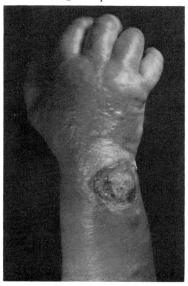

FIG. 8.1  Acute inflammation of back of forearm. Note oedema of hand and fingers.

**Stage 1. Traumatic inflammation.** During this phase the edges of the wound becomes oedematous and matted together with fibrin. Within a few hours of injury the capillaries dilate and fluid leaks through the damaged endothelium and accumulates in the interstitial space. The body temperature may

63

rise to 37·2 to 37·5°C (99 to 99·5°F) as in acute inflammation elsewhere. Lymphangitis and lymphadenitis occur at this stage.

**Stage 2. Destruction,** in which necrotic material is removed. It is characterised by the migration of leucocytes and macrophages into the wound. These cells engulf and destroy dead or dying tissue. It is terminated by the formation of pus. If the destructive stage is very severe the process goes on to necrosis, which is death of a small area of tissue as opposed to gangrene, which may also occur and means gross death.

**Stage 3. Proliferation.** When epithelium and connective tissue develop, new capillaries sprout off the sides of existing wounds. Fibroblasts appear alongside the capillaries. These two together constitute granulation tissue. Fine fibrils soon form in the ground substance and then gradually aggregate into typical collagen fibres. The stage of proliferation starts from the 4th to 14th day. During this phase all the cells forming the surface epithelium undergo rapid division and migrate as a thin film covering the wound. They also grow down as several sprouts into the depth of the wound. It is thought by some pathologists that these tiny growths of epithelial cells stimulate the formation of granulation tissue.

**Stage 4. Maturation.** During this phase the blood vessels gradually disappear and the number of fibroblasts in relation to fibres diminish. The red elevated recent scar is gradually changed into a thin white line.

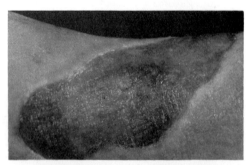

FIG. 8.2   A granulating wound.

*Healing by first intention* (primary healing) and *healing by second intention* (healing by granulation) were in the past considered to be distinct processes. Healing by granulation is essentially the same as primary healing, the only difference being that usually, as a result of infection, the stage of destruction is greatly prolonged and results in a deep cavity which is filled gradually from the bottom by granulation tissue.

*Tissue repair*

Repair is the process by which tissue is replaced—the simpler the tissue the more effective repair can be. As tissue, i.e. cells, become highly specialised repair becomes more difficult. Epithelial surfaces and fibrous tissue will regenerate without too much difficulty, but most other cells, and in particular nerve cells and structures like the glomerulus in the kidney, are not replaced but the space they occupy is filled with fibrous tissue. Some apparently highly specialised epithelial tissue is capable of regeneration and this is seen particularly where liver cells may be destroyed by disease.

If granulation tissue is excessive it is raised above the level of the approaching epithelium and forms an insurmountable barrier to the spread of epithelium. This is corrected by cauterising the granulation tissue to the level of the epithelium with silver nitrate.

**Changes in the other body tissues and body fluids.**

1. *Blood*—leucocytosis (increased number of white cells).
2. *Skin and tissue*—temperature increased.
3. *Urine*—concentrated because of the need to conserve fluid in the body.
4. *Bowels*—constipated.

### FAILURE OF THE INFLAMMATORY REACTION

In severe infection the inflammatory reaction may fail to develop and the patient succumbs rapidly. More commonly the failure is partial and it is important to recognise at once the factors which may be preventing its full development. They are:

1. **Poor arterial blood supply.**
   (a) Age—arteriosclerosis.
   (b) Site—the lower third of the leg—gross scarring.
   (c) Tight dressings. Tourniquets.
   (d) Arterial thrombosis or embolism.
   (e) Shock—A poor blood supply diminishes the supply of leucocytes and allows bacteria to multiply.
   (f) Gas pressure—gas gangrene.
2. **Deficient venous drainage.**
   (a) Venous thrombosis.
   (b) Varicose veins.
3. **Depression or deficiency of the quality of the blood.**
   (a) Anaemia—nutritional.
                    haemorrhage.
   (b) Leucopenia. Steroids suppress the action of the leucocytes.
   (c) Hypoproteinaemia, Plasma protein levels below 5 g per 100 ml are insufficient for a skin graft to take.
4. **Malnutrition and dehydration.**

General.
Vitamin deficiency.
Zinc deficiency.
5. **Excess of fluid in the tissues.**
*Oedema*—cardiac.
　　　　nephritic.
　　　　lymphatic obstruction.
　　　　venous obstruction.
6. **Metabolic.**
Diabetes.
Nephritis.
Uraemia.
Portal cirrhosis.
Jaundice.
7. **Drugs.**
ACTH.
Cortisone.
Metallic poison.
Cytotoxic drugs.

*The signs and symptoms of inflammation*

The constitutional symptoms include malaise, loss of appetite, fatigue and sleeplessness. The temperature is elevated and the pulse rate is increased. The urinary output is scanty and the bowel is constipated. All these symptoms are due to the toxins which are liberated by the invading organism into the blood stream. In overwhelming infection the patient may be in bacteraemic shock.

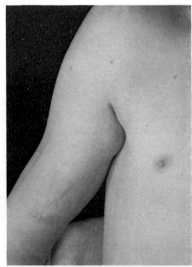

FIG. 8.3   Acute abscess of the arm.

LOCAL SIGNS AND SYMPTOMS

1. *Redness* is caused by dilatation of capillaries in the inflamed area.

2. *Heat* is due to the increased blood flow.

3. *Swelling* occurs because plasma is poured into the surrounding tissues. The degree of swelling is dependent to some extent on the natural laxity or otherwise of the tissues, for example, inflammation below the eyes causes an extreme degree of swelling at a very early stage.

4. *Pain* is due to the accumulation of toxins which irritate the nerve endings and hormones released locally from stretching of the tiny nerve twigs caused by the excess of fluid in the tissues, which increases as tension becomes greater.

5. *Loss of function* occurs as a result of pain, swelling and of the toxic effect on the tissue itself. The patient's natural desire is to rest and to avoid using any painful part.

The termination of inflammation may be:

   (a) Resolution
   (b) Suppuration
   (c) Ulceration
   (d) Gangrene
   (e) Fibrosis

## THE SPREAD OF INFECTION IN THE TISSUES

According to the form of spread which occurs, special terms are used to describe the process.

1. **Cellulitis.** It is the direct spread of infection in the tissues, or more strictly in the extracellular spaces. The term cellulitis is really a misnomer, and resolution may occur spontaneously, or pus may form.

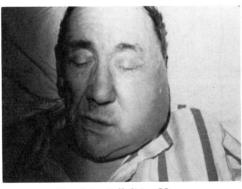

FIG. 8.4   Cellulitis of face.

2. **Lymphangitis.** The lymphatic vessels between the site of infection and the regional lymphatic glands are usually

inflamed. Classically they are best seen as red lines on the arm of a patient suffering from a septic finger.

3. **Lymphadenitis.** The lymphatic glands (syn. nodes) are invaded by organisms carried by the lymph stream in the lymphatic vessels. The lymphatic glands, which become swollen and tender, are structurally well equipped to deal with infection by their complex network, which filters the organisms.

The common sites for lymphadenitis and the areas from which they are infected are:

| Glands | Area of infection |
|---|---|
| (a) The neck | Face, mouth, tongue and scalp |
| (b) The axilla | Breast and upper limb |
| (c) The groin | Lower limb, groin and perineum |

4. **Bacteraemia.** Bacteraemia is the spread of organisms into the blood stream where they are usually destroyed.

5. **Septicaemia.** Septicaemia is the invasion and multiplication of bacteria in the blood steam, and the onset is usually heralded by a single rigor followed by persistent pyrexia.

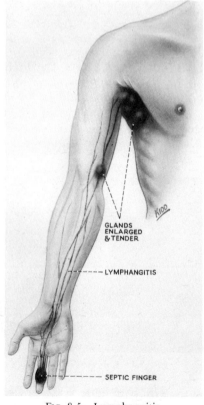

FIG. 8.5   Lymphangitis.

6. **Pyaemia.** Pyaemia is the spread of organisms in the blood stream, with the formation of abscesses at many sites in the body. Although the tissues have failed to contain the process locally, they are still endeavouring to localise it at more distant sites. The great danger is that the abscesses are usually multiple, and are often at sites not only remote from one another but relatively inaccessible to surgical drainage, such as the liver and the brain.

7. **Other forms of spread.** In the body cavities and the lumen of tubed viscera, infection can spread very rapidly.

Two other terms must be mentioned: *toxaemia*, which is the spread of the toxic products of inflammation from the site of infection into the blood stream; and *suppuration*, which is the process of pus formation.

## TREATMENT AND NURSING CARE

1. Rest is a counsel of perfection and has to be interpreted in relation to the function of the part inflamed. It consists of a darkened room to a patient with an inflamed eye, a bland diet in gastrointestinal infection or a sling to rest an infected arm.

2. Analgesics relieve pain and enable the patient to sleep.

3. Restoration of function must be kept in mind from the beginning.

4. Specific measures to counteract the infection, such as the administration of antibacterial drugs and surgical measures like incision or excision, are considered in appropriate sections later.

## CHAPTER 9

# The Specific Surgical Infections

A specific surgical infection is a disease which can be caused only by a particular strain of organism. Tetanus can be caused only as a result of infection with the tetanus bacillus, and anthrax by infection with the anthrax bacillus.

### TETANUS (Lock-Jaw)

Tetanus is commonly known as lock-jaw, because the muscular spasms which characterise it frequently attack the muscles of the jaw. The discovery of an antitoxin and methods of active immunisation as well as control of the preparation of catgut have made tetanus almost a rare disease.

BACTERIOLOGY. The *Clostridium tetani* is the causal organism. It is an anaerobic organism with a drum-stick head, the spore of which is very resistant to the ordinary methods of sterilisation. The bacillus is a normal inhabitant of the large intestine of several animals, including the sheep; for this reason highly manured soil is rich in tetanus spores. Catgut is prepared from sheep's intestine, hence the special precaution necessary in its manufacture. The organism elaborates a powerful toxin which poisons the motor nerve cells, with the result that spasm occurs in the muscles supplied by the corresponding nerves.

MODE OF ACCESS. A small, deep, punctured wound is the most dangerous, but all wounds contaminated with soil, manure, etc. are suitable points of entry.

Wounds may be contaminated in the theatre from:

1. Catgut
2. Improperly sterilised dressings and powders
3. The air. Infected hair used in replacing defective plaster walls is a possible source
4. Outdoor shoes

*Symptoms and signs*

The first symptom is slight stiffness of the muscles, particularly those of the jaw. The patient is anxious, but mentally clear. As the disease progresses the classical picture of tetanus appears.

The back is arched and the head may be thrown back (opisthotonos). The facial muscles are in spasm, and the

70

mouth can be opened only with difficulty (trismus). Drawing up of the angle of the mouth gives rise to the characteristic smile (risus sardonicus).

Spasms may affect every muscle in the body, and in severe cases the muscles rupture. Spasm of the sphincter muscles of the body render swallowing, defaecation, and micturition very difficult. Spasm of the respiratory muscles causes long periods of anoxia until death ensues. The temperature is elevated and the pulse rate is increased.

PROGNOSIS. The longer the incubation period the more hopeful is the outlook.

### Treatment and nursing care

PROPHYLACTIC. Careful surgical toilet and a prophylactic dose of penicillin is the best prevention. If the patient has not been immunised human antitetanus immunoglobulin is the ideal.

If an old accidental wound has to be reopened (perhaps years later) tetanus spores may be lying dormant in its substance. Their reactivation may give rise to tetanus. This danger is described as latent tetanus. The best prophylactic treatment is active immunisation against tetanus.

If one can be certain of the patient's immunity status, a patient who has been actively immunised should be given a booster dose of tetanus toxoid, but within three years of immunisation it can be omitted.

THERAPEUTIC—SPECIFIC TREATMENT

Penicillin is bacteriostatic and is administered in all cases of tetanus. It is also protective if there is an accompanying pneumonia. Human antiserum is given.

*The wound must be excised* and irrigated with hydrogen peroxide, because the tetanus bacillus will not grow in the presence of oxygen. The wound is not sutured.

GENERAL TREATMENT

*Absolute rest and isolation* are important, since the slightest noise or flicker increases the spasms. The patient is nursed in a quiet dark room which must be draught-free. The door should be fitted with suitable closing springs to prevent slamming. The nurse should warm her hands before touching the patient to avoid stimulating further spasms.

Most deaths are due to lack of oxygen and pulmonary infection. The toxin infects the bulbar nuclei so that the muscles of the pharynx and larynx are affected; the larynx is no longer the watch-dog for the lungs. Coughing is ineffective and anything that the patient swallows or regurgitates from the stomach is liable to infect the lungs. The important points in treatment are:

1. No oral feeding. A nasogastric tube is passed in all but the mildest cases and the stomach is aspirated before each feed if nasogastric feeding is permitted.
2. A tracheostomy is performed and suction applied at regular intervals. Controlled respiration using a mechanical respirator should be used as soon as possible. Regular suction produces sympathetic overactivity with resultant fall in blood pressure and tachycardia. The pulse should therefore be checked and any alteration reported.
3. Muscle relaxants relieve most of the symptoms. The eyes are protected if curare is used, otherwise conjunctivitis develops.
4. The maintenance of a fluid balance by intravenous fluids. The relaxant is injected into the drip by the anaesthetist.
5. Sedatives are used very sparingly and are almost unnecessary if relaxants are used correctly.

### ANTHRAX

Anthrax is a disease contracted by handling hides, animal coverings, wool, and hair.

BACTERIOLOGY. The causal organism is the *Bacillus anthracis*, and its importance in causing disease lies in the resistance of its spore, which requires special methods of sterilisation for its destruction. The incubation period is one to three days.

*Symptoms and signs*

A small patch of inflammation develops in the skin and the local lymphatic glands are enlarged. It is similar in appearance to an area of cellulitis, but is usually much less painful. Later, a blister or vesicle forms, and in a day or two several small blisters become confluent and fill with blood; this is known as a malignant pustule.

A pulmonary and gastrointestinal form may occur.

The anthrax bacillus is an organism which is penicillin-sensitive, and this is the treatment of choice. It is usually sensitive to streptomycin.

*Local treatment*

This consists of rest and keeping the lesion covered with an antiseptic compress.

### GAS GANGRENE

Gas gangrene is the occurrence in a wound of putrefactive changes similar to those which occur in the decomposition of the body after death. The more earth-stained and lacerated a wound, the more likely is gas infection to develop.

SOURCES IN HOSPITAL. The organism is most commonly

patient's own intestinal flora. It is particularly significant and, if gas gangrene is to be avoided following amputations or operations on the hip in these patients, the skin should be treated with compresses of Povidoiodine applied for 30 minutes. This reduces the number of organisms and afterwards the skin is swabbed with alcohol—soap and water washing has little effect. Additionally, penicillin is administered intramuscularly at the beginning of the operation.

BACTERIOLOGY. Two organisms are mainly responsible for gas gangrene. They produce powerful necrotising exotoxins:

1. *Clostridium welchii* which destroys glucose and produces carbon dioxide and hydrogen gases;
2. *Clostridium sporogenes*, which destroys protein and produces hydrogen disulphide and hydrogen gases.

These organisms can thrive only in conditions which are devoid of oxygen. The depth of a wound containing lacerated muscle to which the blood supply has been impaired is ideal for their proliferation. The gases produced spread along the muscle sheaths and compress the blood vessels so that the blood supply is still further impaired. A virulent toxin is produced, and finds its way into the blood stream by the small blood vessels which are not yet compressed. This gives rise to the profound toxaemia so characteristic of the disease.

*Symptoms and signs*

Pain in the wound is extremely severe. It is important to remember that the disease may develop in a wound under plaster. Never neglect the pain of a patient in plaster—at least it may indicate a pressure sore or gas gangrene.

The wound, which may be green or black, has a strong 'mouselike' odour. Small bubbles of gas may be seen escaping and the surrounding tissues are swollen and crackle when touched (crepitus). Untreated, deterioration is rapid.

In early cases, radiographic examination may reveal the presence of gas in the tissues.

*Treatment*

Wide excision of all infected tissue must be performed and the wound left open after resuscitation with blood transfusion and the administration of antibiotics. The wound is irrigated with hydrogen peroxide and eusol afterwards, and the danger has passed only when granulations appear. Complete isolation is essential to prevent infection spreading into the wounds of other patients.

Hyperbaric oxygen therapy may save the limb but is of no value until after excision has been performed.

## SURGICAL TUBERCULOSIS

THE ORGANISM. The *Mycobacterium tuberculosis* is an aerobic rod-shaped organism, and, because of certain staining peculiarities, is described by bacteriologists as acid-fast.

MODE OF ACCESS. The organism may be ingested, inhaled or inoculated through the skin.

COURSE OF THE DISEASE. The pathological reaction of tissues to the bacillus is known as a tubercule which consists of a central necrotic mass of caseous or cheese-like material containing giant cells surrounded by a layer of lymphocytes. It may li-

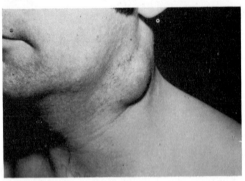

FIG. 9.1    Cold abscess of the neck.

quefy to form what is known as a cold or tuberculous abscess which may point on the surface and become infected with organisms on the skin. The result is that chronic infection with pyogenic organisms results in a persistent discharge and this may cause amyloid disease (p. 559). At any stage of the disease healing may occur by fibrosis of the tubercule, and this is sometimes consolidated further by calcification of its substance.

**Cold abscess.** The tuberculous abscess is described as cold because the skin temperature is not raised. Erythema of the skin and pointing of the abscess develop slowly. Frequently these changes never appear, because resolution occurs and the pus is absorbed.

If pointing is threatened, aspiration is performed through an area of relatively healthy skin. The greatest care is taken to prevent secondary infection. Very rarely are tuberculous abscesses incised, and then only if it is possible to eradicate the underlying focus.

*Treatment*

1. SPECIFIC TREATMENT

Chemotherapy has made tuberculosis at any site a most curable disease. It is almost always treated by a combination of two or more drugs to diminish the risk and time of onset of bacterial resistance. The drugs are:

(a) Streptomycin. The usual dosage is 1 g daily for a period of six to 12 weeks or longer.
(b) Isoniazid (INAH). The usual dosage is 100 mg three times a day for a year.
(c) Para-amino-salicylic acid (PAS). The usual dose is up to 12 g a day for one year.

Antituberculous chemotherapy is used in one form or another for long periods, sometimes as long as one year. Second line or salvage drugs include Pyrazinamide, Viomycin, Ethionamide, Cycloserine, Ethambutal, Rifampicin or kanamycin, and are used only when drug resistance to one of the standard drugs has emerged.

The principal cause of failure is irregular self-medication. The patient is feeling better, unpleasant side effects and forgetfulness lead to irregularity. Careful monitoring of therapy by urine testing for the drugs, frequent interrogation of the patient and home visits are desirable.

2. GENERAL MEDICAL TREATMENT

Measures to improve the patient's health—good food and fresh air are important.

3. SURGICAL TREATMENT

The scope of surgical treatment has greatly diminished since the advent of chemotherapy, but it still has a place in the excision or partial excision of an organ infected with tuberculosis, and the management of a cold abscess is still an important surgical condition.

### THE VENEREAL DISEASES

There are a number of venereal and allied diseases but only two, syphilis and gonorrhoea, are commonly seen in the British Isles. A third disease, chancroid or soft sore, is seen from time to time in the seaports. It is a disease of the tropics caused by Ducrey's bacillus.

Syphilis and gonorrhoea both produce local lesions at the site of infection, usually on the sex organs. The local lesions of gonorrhoea are painful and alarming, and the patient usually seeks advice, while those of syphilis are surprisingly trivial and sometimes so slight that even the patient is unaware of their presence. Both diseases may produce widespread lesions in later years, but the ravages and destruction caused by syphilis in almost every organ of the body culminate in a large variety of lesions which simulate almost every disease. It was for this reason that Osler called it the 'Great Imitator'.

## SYPHILIS

**Congenital syphilis.** The mother may infect her unborn child *in utero*, and, clinically, this may have the following results:

1. Abortion—usually after the fifth month.
2. The child is rarely born with signs of active disease but may develop them in the first two weeks of life.
3. The child appears to be normal at birth and the signs of congenital syphilis appear in later years.

If treatment is given up to the 28th week of pregnancy the child can be born free from syphilis.

*Symptoms and signs*

The signs of congenital syphilis are essentially those of acquired syphilis, commencing at the secondary stage. The most characteristic sign is the typical secondary rash, which usually develops in the course of the first fortnight of life. It is a widespread copper-coloured rash affecting almost the whole of the body. Scars may appear around the mouth, known as rhagades, and infection of the nose causes a thick purulent discharge, the typical snuffles of congenital syphilis.

Other signs are:

1. Flattening of the nose from destruction of the nasal septum.
2. Interstitial keratitis and iritis. The cornea is dull and opaque, due to syphilitic thickening, and if the infection is untreated blindness may result.
3. The permanent upper incisor teeth may have concave lower borders (Hutchinson's teeth, Moon's 'turreted' molars are sometimes seen), and are pathognomonic of congenital syphilis.

Other symptoms, such as painless effusion into the knee joints (Clutton's joints), infantile tabes, congenital deafness, and cerebral deterioration, may all appear at a later stage. The bones may be affected by inflammation of the periosteum, which is so painful that the child is unable to move his limbs, and the condition is described as syphilitic pseudoparalysis.

**Acquired syphilis.** *The primary lesion* of syphilis is the chancre, or septic sore at the site of infection—in men usually on the penis and in women either on the vulva or the cervix of the uterus. Occasionally chancres are found elsewhere, for example, on the lips, or on the nurse's finger from contact with a syphilitic lesion while in attendance on the patient. The primary lesion has an incubation period of one to three weeks and is painless; it is highly infectious, and must never be touched with the naked finger. Untreated, it rapidly heals and gives rise later to almost any symptoms in any part of the body.

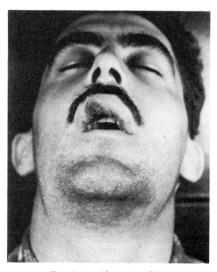

FIG. 9.2    Chancre of lip.

After its disappearance the patient may have no further clinical evidence of syphilis until he develops lesions many years later, or he may pass into the secondary stage two to six months later.

*Secondary syphilis.* An extensive rash is the characteristic symptom. It is usually a dull copper-coloured eruption, particularly on the back and face.

A similar lesion occurs in the throat, and the moisture of that area produces what is known as a snail-track ulcer. The presence of secondary syphilitic lesions in the anal region produces large soggy thicknesses known as condylomata.

All the lymphatic glands are very much enlarged. They are rubbery to the touch and are not tender.

*Tertiary stage.* This may occur years after the primary or secondary lesion. The characteristic lesion is known as a gumma, and may occur in any organ of the body. The tibia and skin overlying it, as well as the palate, are favourite sites. It takes the form of a hard mass which gradually breaks down to form an ulcer, which has a typical punched-out appearance.

*Parasyphilitic lesions.* These are the most dreaded of all manifestations of syphilis, and include tabes dorsalis, general paralysis of the insane, and lesions of the heart and circulatory system, such as aortic regurgitation and aneurysm of the thoracic aorta.

*The diagnosis of syphilis*
The finding of the *Treponema pallidum* in the primary lesion

is the most certain method of diagnosis. A specimen is taken by the doctor by means of a capillary tube and examined immediately under a microscope by darkground illumination unstained.

The Kahn or Wassermann reaction is positive on examination of the blood two to three weeks after the appearance of the primary lesion. The blood collected for this test should not be oxalated, as the test is performed on the serum content. Five millilitres of blood are withdrawn from a vein in the arm.

*Treatment*

Penicillin is now the drug of choice. In the later stages of the disease potassium iodide is still of value, often in combination with penicillin. Few complications are likely to occur, but some patients are allergic to certain forms of penicillin and care is necessary in such cases.

### GONORRHOEA

Gonorrhoea is due to a diplococcus known as the *Gonococcus*. It is an aerobic organism and extremely delicate. The acute symptoms appear after about three days from the time of infection. They consist of irritation of the urethra in the male, followed by a copious, yellow, purulent discharge. The patient is toxic, complains of malaise, and has a high temperature. There is frequency of micturition and the patient finds walking uncomfortable. In the female, Bartholin's glands may be swollen and a local abscess or cyst may form.

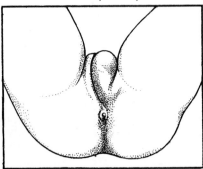

FIG. 9.3   Bartholin's cyst.

In pregnant women there is sometimes surprisingly little evidence of infection.

Gonorrhoea may spread through the whole of the genital tract. In the female, infection of the cervix uteri and of the Fallopian tubes (salpingitis) is not uncommon. In the male, the Cowper's glands, the prostate, and sometimes the epididymis may be affected.

**Chronic lesions of gonorrhoea.** Any of the acute lesions in the urinary tract may become chronic, but, in addition, infection may spread to other regions of the body. Arthritis, particularly of the ankles, is not uncommon. In babies, conjunctivitis and keratitis may be acquired during birth. The treatment of ophthalmia neonatorum is described in Chapter 51. Occasionally gonorrhoea is responsible for infective endocarditis.

The outstanding chronic surgical lesion resulting from gonococcal infection is stricture of the male urethra.

*Treatment*

The most useful drugs in the treatment of gonorrhoea are penicillin, streptomycin, and the sulphonamides such as sulphathiazole or sulphatriad, either alone or in combination, depending on the stage of the disease when first seen. If resistant strains have developed, kanamycin, the tetracyclines or trimethoprim may be used.

Repeated examinations by direct smears and cultures are essential before declaring the patient cured.

It is not very uncommon for a patient to be suffering from both gonorrhoea and syphilis. It is important that this should be discovered by the appropriate serological tests as short-term penicillin therapy will cure gonorrhoea but only mask syphilis.

### NON-SPECIFIC URETHRITIS

This troublesome condition, almost exclusively confined to the male, is becoming increasingly prevalent. It consists of a urethral discharge containing no recognisable organisms and tends, quite often, to run a chronic course. The cause is at present unknown but a virus is suspected in many cases.

It is often associated with various forms of arthritis which may respond to ACTH or cortisone.

Treatment consists of sulphonamides, the various antibiotics, and irrigation of the urethra with a 1 : 8000 oxycyanide of mercury solution.

*Social aspects of venerology.* Follow-up contact tracing and publicity campaigns are important in limiting the spread and prevention of disease. The patient is more likely to continue treatment until a cure is effected and to co-operate in tracing contacts if the doctors and nurses treat him with human understanding, tact and compassion.

# CHAPTER 10

# Sterilisation

To sterilise is to render a micro-organism incapable of reproduction. Efficient sterilisation is fundamental to the practice of surgery, and it is surprising that even today, although so many years have passed since Louis Pasteur and Lord Lister first demonstrated its importance, we should still be quite undecided about the best methods.

The antiseptic era of Lister brought unbelievable change in hospitals and much greater change in surgical practice. Quite apart from the more intimate treatment of the patient, it stimulated a very desirable improvement in cleanliness in the fabric of the buildings themselves. With the labour shortage during and since the Second World War, the standard of cleanliness of most hospitals has seriously deteriorated and the contamination of all objects by micro-organisms has increased. The development of antibiotics opened up a new era in treatment, and the worst effects of increasing uncleanliness of hospitals were, to a large extent, masked by the efficient activities of the antibiotics. However, as more organisms have become resistant to an increasing number of antibiotics, the importance of efficient sterilisation is even greater.

With advances in knowledge, particularly of the viruses, it has been shown that methods once believed to be adequate are far from satisfactory. The equipment for sterilisation in a hospital may be old or suffering from lack of servicing, and in some cases reinfection is an almost inevitable sequel to sterilisation. There are various methods of sterilisation suitable for different objects. The principle of sterilisation is applicable to many forms of treatment, notably the use of chemotherapeutic agents and the antibiotics. Infection in the urinary, intestinal, and respiratory tracts is overcome by what is, in fact, sterilisation of their contents. The process is a slower one than that to which we are accustomed in the case of surgical instruments, but the principle is similar. Another interesting example is the sterilisation of ingested food in the stomach by hydrochloric acid. In 4 per cent of normal subjects who do not secrete acid, there is increased incidence of occasional diarrhoea, which the administration of acid hydrochlor. dil (3·75 ml t.d.s. before meals) will largely overcome.

The first essential in preparation for sterilisation is cleanliness. The objects to be sterilised must be cleansed and washed or laundered as the case may be, and these preliminary processes must be carried out in surroundings which are satisfactory in construction, ventilation, and repair. If they are, then the majority of these objects are already nearly sterile. It must be stressed, however, that there are no degrees of relative sterility. An object is sterile or it is not, and if it is not it is infected—slightly or heavily.

### METHODS OF STERILISATION

The choice of method is determined by the nature of the article to be sterilised as well as by the facilities which are available.

To an increasing degree disposable materials are being introduced into surgical practice and many of these have specialised methods of sterilisation such as ethylene oxide for certain disposable syringes and gamma-ray radiation for certain plastic materials. The common methods in use are:

1. **Chemical.** Chemical sterilisation is one of the oldest methods of destroying organisms. The subject has become very confusing for the nurse because of the infinite number of commercial preparations available. In this book the solutions mentioned will be limited to a few, which have been standardised for use in one hospital. In her own hospital different solutions may be used, and the nurse must familiarise herself with their use and concentration. The following principles should be borne in mind:

(a) The strength of the solution may be altered by evaporation, therefore the plastic or aluminium screw top should be replaced at once after pouring.
(b) They must be used at the correct strength.
(c) Instruments, if sterilised by this method, must be rinsed in sterile water before use.
(d) The whole of the object to be sterilised must be completely immersed in the solution; or exposed in the vapour for the correct time.

Cetrimide (cetavlon) has been discontinued in its present form because it is ineffective against many Gram-negative organisms. It is now combined with hibitane in the solution known as Savlon.

2. **Radiation.** Radiation supplied as high-energy electrons from a linear accelerator or as gamma radiations from cobalt-60 is a useful addition to the methods of sterilisation. It is now used for sterilising heat-sensitive materials such as powders, rubber and plastic goods which are supplied by the manufac-

turers in sterile sealed packages of plastic or other durable material. Its use demands a high standard of packaging as well as effective sealing.

3. **Dry heat.** Dry heat is one of the most efficient methods of sterilisation. The object to be sterilised is sealed in a container and placed in a hot-air oven at a temperature of 160°C and this is maintained for one hour. The destruction of spores is complete. It is suitable only for glassware, all glass syringes, metal instruments, and ointments and powders. In order to prevent reinfection, the materials must be sealed in a container such as aluminium foil. An alternative to a hot-air oven is sterilisation by infrared rays.

4. **Moist heat** (steam under pressure). Moist heat is the most important and most universally applicable method of sterilisation. Instruments and textiles can be sterilised in these ways:

(a) Steam may be fed from the mains, known as a steam steriliser.
(b) Steam may be generated in the steriliser, in which case it is known as an autoclave.

The modern high-vacuum high-pressure steriliser autoclave will after 3 minutes at 143°C, 10 minutes at 126°C and 15 minutes at 121°C and a pressure of 2 kg per sq cm, sterilise its contents. Less modern autoclaves require a longer period, and the nurse must learn the routine in her own hospital. The following points, however, are important.

*Containers.* These must be such that adequate penetration of the steam is possible. Drums which were used for so long as containers have been abandoned as unsuitable. A suitable material must:

1. Allow steam to penetrate it to sterilise its contents;
2. Afford adequate protection against bacterial contamination and infestation;
3. Be light to transport;
4. Be inexpensive;
5. Have a long shelf life.

Paper, metal, balloon cloth, linen and calico are all used. Packs must be stored on slotted shelves, kept free from dust and dated.

*Moist textiles.* If dressings or gowns are damp then they should be regarded as unsuitable for use. Gloves should be sterilised at the same pressure, temperature, and time as dressings and textiles. It has been shown that it is quite unsafe to accept a lower standard. In modern rapid autoclaving at high temperature the gloves are not damaged. Most disposable gloves are now sterilised by gamma radiation.

Objects may be unsterile because of:

1. Incorrect packing
2. Incorrect loading of the autoclave
3. Mechanical defects such as a blocked air ejector.

Daily testing of the autoclave should eliminate objects being unsterile. Water-repellent materials should be used for surgeons' gowns and dressing towels. Water-repellent paper is now available. Brown or charred textiles indicate super heating.

*Sterilisation checks.* The sterilisation of dressings depends on their being completely permeated by dry saturated steam. The efficiency of sterilisation is reduced if the steam is wet or supersaturated. Many sterilisers are inefficient and in some cases recondensation infects the dressings. Again some are efficient only in part so that any tests undertaken are valueless unless the test material is widely dispersed. Therefore the first action in testing a steriliser is an engineer's report on its mechanical efficiency.

The *Bowie-Dick test* is the only satisfactory check that the contents of an autoclave have been sterilised. The test must be carried out in meticulous detail. The principle is that high pressure autoclave tapes are used to fasten a pack of 30 huckaback towels, each folded eight times and wrapped in paper. This is subjected to a standard cycle. After a satisfactory run the tapes will show a colour change which is the same at the centre as at the edges.

5. **Boiling.** Boiling used to be the method in common use and was not an adequate method of sterilisation because it would not kill all spore-bearing organisms. However, it may be the only method available. It is important to ensure:

(a) That the instruments or containers are completely immersed.
(b) That boiling at a temperature of 100°C is maintained for 5 minutes. Boiling for a longer period will be of no further benefit.

The boiling point of water decreases by $1 \cdot 1$°C for every 305 m above sea-level and 5 minutes should be added to the time required for every 305 m of altitude.

## STERILISATION OF EQUIPMENT

All equipment is now supplied already sterilised—it saves the nurses' time, the use of the most effective methods of sterilisation is possible and the efficiency of these methods can be tested and guaranteed.

The nurse's main task will be to select the correct packs or combination of packs and to open them without contamination and dispose of their contents after use, so that there is no spread of infection or waste of recoverable objects.

*Packs can be assembled* to contain anything that may possibly be needed. In practice a simple pack consists of gauze, wool balls or, better, compressed cotton-wool swabs, a dressing towel which may be made of paper and a disposable gallipot. Instruments in tubes or packs are usually supplied separately for ward dressings. After use recoverable materials like surgical instruments should be sealed up and returned for cleaning in the central department. They should not be cleaned in the ward or in the theatre. The cost of cleaning, laundering and returning of materials has stimulated research for disposable materials. Great advances have been made in the fields of paper and plastic manufacture. Longer experience is necessary, however, before it can be decided that all disposable material is suitable. Disposal of disposable materials creates its own problems for a hospital.

Preset trays (Fig. 10.1) are now in use for the operating theatre.

Sterile water is produced by some form of steam distillation, bottled and sterilised in the autoclave.

Everything the nurse may require is better presterilised. All stainless-steel ware and most instruments are best sterilised in the autoclave after cleaning in soapy water or with detergents. The following are unsuitable for autoclaving, the first three be-

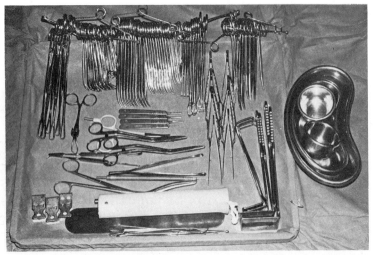

Fig. 10.1   Instrument set for large basic tray for operating theatre (Edinburgh method).

cause of their composition and syringes because autoclaving is ineffective.

1. **Catgut.** Catgut is already prepared in sterile containers, usually double wrapped envelopes of plastic or metal foil, and stored in the sterile pack fluid provided. As an additional precaution against tetanus every batch of catgut has a special number which should be written against the patient's name in the theatre register.

2. **Gum elastic.** The use of gum elastic in practice is almost entirely confined to oesophageal bougies.

3. **Electrical apparatus.** Cystoscopes, laryngoscopes, bronchoscopes, etc. should be cleansed with a detergent, rinsed in water and immersed in a solution of Savlon 1:30 in 70 per cent methylated spirit. Cystoscopes are usually kept in an aqueous solution of cidex. All instruments are rinsed in cold sterile water before use. The instrument should be assembled and tested before and after use. An alternative method for dealing with cystoscopes is a pasteuriser, which is simply a water bath thermostatically controlled at 70° to 75°C. Immersion in this bath for 10 minutes is sufficient to kill vegetative bacteria and in practice has been found not to damage any but the most delicate instruments. A further precaution in using a cystoscope is the instillation of a chlorhexidine (0·1 per cent) gell which also contains as a local anaesthetic 1 per cent lignocaine into the urethra for 5 to 10 minutes before passing the instrument.

4. **Syringes.** Sterilisation of glass syringes is best undertaken in a hot-air oven at a temperature of 160°C maintained for one hour. If this is not available, they have to be autoclaved or boiled.

A disposable syringe sterilised by gamma radiation is now almost standard equipment in most hospitals. Glass syringes, however, are still necessary for the administration of certain drugs such as paraldehyde which can be altered by the plastic material in a disposable syringe.

# CHAPTER 11

# Asepsis and Theatre Technique

Asepsis is the underlying principle of surgery by which organisms are denied access to the patient. It encompasses sterilisation which has been discussed in the previous chapter. It is much easier to check the efficiency of sterilisation and to trace the fault than it is to discover the flaw in asepsis. Asepsis has a discipline all its own. From the beginning of her career the nurse must train herself to recognise at once conditions which are at variance with an aseptic technique.

The problem is that micro-organisms are to be found everywhere. Objects which can be sterilised and wrapped in sterile containers present the least difficulty, provided sterilisation has been adequate, but most objects which come into contact with the patient are either impossible to sterilise or are easily recontaminated. Consideration of the following points illustrates the problem:

1. The air. Air contains organisms and it is an ideal vehicle for their dissemination. It is added to in hospital by organisms from other patients, from visitors and from staff. To lower the bacterial content of the air the following precautions are essential:

    (a) Ventilation. Ideally, air should be filtered, moistened, and warmed or cooled to the regular temperature, Air conditioning plant should be capable of changing the air in the theatre suite 15 or 20 times each hour. When a wound is exposed movement is kept at a minimum. Doors and windows are closed (if a room is air conditioned they will always be closed).

    (b) Speech is limited to the minimum and masks should be worn intelligently.

    (c) Bodily movement should be gentle and unhurried.

    (d) Cleaning procedures are completed one to two hours previously. Floors are sprayed with tego and furniture washed over with a germicide one hour before an operation is commenced. Electric scrubbers are used.

    (e) Flies should never be allowed to survive.

    (f) The patient is transferred from the trolley to the table in the anaesthetic room or at interchange areas and vice versa at the end of the operation. Theatre porters, trolleys and ward blankets should not enter the theatre.

2. Many objects cannot be sterilised. The most important are:

(a) The patient's skin.
(b) The hands of the surgeon or nurse. It has been shown, however, that routine baths before operation tend to increase and not diminish infectivity.
(c) The throat, nose and mouth of the staff.

3. The operating table and floor are easily contaminated from infected discharges during the operation.

4. Blood stains and pus are excellent media for the propagation of organisms, especially as the temperature is usually fairly high and the atmosphere is kept humid. Cross-infection can occur from anaesthetic apparatus, which should be pasteurised. Theatre staff, as all nursing staff, should be very careful in handling blood and its products since pricking of the skin or abrasions of the finger may be an entry for viruses which are sometimes present not only in stored blood but also in patient's blood.

5. Recontamination of sterile objects may occur because of:

(a) Inefficient sterilisers or condensation of steam.
(b) Mishaps with air conditioning.
(c) Cracks in the fabric.

6. Clothing and footwear. Outdoor clothing and footwear, in fact all clothing which has not been recently laundered, is particularly liable to carry infection.

7. Masks give only relative protection and should be renewed after one to two hours and never touched by the fingers.

Because of the importance of maintaining asepsis, operating theatres should be designed so that they have:

(a) Air-conditioned ventilation.
(b) Easily cleanable fabric.
(c) A one-way traffic circulation from 'clean' user space to 'dirty' user space.
(d) Adequate shower baths for surgeons and nurses.

## THEATRE TECHNIQUE

The theatre nurse is a member of a team, and unless she and all the theatre staff carefully observe all the principles and technique of asepsis, infection in the patient's wound is an inevitable result of the operation.

### THEATRE DRESS

The nurse should be clean in her person, her hands kept free from cracks and abrasions, and the finger-nails cut short, rounded and unvarnished. In the theatre she should wear the special uniform provided, which usually consists of an overall-type dress with short sleeves or trousers and top. The material has a smooth surface and is boilable, so that all germs are destroyed in the laundering process. All hair should be concealed under a special cap. Footwear with antistatic and impervious soles should be kept in the theatre cloakroom and never worn outside the theatre. It is possible to carry the tetanus bacillus into the theatre from outside, and this point should always be borne in mind. The nose and mouth are covered with a mask whilst the operation is in progress and whilst the theatre is being prepared. Nurses from the ward must change, like the theatre staff, if they enter the theatre.

Blankets or blanket substitutes from the ward are not taken into the theatre because they are a source of infection. The theatre has its own materials for covering the patient and on arrival these must be used.

## THE WARD NURSE AND THE THEATRE

The ward nurse accompanies the patient to the theatre entrance and takes him back to bed. She must comfort the patient and inspire confidence. Her responsibilities include:

1. *The instruments on the trolley.* A receiver containing an airway and swabs must be taken to the theatre in case they are required on the journey back to the ward after the operation.

2. *Case notes and X-rays.* These must be taken to the theatre. The nurse should also record at what time premedication was given. A form of consent signed by the patient should be in the notes—as well as a report of a urine test made that day (Fig. 11.1 and 11.2). Dentures should have been removed.

3. *Identification* of the patient to the theatre superintendent, who checks his name with the operating list, with the patient's notes, with the patient himself, so that she can satisfy herself that she has the correct patient for the proposed operation.

4. *After operation.* The ward nurse, before she leaves the theatre, should see that she has the case notes which will be written up and include:

   (a) The nature of the anaesthetic.
   (b) The diagnosis and nature of the operation.
   (c) The type of stitches inserted.
   (d) The number and type of drainage tubes or packs inserted.
   (e) Any special instructions from the surgeon or anaesthetist about the postoperative care.

## CONSENT BY PATIENT

I, ....................................................................................................

of .....................................................................................................

hereby consent to undergo the operation of ...........................................

.........................................................................................................

the nature and effect of which have been explained to me by Dr./Mr. ...........................................................................................

I also consent to such further or alternative operative measures as may be found to be necessary during the course of the operation and to the administration of a general, local or other anaesthetic for any of these purposes.

No assurance has been given to me that the operation will be performed by any particular surgeon.

Date .............................. (Signed) ..............................................................
(Patient)

I confirm that I have explained to the patient the nature and effect of this operation.

Date .............................. (Signed) ..............................................................
(Physician/Surgeon)

## CONSENT BY RELATIVES

I, ....................................................................................................

of .....................................................................................................

the *husband/wife/parent of the above-named .......................................

hereby consent to my *wife/husband/child undergoing the operation indicated above.

*delete as necessary.

(Signed) ..................................................................

FIG. 11.1    Consent form.

| Patient's Surname .................... Forenames ........................ D.O.B. ............ |

Ward .............................................  )
                                   )  *To be completed by*
Operation ........................................ )  *Theatre Sister*
                                   )
Date ...........................................  )

|                                   | *Tick* / | *Tick* / |
|-----------------------------------|----------|----------|
| Premedication given ....................  | .......... | .......... |
| Dentures removed ....................  | .......... | .......... |
| Urine tested and recorded ...............  | .......... | .......... |
| Signed Consent Form enclosed ...........  | .......... | .......... |
|                                   | *Signature of Ward Sister or Staff Nurse* | *Signature of Anaesthetist* |

...........................................

FIG. 11.2    Final check form before anaesthesia.

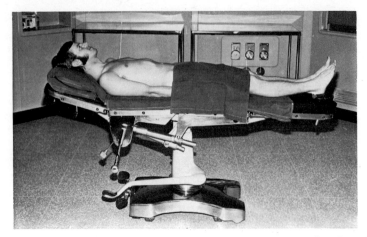

FIG. 11.3   Usual position for operation on abdomen. Note elevation of calves by pads under the heels.

5. *Care of the unconscious patient after the operation.* The patient should be conscious before he leaves the theatre. The ward nurse is entirely reponsible for the patient during transit from the theatre to the ward. She must above all else keep the airway clear and have with her an artificial airway and gauze swab in a receiver. Care must be taken of a blood transfusion if it is to be continued on the journey to the ward. The patient should be kept warm, and special care taken to avoid chilling of the chest and the extremities.

THE DUTIES OF THE NURSE WHO IS A MEMBER OF THE THEATRE STAFF

It is the sister's duty to attend to the instruments. A sterile mask and cap must be worn. The hands and arms are soaped and the nails are scrubbed for two minutes. Because ordinary soap is not as effective as an antiseptic soap, it is now customary to use one containing hexachlorophane. A sterile gown is put on and tied behind by another nurse, who stands clear and does not allow her clothing to come into contact with the hands or gown of the nurse who has scrubbed up. At least the sleeves, if not the whole gown, should be made of a water-repellent fabric such as Ventile. It prevents skin organisms passing through to the wound when the sleeves become wet, as they often do during an operation. The gown should be back-wrapped (Fig. 11.4) and the tape on the front has to be unloosened by someone who is already scrubbed and, in turn, this person's tape has to be unloosened by another who is also 'scrubbed'. Sterile gloves will have been put on to the prepared hands. Gloves are presterilised and disposable. It is illogical not to change one's gown if gloves have been punctured. In general, the less movement and the fewer people there are to move about the operating theatre, the better.

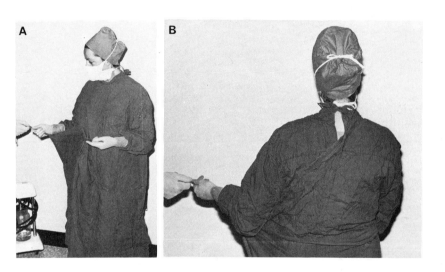

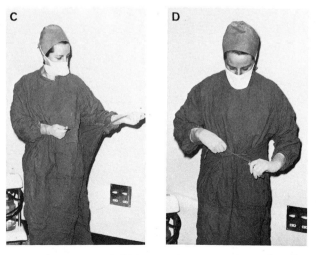

FIG. 11.4  Backwrap tapes held by 'scrubbed' members of staff and tied on front of gown by gowned sister.

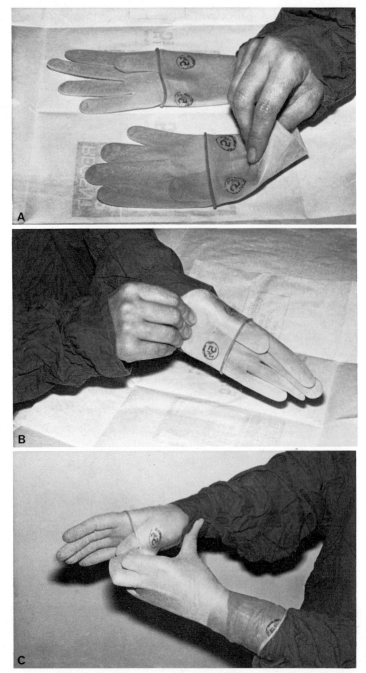

Fig. 11.5 Correct method of putting on gloves: A, Picking up first glove;
B, Putting on first glove; C, Both gloves drawn over cuffs

CORRECT METHOD OF PUTTING ON GLOVES:

1. The hands are first powdered with special glove powder.
2. The first glove is put on, held by the opposite hand on its inner surface (Fig. 11.5 A and B).
3. The second glove is then picked up on its outer surface by the opposite gloved hand.
4. The cuffs of both gloves are drawn up over the gown sleeves (Fig. 11.5c).

The nurse who has scrubbed up now handles only sterilised materials. The hands and arms should always be kept above waist level. Should she inadvertently touch something which is non-sterile she must change her gloves, and gown. She supervises the instruments, threads needles, prepares ligatures, and keeps the surgeon supplied with swabs (which are now wrapped in bundles of five), tubes, or anything else which is needed during the operation. She must be quick to respond to the whispered word or gesture, for unnecessary speech is out of place in the theatre. The instrument nurse does not handle the soiled swabs but she is responsible for the number used by the surgeon.

The exposure of autoclaved supplies to the air in the theatre is minimised by the use of prepackaging. Instruments need not be unwrapped until immediately before the operation.

DUTIES OF OTHER NURSES IN THE THEATRE

The nurse counting the soiled swabs should report to the instrument nurse the number of used swabs recovered before

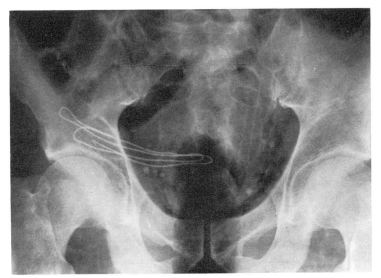

FIG. 11.6 A swab containing a radio-opaque thread. Particular care must be taken to ensure that all dressings are removed from the wound before an X-ray is taken if the retention of a swab is suspected.

the wound is closed. Then both should recount the swabs together to ensure that no swab is left in the wound. All swabs
contain a strip of radio-opaque material (Fig. 11.6) so that if
one is missing it can be checked by X-ray and searched for in
the wound before it is closed. Similarly a check should be
made of the number of needles and instruments used and re
covered.

Other nurses in the theatre are responsible for the collection of lotions, presterilised packs of instruments and dressings. They should be conversant with the working of the
diathermy machine and the electric suction apparatus.

Their duties are many and varied. Although they do not
scrub up they should be familiar with the method used in case
they are required. Each nurse must learn the theatre routine in
her own hospital. Most important of all, she must attend to
detail just as conscientiously when she is alone preparing the
theatre as she does when an operation is in progress.

The theatre nurse is an essential part of a closely working
team, must know her duties and perform them definitely and
correctly. She must maintain her professional standards, be-

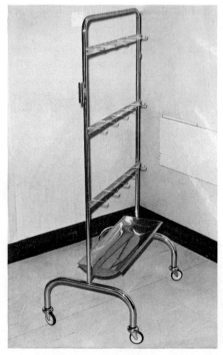

Fig. 11.7　Swab rack on which all swabs should be hung and counted.

have quietly and decorously and never discuss anything which she may see or hear during her theatre duties.

*Prevention of infection from the skin to the open wound.* Because skin cannot be sterilised this remains one of the most important sources of infection in the theatre. The skin is isolated as soon as the wound has been made. There is considerable difference of opinion as to the best method of covering the skin adjoining the wound. The choice would seem to be:

1. Muslin towelling.
2. Semitransparent sheeting.
3. Adhesive surgical film.
4. Ventile water-repellent material.

An additional precaution is to use a separate sterile needle for every skin stitch.

### 'SEPTIC CASE' CLEARANCE OF THEATRE

The dangerous bacteria are confined to the contaminated area during the operation and should be destroyed as quickly as possible before they spread throughout the theatre. At the conclusion of the operation there should be at hand equipment for:

1. Linen ⎫ a strong paper bag.
2. Dressings ⎭
3. Instruments—a container should be at hand and the instruments, with their joints *unlocked*, are sterilised in it.
4. Cleaning the table, floor and sinks—with a germicide solution.

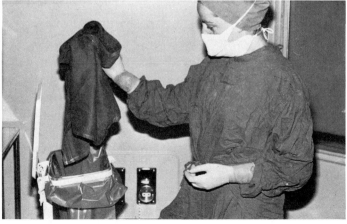

FIG. 11.8   Clearance at the end of the operation.

PREVENTION OF BURNS AND EXPLOSIONS IN THE OPERATING
THEATRE

The patient in an operating theatre is liable to be injured
in the following way:

*Anaesthetic explosions and burns.* When inflammable agents are
used to procure anaesthesia, the presence of a naked flame or
sparks from faulty switches or from static causes can induce
violent explosions, extensive burns, and death to the patient
and his attendants. All metal apparatus is fitted with antistatic
rubber wheels.

Measures to prevent static electrification are:

(a) The use of cotton blankets before commencing anaes-
    thesia.
(b) Ordinary rubber sheeting or plastic materials should
    be replaced by antistatic rubber or the rubber should
    be covered by cotton material.
(c) Sorbo mattresses or cushions should be of anti-
    static rubber or covered with cotton.
(d) All rubber parts of the anaesthetic apparatus should
    be antistatic in type.

Equally important are the following measures to encourage
the dissipation of static charges:

(a) The humidity of the atmosphere should be checked
    and kept above 55 per cent.
(b) Provision of antistatic castors for theatre trolleys and
    tables.
(c) Suitable antistatic footwear.
(d) The investigation of the earthing properties of the
    theatre floors and, if necessary, exploration of the
    various possibilities of making them conform to an
    official specification.
(e) Nylon clothing should not be worn in the theatre.

A spark may be generated from:

(a) A cautery or diathermy.
(b) An electric motor or suction machine.
(c) The electric light of an endoscope, particularly a
    bronchoscope.
(d) Oxygen cylinders. The friction of gases escaping
    causes heat to be generated. The presence of oil or
    dust in the oxygen-rich atmosphere may cause an
    explosion.

## SURGICAL DIATHERMY

When an electric current is passed through a resistance, heat is
generated in the resistance. If the current is of very high fre-

quency, electric shock as commonly understood is avoided. These facts form the basic principles of surgical diathermy:

In practice:

1. The main current is passed into a diathermy machine.
2. A high frequency is generated in the machine.
3. A current is concentrated through a small point (the active electrode of the diathermy) which is controlled by a foot switch.
4. The body cells when they come in contact with this electrode provide the resistance. The result is that the cells in the immediate neighbourhood are destroyed. Beyond this immediate area the current fans out and is insufficient to cause any damage.
5. The indifferent electrode completes the circuit and takes the current back to the machine.

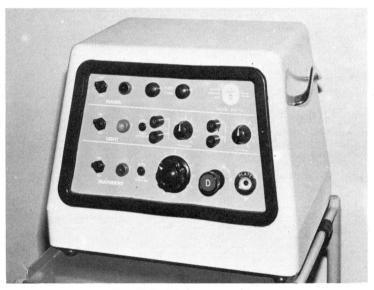

FIG. 11.9   Diathermy machine.

*Care of the patient when diathermy is being used*

1. FIXATION OF THE INDIFFERENT OR PASSIVE DIATHERMY ELECTRODE

This usually consists of a lead foil with an electric flex running back to the machine. The foil is enclosed in lint which has been moistened in hypertonic saline. This electrode has a large surface area so that the activity of the current is fanned out and not concentrated. This avoids the danger of a burn to the skin which should be shaved before the plate is applied. It is important to see that the electrode does not become loosen-

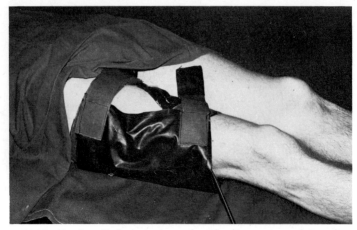

FIG. 11.10  Passive diathermy electrode. The lint moistened in saline or diathermy cream or paste covers the electrode, which is applied to the patient's thigh. Will probably be replaced by a disposable foil.

ed from the patient. Also the electric flex should be firmly attached. The end of the electric flex lying loose from the plate, but in contact with the patient, could cause a burn. Further, if an operation is a prolonged one—that is more than an hour and a half—the electrode should be examined and the lint remoistened, or better, wrapped in rubber to diminish evaporation.

There is now available a disposable metal foil passive electrode which is secured to the patient with crêpe and requires no moistening.

*Point of fixation.* The electrode is strapped to the thigh.

2. THE ACTIVE ELECTRODE

Special care must be taken to ensure that the active electrode is always pointing away from the patient when not in use and properly secured. The foot switch must be conveniently placed for the surgeon and there must be no danger of it being operated accidentally.

3. THE METAL OF THE TABLE

The patient must be insulated from the metal table by adequate rubber or foam cushions treated with antistatic solutions. Metallic objects should have been removed from the patient's body.

The complications of the use of diathermy may be summarised as:

(a) Electric shock which results in burning.

(b) Accidental burning with the active electrode from inadvertent operation of the foot switch.

(c) Infection due to:
   (i) Inadequate sterilisation of the leads. These should be autoclaved.
   (ii) Some infection is unavoidable and is secondary to an aseptic inflammation. On almost dry surfaces, such as the skin, a tiny point of sloughing occurs, but in moist cavities such as the bladder it is usually complicated by bacterial infection.
(d) Explosion. Theatre explosions have been discussed previously, but diathermy may provide the spark.
(e) Lateral popliteal palsy if the diathermy (passive) electrode is strapped to the head of the fibula.

## ELECTRICITY FAILURE IN HOSPITAL

Sudden failure of electric power becomes increasingly significant as the patient's needs become more dependent on its use. Most people think at once of the theatre lighting and the danger which may ensue for a patient undergoing an operation. In practice, however, this is usually very well taken care of by the theatre emergency lighting, provided from a 12-volt wet battery. The danger to the patient arises from:

### 1. MECHANICAL VENTILATORS (ARTIFICIAL RESPIRATORS)

This transcends in importance everything in the hospital. The patient whose life is dependent on an artificial mechanical respirator which is powered by electricity is saved by the fact that all machines can be operated manually, and the nurse needs to know how to use those in her own hospital.

### 2. BLOOD TRANSFUSION

The blood in the refrigerator will usually be safe for some hours but the advice of the blood transfusion officer must be sought. The nurse should consult the medical officer about securing further blood for patients undergoing transfusion or already suffering from haemorrhage.

### 3. SUCTION APPARATUS

For operations such as tonsillectomy, alternative suction should be available in every theatre. This can be provided very simply by siphonage from a water tap or by a foot pump.

Other effects on the hospital are:
(a) Theatre.—Sterilisation, diathermy cautery, endoscopic lights, pump for open heart surgery, heating, and even the water supply may be threatened.
(b) In the laboratory there are no lights, the incubator may be out of action, and microscope lights may be ineffective.

(c) In the maternity department incubators for premature babies are affected.
(d) General.—X-ray department, kitchen, dispensary, general heating, lighting, laundry, and physiotherapy departments are all affected.

Modern units tend to have a self-starting Diesel alternator as an alternative in case of power failure.

# CHAPTER 12

# Surgical Ward Dressings

The provision of a bacteriologically clean atmosphere is one of the greatest of surgical problems. In operating theatres this is attempted at great expense. In the hospital of the future a similar but smaller scale provision will be built on every ward. This would consist of a dressing room which is air conditioned and a 'clean' and 'dirty' room on either side of it. All dressings would be performed in the dressing room, the only exception being infected cases which would be nursed and dressed in their own isolation ward. In the meantime, however, the vast majority of patients will be nursed in large wards and the problems which arise will have to be dealt with as they occur.

It is inevitable that the more patients there are in a ward the greater is the risk of infection, whilst an ideal number of patients from this point of view is one that is economically impossible. However, the situation can be controlled by the separation of clean from infected cases in the ward. A small isolation ward attached to the main ward is a great advantage and glass partitions in the ward diminish cross-infection.

Patients particularly liable to infection are diabetics, amputees and patients on steroid or immunosuppressive drugs.

Most wounds are infected in the theatre. Other sources of wound infection are:

> Dust in the air of the ward
> Infected droplets from the mouths and noses of those near-by when the wound is uncovered
> The hands of the dresser
> Other wounds which are themselves infected.

Dressings should ideally be carried out in a room or cubicle specially designed for the purpose. Where this is not practicable the following points should be observed.

1. *The air in the ward.* The bacterial content of the air in the ward rises to a maximum in the early morning owing, among other factors, to the domestic activities in the ward, including the cleaning of floors, dusting, bed-making, etc. Bacteria are less likely to be scattered if the precautions mentioned on p. 45 are observed with the following additional measures:

(a) When making beds the clothes are handled slowly and gently.

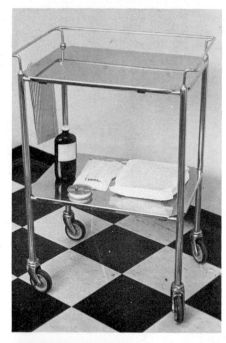

FIG. 12.1 Surgical dressing trolley.

*Top Shelf* is dry and bare. Disposable paper bags clipped on to the rails.
*Lower Shelf:*
  Lotions for cleaning skin and application to wounds
  A dressing pack
  Disposable paper masks
  Adhesive tape
  Sealed containers of instruments.

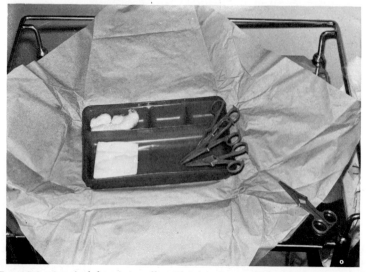

FIG. 12.2 Surgical dressing trolley. The dressing pack has now been opened, its inner wrapping forming the sterile surface on the top of the trolley.

The *top shelf* now contains—
  Four pairs of forceps
  And the contents of a standard dressing pack, namely, gauze, disposable wool balls.

(b) Bed-making, floor-cleaning and dusting cease at least one hour before the first dressing is uncovered.

When dressings begin the ward is closed to all visitors and all unnecessary personnel. Windows and doors are shut.

2. *Droplet infection.* To prevent the spread of infection, surgeons, nurses, students, orderlies and domestic workers with respiratory infections or septic lesions should not be on duty in a surgical ward.

3. *Hands.* Hands cannot be properly sterilised, though thorough washing can remove recent contamination. It is essential, therefore, that during a dressing the hands should not come in contact either with the wound itself or with any material in the vicinity of the wound. The hands should be thoroughly washed, using plenty of soap and water, paying particular attention to the nails, which should be cut short and free of varnish. A Towelmaster or disposable paper towels are used to dry them and the dressing is performed, using sterile forceps.

4. *Masks* should always be worn during dressings, and efficient masks made of paper are now in use. They should be changed hourly, since after that period they only present a further source of infection, and should not be touched with the fingers during use. As soon as the need has passed, the mask should be removed, and to go around all day with a mask covering the nose is to increase the chance of infection because of lack of proper ventilation to the nose.

*Changing a simple dressing—one nurse*

A basic trolley is prepared. The nurse washes and dries her hands, and puts on a mask.

Using Jontex cloth the whole trolley is washed with soap and water and dried. It is then swabbed with a disposable swab soaked in 70 per cent isopropanol.

A basic dressing pack, supplementary pack, adhesive, recommended antiseptic and any other necessary equipment are placed on the bottom shelf. A 'used instrument bag' is attached to one end of the trolley with a strip of Sellotape. Two strips of Sellotape are attached to the rail at the other end.

The procedure is explained to the patient. Privacy is ensured and near-by windows are closed as necessary. The trolley is then taken to the bedside.

Using her scissors the nurse cuts the sealed end of the pack and tips the inner pack on to the top of the trolley. She attaches the outer pack to the other end of the trolley, for receiving soiled dressings. The patient is placed into an appropriate position and made comfortable. The bedclothes and personal clothing are adjusted as necessary. The nurse loosens the bandage or adhesive holding the dressing. She then thoroughly washes and dries her hands. The inner wrapping is then opened and partially spread by pulling on the first three corners. The fourth corner is lifted carefully with one hand and the nurse picks up the first pair of forceps with the other and continues to spread the final corner. Using the pair of forceps she arranges the sterile field and tray, placing the instruments on the side of the tray. The forceps are then placed at the side of the trolley with the points only on the sterile field. She opens any supplementary packs. She pours out the antiseptic. Using the first pair of forceps she removes the soiled dressing, discarding it into the appropriate bag. The soiled forceps are placed into the used instrument bag. She picks up two pairs of forceps. If towels are necessary, they are arranged around the wound.

With the forceps in her left hand she picks up a swab, dips it into the antiseptic and transfers it to the forceps in her right hand. The wound is cleaned and the swab discarded. As many swabs as necessary are used, each swab being used once only. She discards the forceps in her right hand, and transfers those in her left hand to the right hand. In her left hand she picks up the remaining forceps. Using the two forceps the dressing is applied. Both forceps are discarded. The dressing is secured, using adhesive or bandage as indicated. The patient is made comfortable.

Any unused wool or gauze is saved for suitable unsterile procedures. The tray is then placed into the used instrument bag which is disconnected from the side of the trolley. The sterile field, used towels, and the nurse's mask are placed in the soiled bag, which is also disconnected from the side of the trolley and closed tightly by squeezing the top. The trolley is removed and cleaned. The nurse washes and dries her hands. She reports to Sister or Charge Nurse as necessary.

### Protective dressings of the wound

Dressings consist of gauze, lint, cotton-wool, and bandage, Airstrip or Dermicel adhesive dressings, Elastoplast, Tubegauz or Netelast, Sellotape and microporous tape.

The advantages of protective dressings for wounds are many, but one disadvantage is that evaporation from the skin surface is hindered. This may be overcome by:

1. NO DRESSINGS: A little gauze is strapped on the wound for six hours until the edges have become sealed off with exudate. After this all dressings are abandoned.

2. A PLASTIC SKIN DRESSING: Nobecutane is an acrylic resin dissolved in a mixture of acetic esters. When applied to the skin the solvent evaporates, leaving a transparent, adherent, and elastic film. This film is impervious to bacteria but

pervious to evaporation from the skin surface. It must not be used unless haemostasis is perfect. It may be sprayed or spread with a glass rod. A thick layer may be peeled off; a thin layer may be dissolved with ether or acetone.

The advantages are:

(a) The wound is sealed and cannot be infected; this is particularly important if a colostomy or ileostomy is functioning near a fresh wound.
(b) The progress of the wound can be seen without disturbing the dressing.
(c) The patient can take a bath as the dressing is impervious to water.

*Clean wounds* which have been closed without drainage need not be uncovered until it is time to remove the stitches. Pain in the wound or a rise of temperature may necessitate inspection to see if the wound has become infected. Septic wounds require careful dressing.

### The stitches

The skin stitches, mersilene, or nylon, are removed when the wound has healed, usually on the eighth to tenth day. It is advisable to remove alternate stitches on one day and the remainder next day, if the wound is sound. In the neck, to avoid stitch marks, they are removed on the fourth or fifth day. Deep sutures (if inserted) which take up the tension of coughing in the case of an abdominal wound are removed on the twelfth to fourteenth day. When removing skin stitches the cut stitch must be extracted from the skin towards the wound—pulling it away from the wound disrupts its edges.

Michel's clips, Kefa clips or butterfly plasters to hold the skin edges together or Steristrip tape may be used instead of stitches.

A stitch which is cutting through the skin may give rise to considerable pain, and the surgeon's attention should be drawn to this to see if it can be removed earlier than usual.

A stitch abscess is liable to develop if there is slight infection, and to diminish the risk most surgeons paint the skin with antiseptic lotion as they are closing the wound before inserting the stitches. If the patient is running a temperature the wound should be examined for a stitch abscess and the stitch removed to provide drainage.

### Drains

Drains are used—

(i) to drain fluid which has collected or is expected to collect, e.g. blood, serum, pus and bile;

(ii) as a safety valve to an anastomosis or suture lines,
e.g. the duodenal stump after gastrectomy or the
ureter after removal of a stone.

Wherever a drain is inserted it should be covered with an
antiseptic dressing. Shortening and rotation of the open tube
type of drain are undertaken—shortening so that the cavity
can heal from the bottom, and rotation so that the tube does
not become adherent to the tissues. A tube should never be
removed until clear written instructions have been obtained
from the surgeon.

When the original stitch securing the tube has been severed
the tube should be fixed with a large safety-pin to a piece of
Gamgee so that the tube is not lost in the wound.

The following complications may arise if a tube is left *in situ*
for too long a period:

Infection
Intestinal obstruction
Erosion of a blood vessel causing a secondary haemor-
rhage
Perforation of an organ causing a fistula
Adhesions
Incisional hernia.

TYPES OF DRAINS
1. Rubber tubing split or fenestrated.
2. Corrugated rubber sheeting.
3. Firm rubber sheeting.
4. Penrose tubing.
5. Shaped drains such as catheters or T-tubes for the
common bile duct.

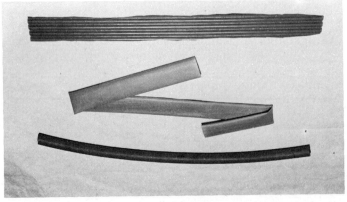

FIG. 12.3   Some types of drains—corrugated, Penrose, tube of rubber or
plastic.

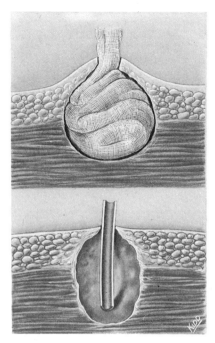

FIG. 12.4 Top: Wrong. Gauze plugs the wound and obstructs drainage. Below: Correct. Tube allows free drainage.

Some varieties of drains are illustrated in Figure 12.3.
Gauze is never a drain.
*Drainage* may be:
1. Open:
   (a) Onto dressings.
   (b) Suction.
2. Closed:
   (a) Catheter into a sealed sterile disposable bag.
   (b) Chest under fluid seal (p. 308).
   (c) Vacuum—such as Redivac.

A Redivac drain (Fig. 42.7) is a small bottle in which a vacuum has been created by a high capacity pump attached to the manometric stopper tube. The antennae on the stopper are 100° apart when the vacuum reaches 600 mmHg. When the antennae are in the vertical position the vacuum is only 40-50 mmHg. At this point another prepared bottle has to be used. The catheter is clamped off at the rubber coupling, the exhausted vacuum bottle is removed, and the clamp is released only when a new bottle has been recoupled.

In closed drainage organisms from the air are excluded, the discharge can be measured and it has the further advantage that the main wound can be kept dry.

# CHAPTER 13

# Haemorrhage

Haemorrhage is the loss of blood from a blood vessel. The blood lost is described as extravasated (outside the vessels) and may lie on the surface of the body, on the patient's clothing or on the floor. Blood which is extravasated into the tissues, a body cavity or the lumen of a hollow organ may in itself be very significant quite apart from any effect which may ensue from loss to the circulation, and the problem is considered at the end of this chapter.

Clotting is the circulatory system's defence mechanism to leakage. Clot formation may be deficient from disease, the absence of essential clotting factors or the use of anticoagulant drugs. To be effective in sealing the leakage the clot has to be inside the lumen of the vessel (intravascular)—clot formation inside a viscus but outside the blood vessels increases the bleeding for reasons given in Fig. 13.5. When bleeding occurs and blood is spilt into a receiver or shed on to the floor it is always worth noting whether clots are forming since in conditions of defective clotting or active fibrinolysis the patient bleeds but clots either do not form or are quickly lysed. Replacement of the missing clotting factors, e.g. by fresh frozen plasma, is necessary when there is defective clotting. In conditions of fibrinolysis it is necessary to give an antifibrinolytic agent such as ε-aminocaproic acid, with or without replacement of any clotting factors which may have been depleted by the lysis.

Blood may be lost from all three types of vessel, the arteries, the veins, or the capillaries, and the type of haemorrhage is named accordingly. Bleeding which occurs as soon as the vessel is divided is known as primary haemorrhage. Should the patient be collapsed the vessel may not bleed immediately, but as recovery takes place the blood pressure rises and bleeding occurs—this is known as reactionary haemorrhage. If infection is present, the walls of the blood vessels may be eroded and burst, causing what is known as secondary haemorrhage.

TYPES:
1. Arterial.
2. Capillary.
3. Venous.

TIME:
1. Primary.
2. Reactionary or intermediate.
3. Secondary.

**Arterial haemorrhage.** The blood is bright red and spurts with the heart beat. The escape is from both ends of the vessel and not only from that nearer to the heart. Blood loss is more rapid than from a vein of corresponding size.

**Capillary haemorrhage.** The blood oozes over the surface and is darkish red in colour.

**Venous haemorrhage.** The blood is dark in colour, there is no pulsation, and the rate of loss is much less severe than arterial haemorrhage. Since the large veins are big cave-like structures, injury to them is a serious matter. A further danger is that air may be sucked into the veins, giving rise to fatal air embolism in which the blood and air may form 'foam'.

**Primary haemorrhage.** Primary haemorrhage is immediate—a cut finger or an operative incision.

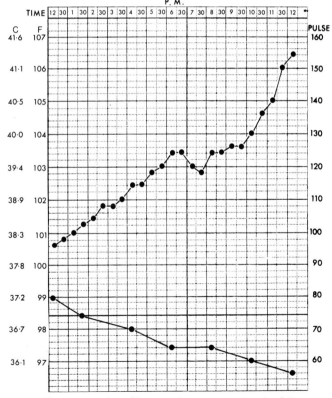

FIG. 13.1    The rising pulse of haemorrhage. Note also the falling temperature.

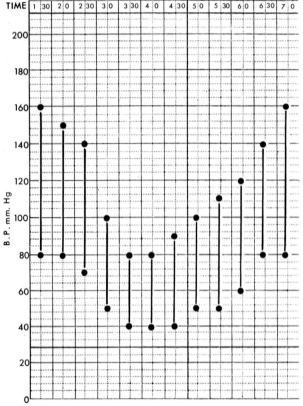

FIG. 13.2   The systolic and diastolic blood pressure is recorded.

**Reactionary haemorrhage.** This type of haemorrhage is important because it occurs in the first 24 hours after operation. The more severe the operation the more likely it is to occur, especially after the patient has recovered from circulatory collapse. Operations on the kidney, the thyroid and the breast as well as total hysterectomy are particularly liable to be followed by reactionary haemorrhage.

**Secondary haemorrhage.** Secondary haemorrhage is due to sloughing of the wall of a blood vessel. The commonest cause is bacterial infection, but in the absence of infection it may be caused by the action of an enzyme, for example acid pepsin on a peptic ulcer. The vessels are eroded. The thinnest walled vessels, the capillaries, burst first and a few specks of blood are found on the dressing, and should be immediately reported. It is a warning that the larger vessels are also being eroded, and in another few days, commonly the tenth after operation, a main artery may burst, giving rise to a torrential, fatal haemorrhage.

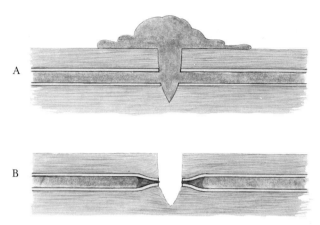

FIG. 13.3   An important part of haemostasis is that the walls of the vessel are able to retract. A, Blood escapes freely from severed artery. B, By retraction and contraction the severed ends are sealed off.

Most symptoms of blood loss complained of by patients at diagnostic clinics are in fact small secondary haemorrhages.

**The severity of haemorrhage in the body of a healthy individual.** There are approximately 5·8 l of blood with 100 per cent haemoglobin concentration 14·6 g per dl. If 1·8 l of blood are lost very rapidly—for example, in half an hour—death usually results, but should loss occur at the rate of 1 litre over the whole day for several days, there would still be very little less than 5·8 litres of fluid in the circulation; the haemoglobin concentration, however may be only 20 per cent, 2·9 g per dl. The fluid lost in the circulation is replaced by fluid from the tissues, so that the volume of blood is restored; but since vast numbers of red blood cells have been shed, the oxygen-carrying power is depleted.

The crucial factor in assessing the result of haemorrhage is the rate of the loss of blood. The body can make tremendous compensation if it is given sufficient time.

*The natural arrest of haemorrhage*

Adequate amounts of calcium and all the clotting factors are essential. The blood in circulation is kept fluid by a fine balance between clotting and fibrinolysis. As a result of a complex series of reactions starting when tissue is damaged, prothrombin is converted to its active form thrombin in the presence of calcium. Fibrinogen is then transformed by thrombin to fibrin, which forms a mesh in which platelets and other blood cells become entangled to form a clot. Alterations of these factors by drugs forms the basis of anti-coagulant and fibrinolytic therapy.

1. *Calcium* may be displaced from blood by:

(a) A 3·8 per cent solution of sodium citrate.
(b) Acid citrate dextrose solution.
(c) Oxalate.
(d) Sequestrene (ethylenediamine tetra-acetic acid, or EDTA).

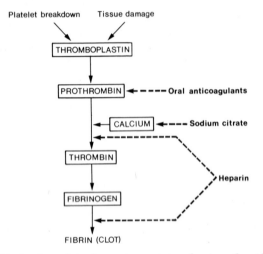

FIG. 13.4    Mechanism of clot formation and site of action of anticoagulants.

Clinically sodium citrate prevents the formation of clots in the bladder; acid citrate dextrose solution is used to prevent clotting in stored blood. Because stored blood has had its calcium displaced, a patient receiving blood requires 10 ml of a 10 per cent solution of calcium chloride with every fourth unit of blood.

Oxalate is used in pathological specimen tubes when it is desired to prevent the clotting of blood.

2. *Prothrombin* is formed from vitamin K, a fat-soluble vitamin absorbed from the bowel. A patient suffering from obstructive jaundice will not absorb vitamin K and therefore is liable to bleed if operated upon. For this reason vitamin K is given by injection until the prothrombin level of the blood has been restored. Oral anticoagulants like warfarin act by preventing the liver utilising vitamin K and so reducing the formation of prothrombin. The dosage is controlled by the prothrombin time. If it is necessary to reverse the process, vitamin K is given, but it may be too slow to act and a transfusion of fresh blood may be necessary.

A more immediately acting anticoagulant is heparin and its action can be easily reversed with protamine sulphate.

3. *Fibrinogen* is the precursor of fibrin. In the absence of fibrinogen severe bleeding may occur. Fibrinolysins are substances which dissolve fibrin and the phenomenon is known as fibrinolysis. The fibrinolytic activity of the blood may be increased:

(a) In complicated obstetric cases associated with haemorrhage.
(b) After severe exercise.
(c) In the presence of some malignant new growths.
(d) Occasionally after operations such as prostatectomy, the fibrinolysin being known as urokinase.
(e) In certain streptococcal infections—streptokinase releases an endogenous activator.

Patients suffering from fibrinolysis will show no evidence of clotting and are treated by neutralisation of the fibrinolysins by the administration of ε-aminocaproic acid or the administration of fibrinogen. Fibrinolysins such as streptokinase are used in the dissolution of thrombi in cases of deep venous thrombosis and pulmonary embolism.

*The signs and symptoms of haemorrhage*

Clinically, haemorrhage may be of two types:
1. REVEALED OR EXTERNAL, i.e. the bleeding can be seen.
2. CONCEALED OR INTERNAL. The bleeding occurs in one of the body cavities, e.g. the abdomen. Since it is less obvious it must be diagnosed on the presence of signs and symptoms alone.

The signs and symptoms are those of a progressive anaemia as well as water and salt depletion when the loss is slow or of acute circulatory collapse when rapid haemorrhage occurs.

EARLY SIGNS AND SYMPTOMS

1. *Restlessness and anxiety.* The patient is conscious that all is not well and feels faint.
2. *Coldness.* The temperature is slightly subnormal, 36·9°C (98°F).
3. *The pulse rate* is slightly increased.
4. *The blood pressure* is lowered.
5. *Pallor* increases.
6. The patient is *thirsty*.

SIGNS AND SYMPTOMS AFTER SEVERE HAEMORRHAGE

1. *Extreme pallor.* The face may be ashen white, and clammy with cold sweat.
2. *Coldness* is profound and the temperature is of the order of 36°C (97°F) or lower.

3. *Air hunger*. The patient literally gasps for breath. The respirations are rapid and sighing.

4. *The pulse* is very rapid in rate, thready in volume and frequently is irregular in rhythm.

5. *The blood pressure* is extremely low.

6. *Thirst* is extreme.

7. Blindness, tinnitus (buzzing in the ears) and coma occur in this order prior to death.

8. The volume of urine secreted is diminished.

9. The central venous pressure is low and often negative.

*The treatment of haemorrhage*

Diminution of the volume of blood in the circulation with depletion of the supply of oxygen to the tissues is the first and most important result of haemorrhage. The problems arising from blood loss may be summarised as those of:

1. Its control.
2. Restoration of the blood volume.
3. The fate of the extravasated blood.

## THE ARREST OF THE HAEMORRHAGE

### EXTERNAL HAEMORRHAGE

Pressure will control all forms of external haemorrhage. According to its severity there is a choice of methods.

1. PAD AND BANDAGE. This simple method is applicable to the vast majority of cases. It is effective and causes no damage.

2. DIGITAL PRESSURE, applied over the pressure point of the artery, will control haemorrhage temporarily. It is particularly valuable in the neck, where other methods are inapplicable.

3. ELEVATION OF THE LIMB will control venous haemorrhage. This is the classical method of dealing with a sudden haemorrhage from a ruptured varicose vein of the leg.

4. APPLICATION OF A TOURNIQUET. This is rarely required except for the control of a torrential haemorrhage from a limb. *It is not without danger.* A temporary tourniquet may have to be devised in a sudden emergency. A pad, e.g. a handkerchief, is placed over the line of the vessel and a tourniquet—which may be a scarf, a tie, or whatever is available—is bound around the limb and tightened if necessary with a small piece of wood. More usually in hospital three types of tourniquet are used:

> The Samway anchor tourniquet
> Esmarch's elastic bandage
> Inflatable cuff tourniquet.

The great danger of a tourniquet, if left on for more than 30 minutes, is that gangrene of the limb may occur. Damage to the nerves is not infrequent, especially if the skin has not been protected before its application. It is essential, therefore, to slacken the tourniquet and tighten it again if bleeding persists.

5. SURGICAL LIGATION is necessary if the bleeding is persistent.

6. COAGULATION of the bleeding point with electrocautery or diathermy may be required.

7. A PACK will temporarily control very severe haemorrhage. This method is used in the theatre to control temporarily a sudden haemorrhage, and the theatre nurse should always have a pack readily available for this emergency.

8. STYPTICS, such as snake venom, adrenaline (1 : 1000), or turpentine, may be used locally in certain cases. Thrombin and Gelfoam have their uses in appropriate cases.

### INTERNAL OR CONCEALED HAEMORRHAGE

Pressure cannot be employed internally except by surgical ligature or packing. Many internal haemorrhages are secondary in nature, and will cease if the infection can be controlled and the vessels encouraged to contract. The following principles are involved in its control:

1. THE ORGAN IS EMPTIED OF BLOOD CLOT IF POSSIBLE. In a case of severe bleeding from the bladder a catheter is passed and the bladder emptied. The blood vessels in a dilated paralysed organ are unable to contract.

2. THE VESSELS ARE ENCOURAGED TO CONTRACT. Warm lotion of saline or sodium bicarbonate, to which a few drops of adrenaline solution (1 : 1000) have been added, is of great value in washing out the organ. This can be repeated every two hours. The use of ergometrine after the birth of the placenta is an example of stimulating the vessels to contract.

Pitressin intravenously is very effective and probably not much safer than the triluminal tube in the control of bleeding from oesophageal varices (p. 330).

3. THE COAGULABILITY OF THE BLOOD IS INCREASED. This is not very valuable unless the mechanism of clotting is deficient, due to the absence of an essential constituent of the blood. The parenteral administration of vitamin K is important to a jaundiced patient who is bleeding, because its absorption from the intestine is deficient. In haemophilia, the administration of AHG (antihaemophilic globulin) is indicated and the administration of fresh blood increases coagulability.

4. PACKING with gauze soaked in adrenaline is effective at certain sites, and Oxycel, which is absorbable gauze impregnated with fibrin, is extensively used.

5. SURGICAL LIGATURE.

6. ANTIBIOTICS. A secondary haemorrhage, whether internal

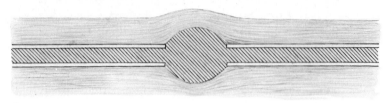

A

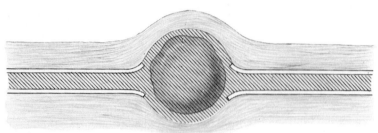

B

FIG. 13.5 Haemorrhage is arrested by clotting inside the vessel but aggravated by clots outside. A, Blood escapes into cavity. B, Cavity distends with blood and prevents severed ends from closing.

or external because it is infective in origin, requires the systemic administration of antibiotics in addition to measures to control the bleeding and restore the blood volume.

7. INTERNAL PRESSURE. May be applied by the balloon of a triluminal tube (p. 330) in bleeding oesophageal varices or by the balloon of a Foley catheter in a prostatectomy cavity.

## BLOOD TRANSFUSION

*Indications*

1. Blood transfusion is undertaken to counteract severe haemorrhage and replace the blood loss.

2. To prevent circulatory failure in operations where blood loss is considerable, such as rectal resection, hysterectomy and arterial surgery.

3. In severe burns to make up for blood lost by burning but only after plasma and electrolytes have been replaced.

4. For severe anaemia from cancer, marrow aplasia and similar conditions.

5. To provide clotting factors normally present in blood which may be absent as a result of disease.

The blood volume can be fairly accurately estimated by a machine using a radio-iodine technique to determine plasma volume and microhaematocrit to estimate red cell volume.

*Technique of blood transfusion*

Blood is collected from healthy donors, 420 ml being collected on each occasion. Blood which is administered in the same form as it is collected, apart from the addition of an anticoagulant, is described as whole blood. In some cases 'packed red cells' are given. This consists of the cellular elements left after siphoning off the supernatant plasma. It is used in cases of chronic anaemia where the volume of blood is not substantially diminished.

## SELECTION OF DONORS

They should be in good general health. The blood Wassermann reaction must be negative, and they must not have had infective hepatitis or malaria.

## BLOOD GROUPING

All humans fall into one of four main blood groups—A, B, AB or O—according to the nature of the blood group antigen which is carried on the red cells. Thus group A persons have A antigen on their red cells, group B, B antigens, group AB both A and B antigens and group O neither A nor B.

A and B antigens have natural antibodies carried in the plasma known as anti-A and anti-B. Anti-A will clump A red cells (and AB) causing a transfusion reaction. Similarly anti-B will clump B cells (and AB). Thus the main groups are made up as follows:

| Group | Red cells (antigen) | Plasma (antibodies) |
|-------|--------------------|--------------------|
| A | A | Anti-B |
| B | B | Anti-A |
| AB | AB | O (none) |
| O | O | Anti-A and anti-B |

In an emergency, where there is doubt as to a patient's blood group, it is safer to cross match a bottle of group O Rh-negative blood than to use another group.

In addition to the main groups there are many rare subgroups which because of their rarity present great difficulties when blood has to be obtained.

The percentage of the population in the various blood groups is:

| | | | |
|---|---|---|---|
| Group AB | 3·0 per cent | Group A | 42 per cent |
| Group B | 8·5 per cent | Group O | 46·5 per cent |

## CROSS MATCHING

The serum of the recipient is matched in tubes against the corpuscles of the donor and the presence or absence of agglutination is noted to determine compatability. To achieve

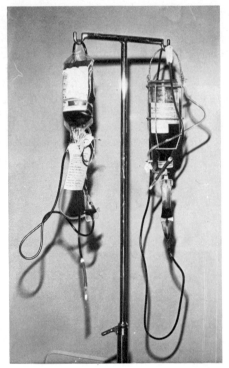

FIG. 13.6   Blood transfusion using the standard gravity drip-giving set.

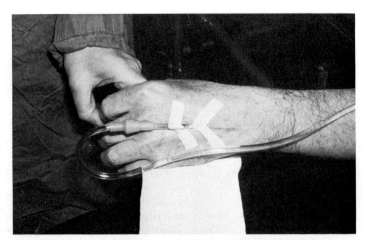

FIG. 13.7   Cannula in the vein.

the high degree of safety necessary in cross matching blood this test is checked under the microscope after two hours incubation in tubes.

*The Rh factor.* There are six antigens involved in the rhesus blood group. The antigen most frequently involved in incompatibility and haemolysis is D, which is present in 85 per cent of the population. These people are known as rhesus-positive. The 15 per cent of people whose blood does not contain D antigen are known as rhesus-negative.

Clarke and others have shown that the production of Rh antibodies in Rh-negative mothers by Rh-positive babies may be prevented by the injection after the baby is born of 5 ml of gammaglobulin containing high titres of antibodies active against the Rh-positive antigen of the foetus.

COLLECTION OF BLOOD

Blood is collected in a sterile flask to which 120 ml of acid citrate dextrose solution has been added. A needle is inserted into a vein at the elbow after the application of a sphygmomanometer to the arm and 420 ml of blood are withdrawn to make a total unit of 540 ml. If the blood is not required for immediate use it is stored in a refrigerator at a temperature from 4° to 6° C.

On the bottle containing the blood is marked the group and the latest date for use. It is important that the blood should not be 'outdated' or haemolysed when given. Another important point is that the blood should not be taken out of the refrigerator more than half an hour before use and not overheated.

Large transfusions of blood may cause citrate intoxication including defective clotting and after every four units (2 l) 10 ml 10 per cent calcium chloride should be injected intravenously. The excess of $K^+$ in banked blood may raise the serum $K^+$ to dangerous levels especially with old blood and, to overcome this, an infusion of dextrose and insulin is given as soon as possible.

TRANSFUSION INTO THE PATIENT

This may be performed by:

1. CLOSED INFUSION (Figs. 13.6 and 13.7), which is the usual method. The blood is given into a vein of the arm or very rarely into a vein of the leg. The arm is the more usual site, because in most cases a cannula can be inserted; in the leg the vein must almost always be exposed and a catheter or cannula inserted. The preparation of the trolley for exposing a vein is shown in Fig. 13.8. A particularly ingenious device is the Medicut.

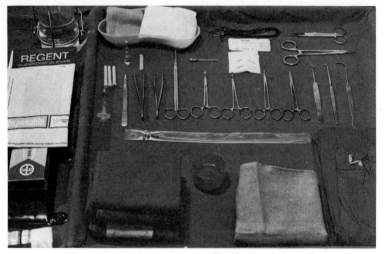

FIG. 13.8   Equipment for 'open' infusion—all sterile.

| | |
|---|---|
| Towels | 2 Straight artery forceps |
| Gallipot with 0·5 % Chlorhexine | 1 Blunt hook |
| Gown | 1 Sharp hook |
| Hand towel | 1 Aneurysm needle |
| Intravenous polythene cannula | 1 Stitch scissors |
| Syringe for local anaesthetic | 1 Needle holder |
| Scalpel | 1 Stainless steel intravenous cannula |
| 1 Toothed dissection forceps | Catgut |
| 1 Non-toothed dissection forceps | Suture material |
| 1 Dissecting scissors | Skin needles |
| 2 Curved artery forceps | Swabs |

*Scalp vein drips in infants.* An area of the scalp selected by the medical officer is shaved and a special fine scalp vein needle with attached polythene tube is held in position with plaster of Paris.

In young children and babies a special drip set with a graduated burette is used to facilitate the accurate administration of small volumes of blood or other fluids.

The most important precautions to take in preparation for blood transfusion is to check that each bottle of blood to be given to the patient is: (a) of the correct group for that patient; (b) that the cross-matching label on each bottle bears the full name, date of birth and ward of the patient to whom it is to be given as well as his unit number; (c) that the expiry date on the bottle has not been reached; (d) and that cross-matching label attached to the bottle matches the label on the bottle.

Blood, like plasma, is not normally heated before use but when rapid transfusions are undertaken it is necessary to take measures to warm the blood. This is done using some form of heating coil which is connected somewhere between the drip set and the patient. There are available drip heaters set at body temperature for this purpose.

The rate of blood flow is carefully regulated on the doctor's instructions by the clip on the delivering tube. The limb is lightly splinted. If the cannula slips out of the vein, blood escapes into the tissues and the patient complains of pain. The tube should be clipped off and the doctor summoned.

In blood transfusion, as in all intravenous injections, the tubing and other portions of the delivery apparatus must be free of air. Air embolism is the danger.

*The drip may fail to run because:*

(a) The vein is obstructed by too tight a bandage.
(b) The outlet of the cannula is against the wall of the vein. This is corrected by adhesive skin strapping.
(c) The head of pressure is too low (corrected by elevating the bottle).
(d) The delivery tube is blocked. This can be tested by disconnecting the tube from the shaft of the cannula.
(e) The air inlet of the bottle is partially obstructed by a fragment of rubber seal or a damp cotton-wool plug
(f) Venospasm. This may be lessened by:
   (i) the injection of 2 per cent procaine around the vein by the doctor.
   (ii) keeping the patient's arm warm. Warmth dilates the vein and is permissible in this strictly localised area.

Other difficulties which may arise are:

1. *An airlock.* An airlock can be cleared by disconnecting the delivery tube from the cannula and running the blood through.

2. *The drip-chamber is too full.* The difficulty can be overcome by turning off the drip and holding the bottle upright, i.e. with the neck upwards. Gentle pressure on the drip chamber will cause air to re-enter this chamber.

The drip that is running satisfactorily *may stop* because:

(a) The cannula has come out of the vein.
(b) The bottle of blood was allowed to empty before it was changed.
(c) Blood has clotted in the cannula.

The blood running into the patient will not clot because it contains an anticoagulant. The clotting occurs because the patient's blood has been allowed to be siphoned back into the cannula. This can be avoided when changing the bottle by:

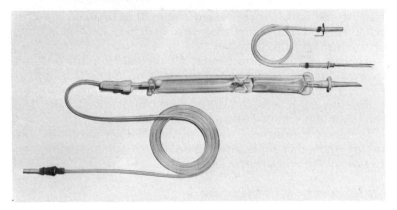

FIG. 13.9  Baxter pressure transfusion set. Note self-sealing rubber (bottom left) to enable intravenous drugs to be given rapidly in to the drip set.

(a) Clamping off the delivery tube as gently as possible.
(b) Turning off the drip set when changing units of blood.

2. PRESSURE ADMINISTRATION PUMP. This should be used only by medical staff. The Baxter transfusion set (Fig. 13.9) permits either a gravity or pressure pump administration.

The inbuilt blood pump permits rapid administration of blood. It is always there when emergency dictates and obviates the necessity to set up ancillary pumping equipment in an emergency. It eliminates the hazards of positive air pressure systems. It cannot pump air.

*Pump instructions.* When pressure transfusion is required, close the regulating clamp and squeeze the (lower) pump chamber to fill completely, so that the float occludes inlet. Open regulating clamp and alternately squeeze and release the pump chamber allowing to fill completely between each action. Pumping action should be discontinued as soon as the container is empty. To return to gravity transfusion remove the bottle from the stand to the upright position and, by squeezing the pump chamber with tubing clamped off, discharge excess fluid back into the bottle. Resuspend the bottle and tap set briskly to disperse any froth.

A second type of pressure pump, the Martin's pump, is in use in many hospitals and is of value when rapid transfusion is required. The pump is clamped to the drip-stand and the drip tubing is inserted into a grooved channel. Manual turning of the handle rollers against the tubing produces pressure to force blood into the vein.

3. **Intra-arterial transfusion.** May be of value very occasionally. It is certainly of value in a patient on the point of death from severe haemorrhage.

*Precautions during transfusion*

Patients and transfusion apparatus must be kept under constant supervision during the entire period of the transfusion.

The medical officer must inform the nurse of the rate at which the transfusion is to be maintained. Forty drops per minute is the usual rate of transfusion, which means that a bottle is transfused in four hours. Patients suffering from haemorrhage may need to be given transfusion at a much greater rate.

Sufferers from cardiac or pulmonary disease, and severely anaemic patients, must be transfused at a slow rate, sometimes as slow as twelve drops per minute or packed cells used (p. 117).

When a transfusion is in progress half-hourly pulse and hourly temperature records should be kept. If the transfusion is for circulatory failure the blood pressure and the pulse should be recorded after each bottle.

Patients receiving transfusions should be kept rather warmer than is comfortable, as this reduces the tendency to febrile reactions and circulatory overloading. All patients should be watched for the symptoms of transfusion reactions. Immediate treatment should be given and the medical officer must be informed without delay. Measurement of the central venous pressure may be of assistance in assessing the amount of blood required.

*Procedure after transfusion*

The details of the transfusion, with serial numbers of bottles given and the time taken for the transfusion, must be entered in the case records. A note should be made of any untoward reactions (p. 124).

The used blood bottles, containing their residues of blood, should be recapped and kept in the ward (preferably in a refrigerator) for 24 hours. These bottles must not be washed out, as the small amount of blood remaining in each bottle may be required in the investigation of transfusion reactions.

When 24 hours have elapsed after transfusion, the bottles should be put out for collection by the messengers, who will return them to the racks outside the blood store. Any unused or partly used bottles of blood which have been left at room temperature for one hour or more should be labelled 'dangerous for patients' and returned to the laboratory.

## COMPLICATIONS OF BLOOD TRANSFUSION

1. Allergic reactions may occur in patients with a previous history of allergic reactions to transfusion or who have a history of asthma or similar allergic conditions. The reaction

tends to occur after about 300 ml of blood have been given. There is no need to stop the transfusion. It is characterised by itching and urticaria. Intravenous antihistamine preparations will usually control it.

2. Pyrexia from pyrogens in the anticoagulant fluid may occur. It is usually due to dirty apparatus and is much rarer since fresh disposable apparatus is used. An infection in the blood is another cause of pyrexia.

3. *Haemolysis* gives rise to rigors at an early stage. The transfusion should be stopped and Mannitol infused.

4. Citrate intoxication may manifest itself by an irregular slow pulse. After every fourth unit of blood 10 ml of 10 per cent calcium chloride is injected intravenously.

5. *Overloading* gives rise to signs of right heart failure. It is very rare if the transfusion is controlled by measurement of the central venous pressure.

6. Transmission of infection of which the most important is hepatitis (p. 385).

7. Air embolism (p. 109) is avoided by keeping air away from the lower portion of the drip chamber and beyond.

8. A thrombophlebitis is an occasional complication.

9. Renal failure is usually caused by mismatched blood.

Finally, after blood transfusion it is advisable to check the haemoglobin to ensure that the patient has received some benefit. Normally a unit of blood should raise the haemoglobin 1 g per 100 ml. In some cases blood is rapidly destroyed and the patient has received little or no benefit from the transfusion.

## CLINICAL USE OF BLOOD AND BLOOD PRODUCTS

Whole blood or some specially prepared constituent of blood may be used in clinical practice.

1. Whole blood is used for replacement in haemorrhage. The usual anticoagulant is acid citrate dextrose.

2. Concentrated red cells (packed cells) replace haemoglobin in anaemia without greatly increasing the circulatory volume.

3. Platelets prepared by concentrating the blood after removal of the red cells may be used in thrombocytopenia.

4. Plasma replaces protein lost in burns and large wounds. At present dried pooled plasma is used, but this is shortly to be replaced by plasma protein fraction (PPF) which will be supplied as a solution. Whereas dried plasma may transmit the virus of serum hepatitis, plasma protein fraction is heated to inactivate the virus.

5. Fresh frozen plasma (FFP) contains all the clotting factors and is invaluable in bleeding states with loss of coagulation.

6. Cryoprecipitate contains a high concentration of antihaemophilic globulin (factor VIII). It is used for treating patients with haemophilia.

7. Fibrinogen is used in conditions of hypofibrinogenaemia such as occur in the defibrination syndrome.

8. Gammaglobulin is used for immunisation against such conditions as hepatitis.

### FATE OF THE BLOOD LOST IN HAEMORRHAGE

At the beginning of this chapter it was noted that all the patient's problems may not be resolved when the bleeding ceases or the blood volume has been restored. In some haemorrhages the amount of blood loss is insignificant, but the actual blood lost is highly destructive in specialised tissues such as those of the eye or small but important areas of the brain or spinal cord. In body cavities such as the skull, the brain may be compressed by extravasated blood lying between the bone and the meninges or between the meninges and the brain. In the chest a large effusion of blood and blood clot may interfere with the action of the heart or lungs. In the pharynx, larynx or trachea, blood may seriously obstruct respiration and give rise to lung infection including an abscess. In more disastrous circumstances the patient may die from flooding of the whole pulmonary field with inhaled blood.

Terms to describe extravasated collections of blood are:

1. *Petechiae* are tiny pinpoint haemorrhages from capillary damage.
2. *An ecchymosis* is a small area of skin bruising.
3. *Haematoma* is a sealed collection of blood and clot. It may be sealed beneath:
   (a) a wound;
   (b) a tissue such as the periosteum (subperiosteal) or beneath the capsule of an organ (subcapsular).
   (c) A tear of a soft organ such as the spleen or liver.

*Complications*

1. *Infection.* 'Stale blood' is an ideal medium for the growth of organisms.

2. *Rupture.* In large haematomas profuse internal 'delayed' haemorrhage may result.

### HAEMORRHAGE FROM SPECIAL SITES

The occurrence of haemorrhage from special sites is designated by special terms.

*Epistaxis*—bleeding from the nose.

*Haemoptysis*—the expectoration of blood from the lungs.

*Haematemesis*—vomiting of blood.

*Melaena*—the passage of dark blood per rectum from a site high in the intestinal tract.

*Haematuria*—blood in the urine.

*Haemothorax*—bleeding into the chest.

*Haemoperitoneum*—bleeding into the peritoneum.

*Haemarthrosis*—bleeding into a joint.

*Menorrhagia*—excessive menstruation at normal intervals.

*Metrostaxis* (metrorrhagia)—excessive irregular or continuous bleeding per vaginam between the periods.

*Haemopericardium* (cardiac tamponade)—bleeding into the pericardium.

*Haematomyelia*—bleeding into the spinal cord.

### THE HAEMORRHAGIC DISEASES

The haemorrhagic diseases are:

1. **Thrombocytopenia.** This may be (a) *primary* or (b) *secondary* to drugs, malignant disease such as leukaemia or to aplastic anaemia.

2. **Anaphylactoid purpura** (Henoch-Schonlein).

3. **Haemophilia.**

4. **Christmas disease.**

5. **von Willebrand's disease.**

6. **Scurvy.**

# CHAPTER 14

# Thrombosis and Embolism

Thrombosis is defined as the formation of a solid or semisolid mass from the constituents of the blood within the vascular system. It is not identical with the clotting of shed blood. Although the incidence of disease is higher in the arteries, thrombosis is commoner in veins where the more sluggish blood flow predisposes to its formation.

A thrombus may:

1. Extend and spread while still attached to the vessel wall.
2. Lyse (dissolve) spontaneously without permanent damage.
3. Organise into fibrous tissue so that the lumen of the vessel is permanently obstructed.
4. Become detached in whole or in part and be swept away into the blood stream until it lodges and blocks another blood vessel. This process is known as embolism, the detached thrombus being the embolus and the area deprived of blood is known as the infarct.

Thrombi may form in any part of the vascular system. The common sites are:

(a) *The veins of the lower limb and pelvis*, and detachment gives rise to pulmonary embolism.
(b) *The left heart chamber* in valvular disease or myocardial infarction. As the heart recovers and its action improves, an embolus may be expelled, lodge in an artery of the leg and cause acute gangrene (p. 231) or in the cerebral vessels causing a hemiplegia.
(c) *On an atheromatous patch in an arteriosclerotic artery*, which results in threatened gangrene in a limb already poorly supplied with blood.

When thrombosis occurs in a vein the condition is known as phlebothrombosis but if there is a concomitant inflammation of the vessel wall the process is known as thrombophlebitis. The former is usually painless, the latter is strikingly painful.

**Factors which predispose to thrombosis.** Certain incidents and disease render the patient more liable to form thrombi.

1. *The vessel wall* may be damaged by trauma including pres-

127

sure during operation. Many substances suitable for intravenous injection may cause disastrous thrombosis if injected into
an artery. Before the administration of intramuscular injections one should always check that the needle is not in a vein
by withdrawing the piston before plunging it in, and in intravenous injections care should be taken to note that it is venous
and not arterial blood that is flowing back into the syringe before administering the injection. The ampoule label should be
checked to ensure that the contents are suitable for intravenous administration.

2. *Structural changes in the vessel wall.* Arteries already the site
of sclerosis may be further obstructed by thrombosis.

On operating tables, particularly when amputating a leg,
the popliteal artery in the opposite limb—often in a parlous
state of health—must be kept free of pressure from the end of
the table which may have been split.

Veins with damaged valves are more liable to form thrombi,
as are heart valves which have been damaged by disease.

3. *Slowing the blood flow* increases the risk. Confinement to
bed in conditions of hypotension and obstruction to the flow
of blood by constricting bandages or bad positioning on the
operating table are to be avoided.

4. *Changes in the nature of the blood.* Dehydration increases the
viscosity of the blood. Other factors which increase its coagulability are leukaemia and splenectomy (because platelet destruction is delayed), drugs such as oestrogens (included in the
contraceptive pill) and malignant disease. In many cases there
is a combination of factors and thrombosis is sometimes the
first clinical feature of malignant disease which even an intensive search may fail to reveal.

## CLINICAL FEATURES

Arterial thrombosis causes loss of function and usually severe
pain. Common examples are coronary thrombosis or thrombosis in the main artery of a leg. In this chapter, however, we
are primarily concerned with venous thrombosis. This may be
present as:

(a) *Thrombophlebitis* more usually affects the superficial veins.
It is painful. The skin over the vein is reddened and the vein itself is usually palpable as a tender, firm cord.

(b) *Massive thrombosis* in a large vein may be relatively painless. There is swelling of the limb, which increases rapidly, and
the foot particularly is usually oedematous. The limb feels
heavy and the superficial unaffected veins may be very prominent.

(c) *Quiet formation* is suggested by a slight rise in the patient's temperature; some aching pain in the calf of the leg; pain in the muscles of the calf on dorsiflexion of the foot (Homan's sign); slight oedema of the foot.

(d) *Pulmonary embolism* (p. 131) may be the first sign that thrombosis has occurred.

## MANAGEMENT

*Prevention*

Large varicose veins may be temporarily controlled by crêpe bandages or ligated if the patient is undergoing a severe operation or one necessitating prolonged bed-rest.

Drugs liable to produce thrombosis such as oestrogens should be stopped four to eight weeks preoperatively. Previous venous thrombotic upsets may be an indication for prophylactic anticoagulant therapy commencing 48 to 72 hours postoperatively or even subcutaneous preoperatively. The risk of bleeding has of course to be carefully considered.

Much thought has been given to the prevention of thrombosis.

Factors which diminish thrombus formation are:

1. Analgesics. Relieve pain and make movement easier.
2. Adequate fluids. Prevent 'increased' viscosity of blood.
3. No knee pillow. The patient should be operated on with the foot of the operating table elevated slightly and the heels supported by padded rings so that the calves of the legs are lifted off the table. Postoperatively the foot of the bed should be elevated and when out of bed the patient should not be allowed to sit with his legs dependent.
4. Breathing exercises.
5. Leg exercises.
6. Early rising after operation.
7. Subcutaneous heparin preoperatively is used prophylactically on high-risk patients.

*Established thrombosis* may be obvious or only suspected. In either case further investigation may be advisable to establish the diagnosis, the extent, the type and the number of thrombi, or to gauge the response to treatment. These include:

RADIOGRAPHY

Phlebography will outline the vein or show a block by a thrombus in the veins of the leg or iliac veins.

$^{125}$I-labelled fibrinogen, when injected intravenously, becomes incorporated in a firm thrombus (if present) and may be detected by Geiger-counter scanning of the legs.

THE ULTRASONIC DOPPLER.

The ultrasonic response to an increased venous flow against an obstruction has been termed the A-wave. It can be repeated as frequently as desired to assess progress without any discomfort to the patient and therefore has an advantage over radiographic and isotopic measures, but is not as accurate.

*Treatment*

The objects of treatment are:
1. To prevent extension of the thrombus.
2. To remove or lyse (dissolve) the thrombus.
3. To prevent detachment with embolus formation.

This is achieved in an established case by rest in bed, the foot of which is elevated, and the administration of anticoagulants until an adequate prothrombin time has been achieved. Heparin 10,000 units intravenously is given at once, followed by 10,000 units six-hourly. If it has been decided to use oral anticoagulants, which are slower in achieving their effect, these are commenced when ordered and the dose is controlled by estimation of the prothrombin time. When effective their administration is continued and heparin therapy ceases. The dosage varies with the preparation used. Warfarin has an initial dosage of 30–40 mg on the first day, none on the second day and a maintenance dose of 2–20 mg daily, depending on the level of the prothrombin time which is estimated daily. The prothrombin time should be taken at midday, and the anticoagulant given before midnight each day.

In addition to watching for signs of excessive dosage, delayed haemorrhage, pyrexia, a skin rash, albuminuria and jaundice may develop because of drug sensitivity. Granulocytopenia and diarrhoea have also been noted. The fifth week is the time these symptoms may occur. The drug dosage is regulated according to the prothrombin time and steroid therapy instituted.

If at any time it is desired to reverse or diminish the effects of anticoagulants this can be achieved by 1 ml of protamine sulphate which will neutralise 1000 units (10 mg) of heparin. Warfarin is neutralised by vitamin K 500 mg by mouth, but as it is rather slow a transfusion of fresh blood may be advisable.

Anticoagulants prevent further thrombosis and their extension, but they may not dissolve an established clot. For this reason fibrinolytic agents such as streptokinase 500,000 units may be given over 30 minutes, followed by 100,000 units hourly. Newer fibrinolysins will undoubtedly be developed. As in anticoagulant treatment, fibrinolytic treatment requires close observation, particularly for signs of haemorrhage.

The action of streptokinase may be much neutralised by the administration of ε-aminocaproic acid.

Surgical removal, thrombectomy, may be undertaken with a Fogarty venous catheter and the operation is similar to removal of an embolus from an artery (p. 231). Delaying treatment, or failure to remove the thrombus by drugs or surgery, may result in a permanent white leg by organisation of the clot. Venous bypass operations may be attempted to re-establish the blood flow.

## A NEW ANTICOAGULANT

Arvin, an enzyme separated from the venom of the Malayan pit viper, shows many of the characteristics of the ideal anticoagulant. It acts by reducing fibrinogen (the soluble precursor of fibrin) unlike the oral anticoagulants which depress the synthesis of clotting factors in the liver, and heparin (p. 112) which inhibits thrombin.

## EMBOLISM

An embolus is a foreign body momentarily free in the blood stream. The most common source is a detached thrombus from a vein which gives rise to pulmonary embolism. Detachment of a thrombus from the left side of the heart may cause gangrene of a limb (p. 231). It used to be thought that pulmonary embolus, apart from the immediate postoperative period, was rare, but more careful observation has shown that it is not uncommon at other times. Other forms of embolus are considered and mentioned at the end of this chapter.

### PULMONARY EMBOLUS

Since embolism is a complication of thrombosis, prevention depends on avoiding thrombosis and in detecting established thrombosis as early as possible. The effect of an embolus is entirely dependent on its size. Three syndromes are recognised:

1. A relatively small embolus occludes a peripheral pulmonary artery and produces the classical picture—pleural-type pain, haemoptysis and a shadow of infarcted lung on the X-ray.

2. Repeated embolism without pain initially but gradually increased breathlessness, fatigue and a feeling of collapse on exertion.

3. A massive pulmonary embolism from a large embolus occluding about two-thirds of the circumference of the pulmonary artery. The onset is sudden, there are signs of right heart failure, the patient is clammy, anxious and cyanosed and the veins in the neck are outstanding. The diagnosis from myocardial infarct is often difficult but vital since it is in this form

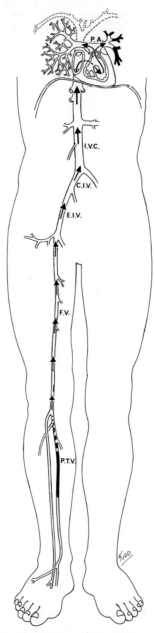

FIG. 14.1   Pulmonary embolism. The thrombus has formed in the posterior tibial veins and passes via the femoral, external iliac and common iliac veins to the inferior vena cava and thence to the right atrium of the heart. From the right atrium it passes to the right ventricle which pumps it in this case into the left pulmonary artery with infarction of the left lung.

that pulmonary embolectomy may be the only hope and such a procedure would be rapidly fatal in a patient with coronary thrombosis. Electrocardiography and lung scanning with radioactive xenon may be advisable. Pulmonary angiography may confirm the diagnosis with certainty—the patient may be too ill for it to be undertaken. Blood gases should be estimated—hypoxia and hypocarbia may be diagnostic of pulmonary embolism. Electrocardiography may help to confirm the diagnosis.

*Treatment*

*Major embolism* presents great difficulties in the choice and timing of treatment. The patient is kept absolutely still and oxygen is administered. If the condition is improving, treatment is conservative. Conservative treatment entails lysis of the pulmonary embolism and the prevention of further embolism by the administration of anticoagulants or fibrinolysins (p. 130).

A large loose thrombus can be removed or the vein above it ligated so that it cannot escape, e.g. the inferior vena cava may be plicated to narrow it so that the embolus cannot pass. Smaller thrombi will lyse with streptokinase given for three days, followed by anticoagulant drugs. The real anxiety is that some hours are necessary before the effects of fibrinolysis or anticoagulants become apparent. If the patient is deteriorating, pulmonary embolectomy may be undertaken as a last desperate measure.

*Lesser degrees of embolism* are always anxious situations since they may be the forerunner of a massive embolism. Movement is reduced to a minimum and anticoagulant treatment is instituted at once. Investigation of the state of the deep veins is undertaken by bilateral ascending and ileofemoral phlebogram by percutaneous or perosseous routes. A decision is made as to whether further measures such as thrombolytic therapy or removal of the thrombus may be advisable.

## OTHER FORMS OF EMBOLISM

**1. Fat embolism.** Fat embolism (pp. 542) is caused as a result of fractures and in severe cases causes respiratory distress due, not to the emboli in the lungs, but to their effect on the brain which may cause death. Assisted respiration is advisable.

**2. Air embolism.** Air embolism is a risk of venous haemorrhage in which air is sucked into an open vein. The air causes frothing of the blood. It is avoided in intravenous injections, including transfusion, by ensuring only fluid and no air is injected (p. 124).

3. **Bacteria spread by emboli.** This may be recognised by the presence of purpuric spots on the skin, tiny splinter haemorrhages under the nails, retinal haemorrhages, or from the presence of red blood cells in the urine of such patients, in cases of infective endocarditis.

4. **Malignant cells.** Spread by the bloodstream (p. 214).

5. **Foreign bodies.** The most important to avoid clinically is detachment of an intravenous catheter.

CHAPTER 15

# Acute Circulatory Failure

The supply of oxygen to the tissues is the first essential in the maintenance of life, and this can only be ensured when the circulatory system is functioning normally. Sudden collapse of the circulation is one of the commonest and most formidable conditions encountered in surgical practice. The circulation may fail from:

1. **Sudden damage to the heart.** This may occur because of:

(a) *Coronary arterial occlusion.*
(b) *Toxaemia*, which may be (i) bacterial (originating elsewhere in the body), (ii) chemical, including drugs and anaesthetic agents.
(c) *Trauma.*

Complete cardiac arrest is the most urgent of all conditions, and death is an inevitable sequel unless the heart can be restored within three minutes. Cardiac massage may be the only hope, and is discussed in detail at the end of this chapter. In certain arrhythmias such as ventricular fibrillation, a defibrillator is required.

2. **Deficient oxygenation of the blood in the lungs.** Amongst the many causes the following are the most important surgically:

(a) *Obstruction of the pulmonary artery by an embolus.* If it is complete sudden death occurs.
(b) *Thoracic injuries*, particularly 'stove in' chest, tension pneumothorax, bruising and laceration of the lungs.
(c) *Postoperative atelectasis* (collapse of a large segment of lung).

The complicated issues involved in this form are discussed in the chapters on Respiratory Failure and Diseases of the Lungs and Thorax.

3. **Reduction in the blood volume (oligaemia).** This may occur from loss of:

(a) *Whole blood*—haemorrhage.
(b) *Plasma.* This is particularly significant in burns.
(c) *Water and electrolytes*, which occurs in (i) peritonitis, (ii) intestinal obstruction and paralytic ileus, (iii) acute

dilatation of the stomach, and (iv) severe diarrhoea and vomiting.

4. **Loss of arterial tone.** This may occur in:

(a) *The common faint.* The arterioles in the muscles relax.
(b) *Acute anaphylaxis* (p. 44).
(c) *Acute hormone deficiency*, notably of the adrenal gland.
(d) *Absorption of metabolites or materials resulting from tissue injury.*
(e) *Overdosage of drugs, for example, analgesics like pethidine.*

Shock is a word with so many different meanings that its use as a descriptive term serves only to confuse.

*Compensatory mechanisms*
    Whatever the cause of sudden collapse there are certain compensatory physiological mechanisms which occur.
    1. POSTURE: A patient in acute circulatory failure falls down. He should be left flat or, better, kept in the head-down position to an angle of 5°. This helps to supply more blood to the brain but an angle of more than 5° is harmful because it causes venous congestion.
    2. CONTRACTION OF THE SKIN VESSELS. Contraction of the arterioles and venules of the skin is usual so as to conserve the blood supply to the more vital centres. The application of heat dilates the skin vessels, thereby aggravating the condition, and should not be used.
    3. INSENSITIVITY. A very collapsed patient usually has little pain. Large quantities of pain-relieving drugs are unnecessary and, in any case, are ineffective because they cannot be absorbed unless given by the intravenous route. Administered subcutaneously they may result in cumulative overdosage as the circulation recovers. Because the patient with acute circulatory failure is insensitive his skin is more easily damaged, so he has to be handled very gently.
    4. URINARY SECRETION is diminished to conserve fluid in the body, but it is also a sign that tissue perfusion (the circulation of blood through the kidney and other tissues) is inadequate.
    5. THE HEART RATE ACCELERATES in most forms of circulatory failure with the important exception of the common faint. It is an attempt to ensure that the remaining fluid is circulated as rapidly as possible.
    6. THE TEMPERATURE IS SUBNORMAL. This reduces the requirements of the tissues for the diminishing amount of oxygen available.
    All these compensatory factors are temporary in their beneficial effects and, if the condition of the circulation is not restored to normal without delay, irreversible changes set in.

*Clinical causes*
1. Haemorrhage.
2. Severe burns.
3. Severe wounds, particularly with extensive skin or muscle laceration.
4. Multiple fractures or single fractures of a large long bone.
5. Perforation of any viscus into the peritoneal cavity.
6. Operative intervention.
7. Adrenal failure.
8. Pulmonary embolism.
9. Myocardial infarction.
10. Severe infection, particularly bacteraemia.

## CLINICAL APPEARANCES OF CIRCULATORY FAILURE

*The face* is ashen pale and expressionless. The eyes are still and the patient takes little or no interest in his surroundings, although he may answer, slowly, questions which are asked. He makes no complaint of pain.

*The skin* is cold, white, and clammy. The respirations are shallow. The pulse is usually rapid and thin, although sometimes it is below normal in rate, and the temperature is always subnormal.

If bacteraemia is suspected, a blood culture is performed.

The most constant finding is a low systolic and diastolic blood pressure.

*Clinical management*

Of the many disturbances which occur in acute circulatory failure, oligaemia is the one best understood and most easily remedied. Its control requires observation of:

1. THE CENTRAL VENOUS PRESSURE which is the best guide to the effective circulating volume. It may be measured by passing a PVC or Teflon catheter into a peripheral vein and threading it up until it is estimated to lie within the thoracic cavity. The veins used are those on the medial side of the arm, the subclavian or the internal jugular. The cannula must be firmly fixed to the skin. Correctly sited there will always be a free rise and fall on the attached manometer.

This catheter is connected to a special venous pressure measuring drip set (Fig. 15.1).

This is distinguished by having a long side-arm. It is provided with a centimetre scale. In use, the side-arm is filled with fluid and is then connected to the patient's venous system. The

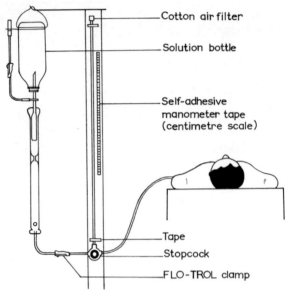

Cotton air filter

Solution bottle

Self-adhesive
manometer tape
(centimetre scale)

Tape
Stopcock
FLO-TROL clamp

FIG 15.1    The estimation of central venous pressure using a
special Baxter drip set.

level above the manubrium sternum at which the fluid in the
side-arm comes to rest is a measure of the central venous pressure. In the normal subject the value will be from 0 to 2 or
3 cm of water.

In the shocked or hypovolaemic patient it will be negative
while in patients who are in heart failure or who have been
overtransfused it may be very high (10 to 25 cm of water).

2. HAEMATOCRIT READING of over 55 indicates the need for
saline or plasma or its substitutes rather than blood.

3. URINARY OUTPUT is the best guide that tissue perfusion is
occurring and an indwelling catheter is inserted in all severe
cases. The specific gravity of the urine should be recorded
hourly, and an output of urine below 60 ml per hour is considered unsatisfactory. Tissue perfusion means that the blood
flow to the kidney is sufficient not only to keep the organ alive
but also to function, and indirect evidence that the circulation of blood in other organs is improving and becoming
adequate.

4. HEART RATE is rapid and diminishes as replacement becomes adequate.

5. THE BLOOD PRESSURE. The reversal of hypotension is in itself an unreliable sign unless accompanied by reversal of the
other signs of oligaemia.

*Taking the blood pressure.* The patient should be at rest lying in
bed, or sitting in a chair. The sleeve of the gown/jacket is

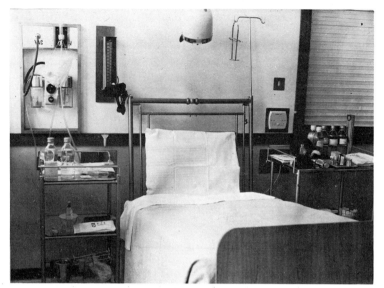

FIG. 15.2    Preparation of bed for acute circulatory failure.

rolled back or removed as necessary. The arm is extended and supported. The cuff of the sphygmomanometer is wrapped firmly and smoothly round the upper arm well above the elbow flexure. The manometer is placed level with the patient's arm, the scale being visible to the nurse. It is connected to the cuff. The nurse palpates the radial/brachial pulse, she inflates the cuff and notes the point on the manometer at which the pulse disappears. (N.B. Care should be taken to avoid discomfort to the patient by the cuff being overinflated or inflated for too long a time.) The cuff is deflated. She adjusts the ear pieces of the stethoscope, and places the other end over the brachial pulse (artery). The cuff is reinflated to above the previously noted point on the manometer. It is slowly deflated. When a tapping sound is heard, the nurse notes the point on the manometer—this gives the systolic pressure. As the cuff is deflated further, the sounds become louder, suddenly they change to a muffled sound, and then cease altogether. The point at which the sound changes from loud to muffled is noted—this gives the diastolic pressure. The manometer is disconnected. The cuff is removed and folded away into the manometer box. The patient is made comfortable.

The result is charted immediately, e.g.

BP $\frac{120}{80}$

Any significant change from previous recordings is reported to the nurse in charge. When there is difficulty in hearing the sounds or in obtaining the readings, the nurse in charge should be asked to help.

6. TEMPERATURE. Observations of differences between the peripheral skin temperature and the rectal temperature (measured by electrical thermometers) are helpful in estimating the peripheral circulation. If the temperature in the rectum is recorded on one chart and compared with the temperature on the big toe it is found that the big toe temperature drops or fails to rise sooner if all is not well. It is an even finer guide than urinary excretion to the state of tissue perfusion.

7. Expansion of the circulatory volume until it is adequate as shown by reversal of the signs of failure. It remains the most hopeful method of treatment whatever the metabolic disturbance, since restoration of normal tissue perfusion is essential.

DRUGS

Vasoconstrictors are contraindicated. Drugs which may be of value if the patient fails to respond to adequate restoration of the blood volume are:

*Hydrocortisone* 100 mg or more in the drip may be effective. It probably acts by stabilization of the cell membranes.

*Vasodilators* may be of value after the blood volume has been restored on the basis that prolonged splanchnic vasoconstriction (constriction of the arteries to the stomach and intestine causes irreversible changes). Phenoxybenzamine has been reported to be of value as has isoprenaline which has a direct inotropic effect as well as being a vasodilator.

*Correction of acidosis.* A solution of 8·4 per cent sodium bicarbonate may be advisable and arterial blood-gas estimations are of value in making this decision.

*Diuretics.* Mannitol (a 6-carbon sugar) is an osmotic diuretic which is neither absorbed in the renal tubules nor metabolised. It may be given when acidosis and oligaemia have been corrected but if oliguria persists Lasix may also be given. If diuresis does not occur with 25 g over half an hour severe renal damage has occurred and fluid should be restricted on this account.

*Antibiotics* are essential if a bacterial element is present.

*Anticoagulants* may occasionally be indicated if microcirculatory thrombosis is suspected.

*Electrolyte imbalance* must be corrected.

*Oxygen lack* is corrected by administration with Argyle spectacles.

*Analgesics* are rarely necessary until the patient's condition has ben restored.

Internal haemorrhage from a ruptured organ may occur so rapidly that the risk of operating on a patient suffering from circulatory failure has to be accepted and rapid transfusion should be performed until the haemorrhage has been controlled and continued until the blood volume has been restored. The shorter the period the patient is collapsed with a low blood pressure, anoxia and loss of tissue perfusion the better, otherwise there is a risk of irreversible damage to the kidneys, the liver, and the brain, especially in the elderly.

Whatever the cause of circulatory collapse the following general principles evolve:

1. Treatment must be instituted without delay and continued until the condition has been reversed.

2. In difficult cases, where the response is slow or inadequate, the diagnosis of the cause may have to be revised.

3. Once the patient's condition has improved every precaution must be taken to see that circulatory failure does not recur. Observation of the pulse, temperature, colour and urinary output is important. Examination of the blood and urine should be continued and the return to a sitting-up position should be instituted gradually and observantly.

Circulatory collapse should be avoided by strenuous measures if at all possible. Preoperatively the patient should be as fit as possible, and from the point of view of the circulatory system:

1. His blood should be adequate in quality and in volume.
2. His tissues should be adequately hydrated.
3. He should be mobile so that there is no stagnation in the circulatory system.

## THE PREVENTION OF CIRCULATORY COLLAPSE

Every operation is an injury, but operative trauma differs from all other injuries in that the surgeon and nursing staff know its nature in advance. Further, we know the early signs of circulatory collapse.

1. The patient is kept warm on his journey from the ward to the theatre and back. Blankets should be warmed. Fear is allayed and tranquillising drugs are commonly used preoperatively.

2. The blood pressure is recorded, and in serious cases is monitored continuously, and blood replacement commenced in good time. Severe operations are commenced only after satisfactory infusions have been established.

3. The head of the table is lowered if the blood pressure falls (the Trendelenburg position).

4. The anaesthetist deepens the anaesthesia temporarily

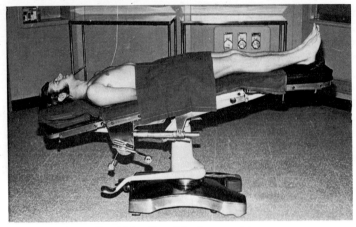

FIG. 15.3   Trendelenburg position.

as specially sensitive tissues are handled. Oxygen is freely provided and cyanosis is avoided.

5. Postoperatively, fluid and electrolyte replacement (saline, 5 per cent, dextrose, Ringer's solution, Lactate, plasma
or blood as indicated), rest and relief from pain are continued.

6. Gentle handling of the patient by the nursing staff is very
important in the prevention of acute circulatory failure.

There are few conditions in which a patient can improve or
deteriorate so rapidly as in circulatory failure. Its treatment
calls for the best organisation of the resources of a hospital
and the most painstaking care from the nursing staff.

### CARDIAC ARREST

The interval between 'clinical death' which occurs with
cessation of the heart beat and respiration and biological
death is three to five minutes. This may be prolonged by:

1. Cardiac massage (external cardiac compression).
2. Hypothermia.
3. Extracorporeal circulation with artificial oxygenator.

Sudden stoppage of the heart requires immediate action on
the part of the nursing staff, as only three minutes of cessation
of blood flow to the cerebrum is permissible before cerebral
damage is permanent and is irreversible.

Pulmonary inflation by a bag and face mask with air and
oxygen should be started immediately so that what little blood
circulating through the lungs is fully oxygenated. If no bag
is available mouth to mouth or mouth to nose breathing
should be carried out continuously, and medical help must be
summoned immediately.

Cardiac massage or, more correctly, intermittent cardiac pumping or intermittent cardiac compression has to be carried out. This may be performed by the nurse while another nurse continues mouth to mouth breathing simultaneously. The patient is laid flat on the floor (a mattress is too soft) or, better, a fracture board on a bed, and regular manual compression is exerted against the lower sternum at a rate of 60 times per minute. Properly performed it can be a very exhausting effort and the rib cage may be damaged. A machine has been designed for the purpose but it is not generally available. The patient's legs should be slightly elevated to aid venous return and the head should be supported.

As soon as possible an ECG machine should be attached to the patient in order to establish what heart rhythm is present. An intravenous infusion should be set up and a sample of heparinised arterial blood is sent for blood gas analysis. 100 mEq sodium bicarbonate should be infused.

Solutions of 1 : 1000 adrenaline and 10 per cent calcium chloride should be immediately available for intracardiac injection.

Cardiac arrest produces a severe metabolic acidosis and solutions of sodium bicarbonate will need to be infused before satisfactory cardiac action can be restored.

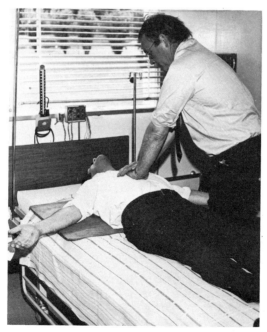

FIG. 15.4   External cardiac compression.

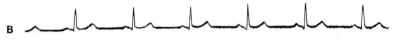

FIG. 15.5   Electrocardiograph. A, Ventricular fibrillation tracing. B, Normal tracing showing P Q R S and T waves.

The provision of a cardiac arrest resuscitation trolley is now a regular feature in many blocks of wards. In addition to an oxygen cylinder with a regulator it should be furnished as follows:

*Top shelf—*
Ambu suction pump
Dunedin emergency inflating bellows
Facepiece and tubing
Catheter mount
Electrocardiograph
Defibrillator
Two Magill cuffed endotracheal tubes
Mannitol 12·5 per cent 100 ml

Mackintosh laryngoscope and spare battery
Adrenaline, 1 : 1000 ampoules
Calcium chloride, 10 per cent
Sodium bicarbonate, 8·4 per cent
Sterile water, 10 ml ampoules
20-ml syringe for inflating endotracheal tube, artery forceps and clip
Ureaphyl

*Attached to trolley—*Solid blade scalpel in pyrex tube

*Lower shelf—*A pack containing—
Swabs, two packets
Towels, six
Syringes, two each of 20, 10 and 5 ml, and spare needles
Water-seal drainage with tube-clip
Intercostal catheter with connection
Rib spreader
7-in Moynihan artery forceps (nine)
BP no. 4 blade handle and blades

Mayo curved and straight scissors, one pair of each
One plain, one toothed dissecting forceps
One needleholder
Two sponge forceps
Two towel clips
Needles and ligatures (linen thread and Mersilene)
Heparinised syringe for arterial blood gases

If ventricular fibrillation is present an electrical defibrillator will be required to administer an electric shock to restore normal rhythm.

Observations which should be made whilst the patient is receiving treatment are:

1. Feel for the pulse in the groin. If the circulation is maintained the pulse will be palpable.

2. Note if the pupils constrict. The pupils always dilate with circulatory arrest.

3. ECG.

4. Arterial blood gas analysis.

*Aftercare.* If normal cardiac function is restored these patients should be treated in an intensive care unit and be carefully monitored.

ECG control for 24 to 48 hours is desirable. Occasionally measures for cerebral dehydration may be necessary and renal failure may follow a period of hypotension.

A useful aid to memory in the sudden emergency of the management of cardiac arrest is:

A Airway
B Breathing
C Cardiac compression
D Drugs and drip
E Electricity.

# CHAPTER 16

# Fluid and Electrolyte Balance

The method and forms of administration of fluid together with its complications are discussed in Chapter 17. Since fluid and electrolyte balance is a subject of great complexity and much still requires to be known, this separation is deliberate. The present discussion is a subject for the senior student.

Before abnormal states are considered an outline of the normal processes is essential.

## THE FLUID

Water is the basis of all body fluids and the total quantity of body water is approximately 42 litres. This is divided into:

1. Water inside the cells (intracellular water) and amounts to 30 l.
2. Extracellular water 12 l.
   Of which:
   (a) the plasma constitutes 3 l
   (b) the water in the tissue spaces 9 l.

The intracellular water is the fluid in which the essentials of nourishment are consumed and metabolites accumulate. The water in the tissue spaces is outside the blood stream and outside the cells. Its electrolyte composition is almost identical with that of blood plasma.

Examination of the various substances in the plasma will provide information about the composition of the fluid in the

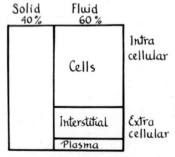

FIG. 16.1   Composition of body.

tissue spaces, but it will not tell us what the position is inside the cells.

## THE ELECTROLYTES

An electrolyte is a substance which when dissolved in water splits (dissociates or ionises is the correct expression) into electrically charged particles known as ions (*ion*, Greek= wanderer). Each electrolyte splits into an equal number of positively (+) charged ions (known as anions) and negatively (−) charged ions (known as cations).

In food an electrolyte is consumed as an independent substance, for example, common salt. To be an independent substance, which can be seen and handled, it must exist in molecular form as NaCl (its chemical formula)—but in the body it exists as $Na^+$ (sodium ions) and $Cl^-$ (chloride ions). Because electrolytes exist as particles, they used to be measured in terms which expressed their biological activity, namely milliequivalents per litre (mEq/l) but in the international system (SI) are now expressed as millimoles per litre (mmol/l).

The principal electrolytes are sodium ($Na^+$), potassium ($K^+$), chloride ($Cl^-$) and bicarbonate ($HCO_3^-$). There are many others like calcium, magnesium, phosphate, and sulphate.

DISTRIBUTION OF ELECTROLYTES

The extracellular and intracellular fluids show a marked difference in concentration of electrolytes. The most striking are:

1. Potassium ($K^+$) is the dominant cation inside the cell. Its concentration is about 144 mmol per litre (144 mEq/l) against 8 mmol per litre (8 mEq/l) for intracellular sodium ($Na^+$).

2. Sodium ($Na^+$) is largely concentrated in the extracellular fluid and plasma with a concentration of 140 mmol per litre (140 mEq/l) against 5 mmol per litre (5 mEq/l) for that of potassium ($K^+$).

Normal metabolism tends to a production of an excess of anions over cations in the blood with the result that there is a tendency to acidosis. This state of affairs is corrected in health by the production of an acid urine. The glomeruli of the kidneys filter 170 l of fluid from the blood in 24 hours, but 168·5 l are reabsorbed by the tubules allowing 1·5 l to be passed as urine.

*Normal control of water and electrolytes*

INTAKE or GAIN is by mouth, followed by absorption from the gut.

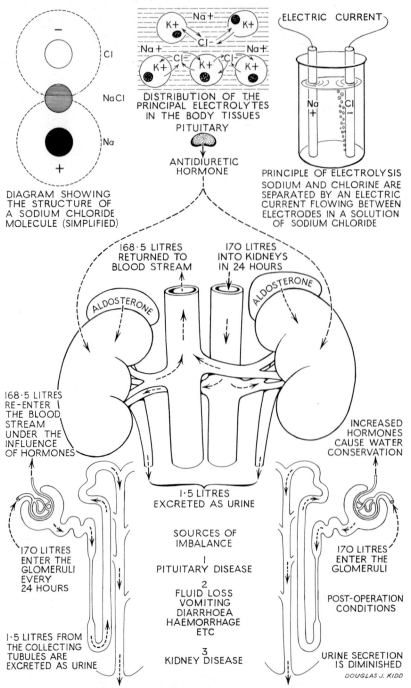

DIAGRAM SHOWING
THE STRUCTURE OF
A SODIUM CHLORIDE
MOLECULE (SIMPLIFIED)

DISTRIBUTION OF THE
PRINCIPAL ELECTROLYTES
IN THE BODY TISSUES

ELECTRIC CURRENT

PRINCIPLE OF ELECTROLYSIS
SODIUM AND CHLORINE ARE
SEPARATED BY AN ELECTRIC
CURRENT FLOWING BETWEEN
ELECTRODES IN A SOLUTION
OF SODIUM CHLORIDE

PITUITARY

ANTIDIURETIC
HORMONE

168·5 LITRES
RETURNED TO
BLOOD STREAM

170 LITRES
INTO KIDNEYS
IN 24 HOURS

ALDOSTERONE

ALDOSTERONE

168·5 LITRES
RE-ENTER
THE BLOOD
STREAM
UNDER THE
INFLUENCE
OF HORMONES

INCREASED
HORMONES
CAUSE WATER
CONSERVATION

1·5 LITRES
EXCRETED AS URINE

170 LITRES
ENTER THE
GLOMERULI
EVERY
24 HOURS

SOURCES OF
IMBALANCE

1
PITUITARY DISEASE

2
FLUID LOSS
VOMITING
DIARRHOEA
HAEMORRHAGE
ETC

3
KIDNEY DISEASE

170 LITRES
ENTER THE
GLOMERULI

POST-OPERATION
CONDITIONS

1·5 LITRES FROM
THE COLLECTING
TUBULES ARE
EXCRETED AS URINE

URINE SECRETION
IS DIMINISHED

DOUGLAS J. KIDD

FIG. 16.2    Fluid and electrolyte balance and imbalance.

EXCRETION or LOSS is from:

1. *Extrarenal sources*—the skin, respiration, and faeces. This amounts to about 1 l. per day.

2. *The kidneys.* Five hundred millilitres of water is the minimum in which a healthy kidney can excrete the body's metabolites. The daily amount is, therefore, this quantity in addition to fluids consumed in excess of $1\frac{1}{2}$ l.

RENAL CONTROL

For the kidney to function adequately it must have:

1. AN INTACT BLOOD SUPPLY and the blood must be supplied at adequate pressure. Its blood vessels must be intact to filter the enormous quantity of 170 l. per day. In any condition of *hypo*tension the mechanism fails. In acute nephritis the glomeruli are swollen and diseased so that they allow blood to pass into the urine. In chronic nephritic conditions the glomeruli are inadequate in number and structure.

2. NORMAL ACTING TUBULES. To function normally and concentrate the glomerular filtrate from 170 to 1·5 l. the tubules must be intact. More than this, they are under the control of hormones, viz:

(a) *The antidiuretic hormone of the pituitary.* If this is inadequate in amount the glomerular fluid is not concentrated and large quantities of water are lost; the condition known as diabetes insipidus in which a vast quantity of pale urine is passed is an extreme example of this failure. Pitressin by injection or by 'snuff' controls the condition.

(b) *Aldosterone.* This is a hormone which is secreted in the adrenal cortex and increases the reabsorption of sodium ($Na^+$) from the filtrate. This is present in such large quantities in the blood and hence also in the glomerular filtrate.

### THE METABOLIC RESPONSE TO INJURY

When a patient is injured, using injury in the widest sense and including bacterial infection and surgical operation, the two hormones acting on the renal tubules are excreted in excess. This is a physiological protective mechanism. The result is:

1. Water is conserved in the body. It is an everyday observation that in the first 24 to 48 hours postoperatively there is oliguria.
2. Sodium ($Na^+$) and chloride ($Cl^-$) are conserved in the body and not excreted in the urine.
3. Potassium ($K^+$) is lost in the urine. Potassium increases in the blood from breakdown of cells, which is just what occurs in trauma.

The kidney allows potassium ($K^+$) to pass more freely, since potassium in excess is lethal, but gross lack, too, can be serious.

Once the blood volume has been restored, that is, once circulatory failure has been adequately treated, further fluid in the 24 hours postoperatively is unnecessary and may be harmful.

ESTIMATION OF ELECTROLYTES

Electrolyte estimations are determined by the laboratory on specimens of plasma from blood which has been collected in tubes containing lithium heparin. Care must be taken not to haemolyse the specimen by using a wet syringe, spirit, shaking the blood or squirting it through a fine needle. If the red cells rupture (haemolysis) they liberate enormous amounts of potassium into the plasma and render this determination completely valueless.

## PATHOLOGICAL STATES

Depletions of fluid and electrolytes rarely occur in 'pure' forms. Sodium and water depletions except in conditions like miner's cramp (where water has been taken without salt) usually occur together.

SODIUM

*Depletion* occurs in:
1. Vomiting.
2. Gastric aspiration.
3. Intestinal obstruction.
4. Addison's disease.

The clinical features are those of 'dehydration', namely a dry tongue, dry wrinkled skin, sunken eyes, and a rapid, thin pulse.

It is corrected by adequate quantities of isotonic saline.

*Retention* is due to deficiency in the mechanism of elimination and is common in oedematous conditions. In addition, drugs such as cortisone, testosterone and stilboestrol tend to cause retention. The treatment is restriction of fluid intake and the use of diuretics.

POTASSIUM

*Depletion* occurs in any illness in which there has been prolonged discharge like a fistula, paralytic ileus, or severe diarrhoea.

THE CLINICAL PICTURE is one of apathy, drowsiness, loss of muscle power. The pulse is slow and full. The electrocardiogram shows characteristic changes.

THE TREATMENT is the administration of potassium salts.

They must always be given with caution and, if by the intravenous route, very slowly. There must be an adequate urinary output (at least 500 ml) before they are given at all.

*Excess* is particularly dangerous and is usually due to failure of elimination by the kidney. It occurs in conditions of:

Uraemia
Acidosis

THE TREATMENT is that of anuria (p. 450).

**Fluid requirements.** The amount of fluid the patient requires is:

| | |
|---|---|
| Extrarenal loss | 1000 ml |
| *Add* urinary loss | |
| *Add* pathological loss: | |
|    1. Aspiration | |
|    2. Fistula | |
|    3. Drainage | |
|    4. Diarrhoea | |
| | ———— |
| Total fluid required in 24 hours | |
| | ———— |

Fluid balance charts may be quite simple and all fluid must be measured in millilitres and totalled every 24 hours. The precise type of fluid to be given is determined by the clinical condition and nature of the fluid lost. The state of the blood chemistry is only a rough guide in treatment and by no means helpful as a constant check. The more important normal levels are:

| Serum | mmol/l | mEq/l |
|---|---|---|
| $Na^+$ | 136–144 | 136–144 |
| $K^+$ | 3.4–4.5 | 3.5–4.5 |
| $Cl^-$ | 95–105 | 95–105 |

**Solutions.** The more important solutions used in maintaining or correcting fluid and electrolyte balance are:

1. *Sodium chloride* (0.9 per cent)—Isotonic saline.
   Replaces $Na^+$ and $Cl^-$.
   150 mmol $Na^+$ and 150 mmol $Cl^-$ in a litre.
2. *Glucose* (5 per cent)—Isotonic.
   Replaces water.
3. *Hypertonic saline* (1.85 per cent).
   Replaces $Na^+$ and $Cl^-$ without water.
   Hypertonic saline (1.8 per cent) contains
   $\left.\begin{array}{l} 154 \text{ mEq } Na^+ \text{ of sodium and} \\ 154 \text{ mEq } Cl^- \end{array}\right\}$ in 500 ml.

4. *Potassium*—5 ml 10 per cent pot.chloride w/v (13 mEq)
   Added to 500 ml glucose (5 per cent).
   Replaces K⁺.

5. *Hartman's solution.*—Na⁺ 131 mEq, Cl⁻ 111 mEq, K⁺
   5 mEq and calcium lactate.
   
   Replaces Na⁺, K⁺, Cl⁻, and corrects acidosis. It should
   be given slowly and not at all unless there is a
   satisfactory renal output.

CHAPTER 17

# Fluid Administration

The administration of fluids is amongst the most arduous tasks the nurse can undertake. The safest and simplest route of all is by drinking. This requires:

A co-operative conscious patient
A normal alimentary tract
Adequate renal function.

In these circumstances no real problem arises although occasionally gentle persuasion is required. Fluids are consumed by drinking, absorbed in the lower small intestine and proximal colon, and normal excretion occurs from the kidney.

There are two main routes by which fluids may be given:

1. Enteral (by the gut). This includes:

    (a) Drinking.
    (b) By nasogastric tube; the lower end of the tube is in the body of the stomach.
    (c) By gastrostomy or jejunostomy.
    (d) Rectal administration.

2. Parenteral (by the side of the gut—which means that the fluid does not traverse the intestinal mucous membrane to reach the circulation). This includes the following methods of administration:

    (a) Subcutaneously.
    (b) Intravenously.
    (c) Intra-arterially.
    (d) Intramedullary.

## ENTERAL ADMINISTRATION

DRINKING
Provided the patient is conscious the nurse can do much to increase the intake if this is desirable, but she must never attempt to pour fluid into the mouth of a patient whose cough reflex is absent. It will flow into the lungs with disastrous effects.

NASOGASTRIC TUBE
May be used for a patient who has difficulty in co-opera-

153

ting but one must be sure that the stomach is emptying satisfactorily, otherwise dilatation may be induced or aggravated.

## GASTROSTOMY AND JEJUNOSTOMY

Gastrostomy is performed in the management of infants
with oesophageal atresia. A temporary jejunostomy is a little
commoner. The advantage is that a wider variety of nourishment may be given than is possible by parenteral routes.

The jejunum will absorb large quantities of fluid which have
been withdrawn by gastric or duodenal suction, but the extra
volume of fluid which can be given should be limited to 1500
ml in 24 hours. The best method of feeding is by a continuous intrajejunal drip. Aspirated fluid should be filtered
before being replaced and additional fluid which is given
should be rich in carbohydrate, contain fat emulsion of small
particle size, and ordinary salt is best avoided. Considerable
trial and error has to be undertaken with the exact mixture of
the food if severe diarrhoea, which is one of the great troubles
of this type of feeding, is to be avoided.

### RECTAL FLUIDS

Rectal fluids which may be administered as a single injection of 400 ml or repeated injections of 200 ml four-hourly
have been largely abandoned. They may be of value in exceptional conditions where medical assistance is not available.

## PARENTERAL ROUTES

The intravenous route is the usual one for parenteral administration. The intramedullary or subcutaneous ones are used
only very occasionally while intra-arterial methods demand
the continued presence of the doctor for the short time they
are used. Their use is quite exceptional.

Blood, plasma, plasma substitute, saline, or glucose saline
are administered by an intravenous cannula.

The type and amount of fluid required is discussed in detail
in Chapter 16. This is a complex and comparatively advanced
study but in this section discussion is confined to the care
necessary during administration and the complications which
may arise. It should be read in conjunction with the section on
blood transfusion (p. 116).

The infusion is usually given into a vein in the forearm or
hand by using the standard blood transfusion gravity set. If intravenous therapy is to be prolonged, or highly irritant solutions have to be used, a PVC catheter is passed into one of the
vena cavae. This may necessitate open infusion and the preparation described on page 119 is necessary but more often percutaneous puncture is used.

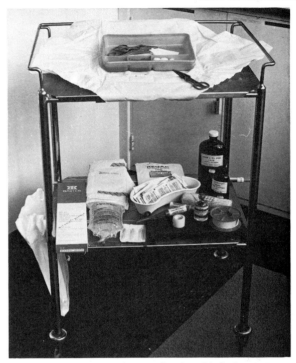

FIG. 17.1   Equipment for closed infusion.
*Upper shelf:*
Basic pack
*Lower shelf:*
Intravenous-giving set
   I.v. fluids
   Cannula
   Local anaesthetic
   Sellotape and strapping
   Antiseptic lotion
   Kidney dish containing disposable syringes
   Disposable needles
   Splint
   Bandage
Disposable bag on side of trolley.

The veins of choice are those near the hand and this has the following advantages:

(a) The patient's joints, particularly the elbow, are not immobilised.
(b) The more proximal veins are intact should further infusion be necessary.

All flasks for use should be sealed and labelled with the nature and strength of the solution. If full volume is not present, then a crack must be suspected and this, as well as debris or so-

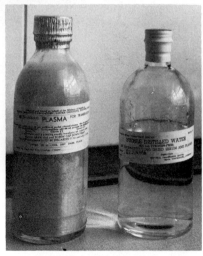

FIG. 17.2    Distilled sterile water is added to the dried plasma for use.

lid matter in the flask, is an indication to abandon it. Modern practice tends to rely more on fluids supplied in flexible plastic containers. The batch and the container number should be noted in the case sheet.

Plasma, unlike whole blood, requires no grouping or cross-matching. The danger of plasma, however, is that hepatitis due to a virus may be transmitted to the patient (p. 385).

To overcome the disadvantage of the danger of hepatitis from plasma, many plasma substitutes have been developed. They include:

(a) Dextran, a polysaccharide of high molecular weight.
(b) Rheomacrodex, which has the property of preventing 'sludging' of red cells and increases blood flow through the capillaries. It is a dextran of medium molecular weight.

Dextran maintains blood pressure if blood is not available, and the number of patients surviving when it is given instead of plasma closely approximates. The amount should be limited to three bags or bottles (540 ml each). Because of its anti-coagulant effect, it is liable to cause some aggregation of the red corpuscles and 10 ml of blood should be withdrawn and kept from every patient about to receive dextran. This enables blood grouping and cross-matching to be carried out with the usual technical ease should blood transfusion be called for in the next few days.

If the cause of circulatory failure is blood loss, blood has to be administered instead of plasma.

## Intravenous infusion

*Equipment required:*

I.v.-giving set
Mediswabs
Selection of i.v. needles and cannulae
Syringe and needles
Sterile towels
Gauze swabs
Adhesive tape, Elastoplast
Appropriate fluid, e.g. normal saline
Splint
Crêpe bandage
Receiver
Fluid balance chart
Local anaesthetic, syringe and needles
Drip stand
Tourniquet
Sphygmomanometer

The patient is informed of the procedure and his co-operation obtained. Privacy is ensured. He is given an opportunity to empty his bladder. The site is shaved if necessary.

The apparatus is taken to the bedside, preferably on a trolley. The site is exposed, usually the arm the patient uses least frequently. The arm is removed from the pyjama/gown sleeve. The patient is made comfortable and kept warm.

The doctor or nurse primes the giving set, fluid being caught in the receiver. He applies the tourniquet, perhaps using the sphygmomanometer for this purpose. Using the aseptic technique, he introduces the needle and cannula into the vein. He attaches the giving set to the cannula and ensures the fluid is flowing. The cannula is secured in position by adhesive tape. The limb may be lightly bandaged to a splint, taking care not to obstruct the flow.

The patient is made comfortable and the used equipment cleared away. The doctor prescribes the fluid to be given and the rate of flow. Whilst the infusion is in progress the nurse observes the rate of flow, the presence of fluid in the drip chamber/airlock, the amount of fluid remaining in the container, the giving set, the position and coverings of the cannula, the patient's arm and his general condition.

When the container is changed, two nurses check the fluid to be given. The guidelines on administration of parenteral infusion fluids are as follows:

THE RATE OF INFUSION. This is determined by the doctor. The amount is determined by the size of the drops and the nurse should read the graduation of drops per millilitre on the

package supplied with the set. In many sets 15 drops make
1 ml. Therefore a rate of 30 drops per minute will infuse
just under 3 litres in 24 hours.

### Complications

*Thrombophlebitis.* All solutions are mildly irritant to the wall
of the vein. Its incidence is diminished by:

(i) Atraumatic vein puncture.
(ii) Maintaining asepsis.
(iii) Limiting the time any one vein is used, ideally not more
than eight hours but in practice usually 24–48 hours.
(iv) Giving specially irritant solutions by caval catheter.
(v) Changing the giving set regularly.

*Extravasation* of fluid into the tissue is due to the point of the
cannula slipping out of the vein. The drip usually stops and
some swelling of the tissues occurs. The cannula is removed
and the puncture wound dressed. There is, however, one solution with which it must not be allowed to occur, namely noradrenaline. If this is being administered the nurse must not
leave the patient *for a single moment.* Extravasation causes necrosis of the tissues. Some antibiotic solutions such as the tetracyclines and cytotoxic agents may produce a similar effect.

As soon as possible fluids are taken by mouth, which is the
natural and best route of all. If the patient is co-operative he
takes just the right quantity. The dangers of the artificial
routes are:

(a) Excess of fluid may be given, resulting in pulmonary
oedema.
(b) Too little fluid is taken, causing water depletion.
(c) The wrong type of fluid may be given.
(d) Infection may be introduced or thrombosis may occur in
the vein.

*Contamination of intravenous fluid* was extensively investigated
by the Clothier Committee, and the fundamental cause of disease was found to be human failing ranging from simple care-
lessness to poor management of men and plant. In particular:

1. A bottle or bag which looks suspicious should not be
accepted.
2. Defaced labels, loose collars, weeping from the bung, and
turbidity or opalescence in the fluid render the contents
suspect.

The Control of Infection Officer should be informed and
stocks in the pharmacy should be immobilised pending
investigation if any of the above defects are discovered in a
single container.

UNIT OF MEASUREMENT OF FLUID. This is expressed in the metric system. A one-thousandth part of a litre is a millilitre (ml).

## THE MAINTENANCE OF NUTRITION

The maintenance of a good nutritional state presents a problem in patients who are unable to take ordinary diets by mouth. For short periods in patients who start off fit the problem is not important, as long as fluid and electrolyte balance is attended to, but the longer the inability to eat continues the more important it becomes. Amongst the sort of cases which we must consider are long-term respirator cases, head injuries, postoperative laryngopharyngeal operations, poisonings, and major abdominal surgery with prolonged ileus or other complications.

It must also be remembered that while the normal adult human requires 2500–3000 calories per day, the response to the stress of surgery on certain diseases and burns produces a hypercatabolic state which requires up to 8000 calories per day.

Two methods of feeding other than by mouth are available.

1. *Intravenous*

Until recently the only method of intravenous feeding was by the use of 5 per cent dextrose solution. In order to give enough calories excessive quantities of fluid are required and hence this was not entirely satisfactory. Emulsion of fats and solutions containing protein hydrolysates have been developed for intravenous use. These are much more satisfactory.

More recently fluids have been developed which are capable of providing a 3500 calorie diet within a fluid output of 2·5 to 3 l per day. The various solutions used include:

Aminosol 10 per cent (casein hydrolysate)
Aminosol/glucose
Aminosol/fructose/ethanol
Intralipid. Fat emulsion which is derived from soya beans for intravenous use (10 and 20 per cent).

It is important when patients are maintained on these solutions for long periods that vitamins and potassium (6 g/day) are added to the intravenous diet.

Finally the use of blood plasma as a means of restoring plasma proteins should not be forgotten. It may be used in above normal concentrations for this purpose.

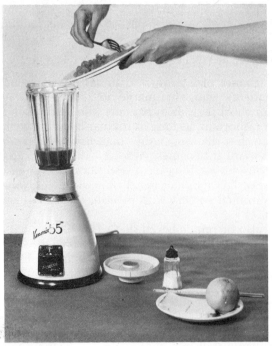

FIG. 17.3   The whole meal is put into a liquidiser. (Dr J. C. Richardson's method.)

2. *By gastric tube*

While the recent innovations in intravenous feeding have produced satisfactory methods they still involve intravenous infusions which have many hazards (upsets of fluid balance—infection—thrombosis of vessels). Therefore intragastric feeding has become popular for any patient who is unable to take oral food, but who has an intact and functioning gut. In this form of feeding a tube is passed via the oesophagus into the stomach and 60 ml of water are put down it hourly until it is established that the stomach is emptying normally. Then fluid diet is passed into the stomach at appropriate intervals—usually two, three or four hourly.

Diets may be made up of eggs, milk, protein, hydrolysates and sugar, but unless great care is taken these tend to cause intractable diarrhoea.

A satisfactory method is to take the ordinary ward meals, complete with bread, butter and fish and chips not forgetting the salt and the sugar in the tea, and put it all into a liquidiser (Fig. 17.3) together with an appropriate amount of water. The resultant thin gruel is then passed down the intragastric tube using a funnel. Three main feeds a day (or more if required) may be given. Volumes of 300 ml per feed are acceptable to most patients. Additional in between feeds of fluids will bring the total fluid intake up to $2\frac{1}{2}$ to 3 litres. Following severe trauma this method may fail to supply the very high calorie requirements of such patients. If this is so, intravenous feeding will have to be resorted to.

## CHAPTER 18

# Respiratory Failure

Respiration is the process whereby the tissues are provided with oxygen $(O_2)$ and carbon dioxide $(CO_2)$ is eliminated. There are certain basic requirements:

1. A MECHANICALLY EFFICIENT bellows consisting of the ribs, and the muscles of respiration (i.e. the intercostals and diaphragm) with an airtight chest wall and a clear passage to the outside air through the trachea, mouth and nose.

2. ENOUGH SOUND LUNG to oxygenate the blood which passes through it and at the same time to eliminate all the carbon dioxide $(CO_2)$ from the blood.

3. AN ADEQUATE CIRCULATION OF BLOOD through the lungs and the rest of the body to carry the gases.

4. THE CENTRAL MECHANISM IN THE BRAIN which controls respiratory efforts must be working and the nervous pathways from this to the muscles it controls must be intact. This centre initiates rhythmic impulses which drive the muscles of respiration and is situated in the medulla oblongata. It is sensitive to chemical changes in the blood (e.g. excess of carbon dioxide and lack of oxygen) and adjusts the rate and depth of respiration to maintain normal blood levels of those substances.

### RESPIRATORY FAILURE

Respiratory failure may occur if any or all of these mechanisms are destroyed or deranged to a sufficient extent to prevent them carrying out their function.

**Defects of the bellows mechanism.** The bellows mechanism may be put out of action. Causes of this are:

1. Extensive fractures of the bony thoracic cage.

2. Tears in the chest wall, allowing the pleural cavity to communicate with the atmosphere and hence preventing the normal lowering of intrathoracic pressure associated with inspiration which sucks air into the lungs.

3. Paralysis of the muscles of respiration may occur due to overdosage with muscle relaxant drugs (often used in anaesthesia), poisoning with organic phosphorus insecticides, or in myasthenia gravis.

162

4. Obstruction of the airway may prevent the bellows from sucking in air. This is often due to foreign bodies, sputum, secretions or trauma to the air passages or face.

**Inadequacy of lung tissue.** An inadequacy of lung tissue is due either to disease, chronic bronchitis and emphysema, pneumonia, tuberculosis, carcinoma of the bronchus, pneumoconiosis, etc., or to destruction of lung tissue by surgery, irritant gases or chemicals. An example of the latter is the destruction of lung tissue caused by poisonous gases such as chlorine.

**Inadequate circulation of blood.** Inadequate circulation of blood may occur from heart failure or sometimes due to vascular accidents such as emboli or thrombosis within the lungs themselves.

**Central failure.** The central mechanism may fail from a number of causes—trauma to the skull, narcotics or toxins. The nervous pathways from the centre to the muscles may be interrupted either by injury as in cervical fractures or by disease such as poliomyelitis.

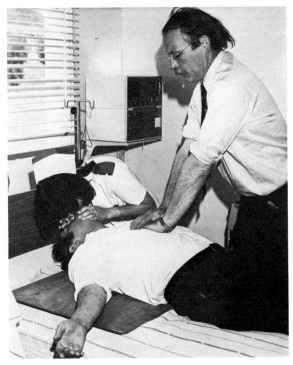

FIG. 18.1   Mouth to mouth respiration combined with manual compression.

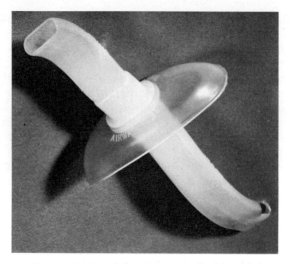

FIG. 18.2   Brooke's airway. A double-ended
airway to facilitate mouth to mouth respiration.

## TREATMENT

The principles underlying the treatment of all forms of respiratory failure are the same. The cardinal rule is to ensure that
the lungs are ventilated efficiently by whatever means are
available.

First in order to ventilate the lungs a clear airway via the
mouth or nose and trachea to the lungs must be ensured.
Therefore foreign bodies, secretions, etc. are removed and
the tongue and jaw must be held forward in the unconscious
patient. Artificial respiration is commenced. The most
efficient and only really satisfactory method of doing this as a
first aid measure is by mouth to mouth or mouth to nose respiration. By this method the patient's lungs are inflated by
the nurse blowing through his mouth or nostrils—then they
are allowed to deflate again by their own elasticity.

*Mouth to mouth or mouth to nose breathing*

Firstly the air passages must be cleared of any obstruction.
The occiput should rest on a surface in the same plane as the
patient's shoulders and buttocks and the patient's neck is extended from the normal lying position so that the tongue does
not fall back and close the glottis. A special airway (Brooke's),
or, alternatively, a handkerchief to fit over the lips can be used
if contact with the patient's mouth is undesirable.

Many favour mouth to nose instead of mouth to mouth, but
for the less expert it is probably easier to nip the nose than to

keep the patient's mouth closed. If a 'bag mask' type of inflating unit is available it can be used only if the operator is quite sure that she has the necessary skill.

As soon as possible this method of maintaining gaseous exchange ought to be replaced by some sort of formal artificial ventilation of the lungs.

### Artificial ventilation

This may be accomplished by passing an endotracheal tube into the trachea and inflating the lungs with air or oxygen either manually, using a rubber bag, or, better, by one of the many machines available.

All mechanical lung ventilators work by intermittently blowing respirable gases into the patient's lungs. The lungs deflate by virtue of their own elasticity. Such a machine is the Manley ventilator which is driven by compressed gas. Other varieties are powered by electric motors.

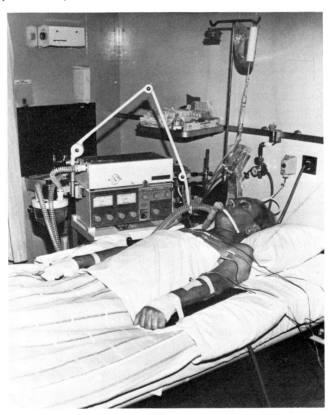

FIG. 18.3    Respiratory failure treated with Elema-Servo ventilation.

The more sophisticated machines not only blow air or oxygen into the lungs but may also suck it out actively. Some of these more advanced machines, such as the Elema-Servo ventilator, have what is known as a patient-triggering device which enables them to assist the inadequate efforts of a partially paralysed patient without his attempts to breathe conflicting with the work of the machine.

All mechanical ventilators must be equipped with efficient humidifiers so that the inspired gas is saturated with water vapour. These may be devices rather like an electric kettle in which the gas is passed over hot water or may be nebulisers, either mechanical or ultrasonic. The newer and better type such as the Bennett cascade may also be heated. The Radcliffe humidifier is an example of the first type (Fig. 18.3). If the inspired gases are not rendered wet the patient's tracheal and pulmonary secretions dry up and are difficult to remove and may even crust on the tracheal mucosa.

It is essential that all equipment used in mechanical ventilation should be sterile before use. Accessories such as endotrachealtracheostomy tubes are sterilised by steam or radiation. (Ethylene oxide should not be used as it may become trapped between the layers of rubber—only to be liberated later when the tube is in use.)

The ventilator itself should have its working parts sterilised by ultrasonically nebulised alcohol (70 per cent solution), ethylene oxide gas or Resiguard, or should be autoclaved.

Ventilators should be fitted with bacterial filters on both their inspiratory and expiratory tubes. These should be autoclaved frequently and always before the machine is used on a new patient. It is important to ensure that these filters do not become waterlogged during use as this may give rise to respiratory obstruction. Waterlogging may be avoided by siliconising the filter or by heating it.

If the use of a mechanical ventilator is expected to last for more than 48 hours it is often considered desirable to carry out a tracheostomy and inflate the patient's lungs via this route.

The reasons are:

1. Prolonged presence of an endotracheal tube in the larynx may cause sloughing with subsequent stenosis.

2. It enables the attendant to remove secretions from the bronchial tree with great ease. This is accomplished with the aid of a suction machine and catheter (Fig. 18.8).

3. The shortening of the air passages which accompanies tracheostomy lowers their resistance to respiration and helps the elimination of carbon dioxide ($CO_2$).

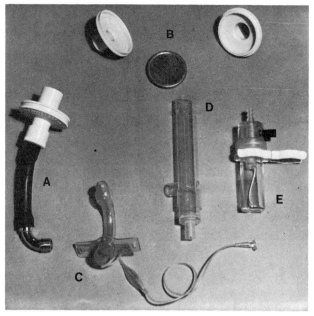

FIG. 18.4 Tracheostomy accessories. A, Catheter mount with a Swedish nose. B, Swedish nose exploded. C, Curved plastic tracheostomy tube. D, A T-piece. E, Nebuliser.

4. The patient may in fact find a tracheostomy less distressing.

It is important that the nurse should understand the care of a tracheostomy (p. 168). The tube which will be used for this type of patient is of plastic and has an inflatable cuff which prevents leakage of air from the trachea. The mechanical ventilator is attached to a swivel connection at the end of this tube. Whenever secretions accumulate in the tube or air passages they should be removed at once. The attendant should scrub her hands and put on clean plastic gloves. She should wear a mask. A sterile towel is spread round the tracheostomy opening and an assistant disconnects the ventilator or preferably removes the bung from the connection. A sterile catheter (Toronto type) should be moistened with sterile saline and then passed into the trachea. The catheter is now connected to effect suction and the catheter should be moved about continuously with a rotating motion as it is withdrawn. The more the patient coughs the better, as this tends to bring secretion up from the depths of the lungs. The catheter should be discarded and a fresh sterile one used for the next bronchial toilet. After a suction session it is desirable to inflate the patient's lungs using a rubber bag as an inflating device.

This avoids leaving collapsed segments of lung. If possible, suction sessions should be attended by a physiotherapist who will help in the production of an artificial cough.

It is impossible to overemphasise the importance of two factors in the care of a tracheostomy.

Firstly, every effort should be made to avoid introducing infection into the bronchial tree during the repeated bronchial toilets which must be carried out and, secondly, at all costs the inspired gases must be prevented from drying out the tracheal and pulmonary secretions.

Because the nose, which normally moistens the inspired air, has been bypassed patients breathing through a tracheostomy tube tend to get tenacious and viscous sputum which is hard to remove. This evil can be mitigated by humidifying all gas used in machines. Some rely on heat to saturate the gas with water vapour while others introduce an extremely finely divided spray of water into the gaseous stream. The Radcliffe humidifier is a good example of the first type. A more modern one is the Bennett cascade.

It is important to remember that whilst artificial ventilation by a machine will keep the patient alive almost indefinitely, machine failure which goes unobserved will kill him within minutes. Therefore machines should never be left unattended and manual means of inflation should always be immediately available for use in emergency.

Whilst mechanical ventilation is in progress the cause of the respiratory failure should be treated if this is possible. Infection is treated with antibiotics or the pressure on nerves caused by fractures is relieved.

Where a mechanical ventilator is in use the patient requires feeding. Some are able to take ordinary light diets, others need intragastric feeds. If they are lying very still in bed they ought to be gently rolled from one side to the other every two hours to prevent hypostatic pneumonia of the dependent parts of the lungs. Care of the pressure areas is important.

*Tracheostomy*

Tracheostomy, or an artificial opening in the trachea, is necessary to relieve sudden laryngeal obstruction. In the very young nasotracheal intubation with a plastic Jackson-Rees tube is used rather than tracheostomy.

INDICATIONS FOR TRACHEOSTOMY
**Obstructive conditions of the larynx**
1. Acute oedema of the glottis. This may occur as a result of Ludwig's angina, carcinoma of the tongue, or as a result of a radium reaction inside the mouth.

2. Carcinoma of the larynx.

3. Foreign bodies impacted in the larynx.

4. Trauma.

5. Burns of the mouth or larynx.

6. Acute laryngitis particularly diphtheria; the diphtheritic membrane may block the airway completely.

**Paralysis or spasm of the respiratory muscles and respiratory failure**

1. Bulbar paralysis including poliomyelitis.

2. Tetanus and certain stages of coma, including some head injuries (p. 513).

**Some types of inability to maintain satisfactory blood gas levels during prolonged artificial ventilation.** Such as respiratory failure due to lung damage—chronic bronchitis.

Haemorrhage into a cystadenoma of the thyroid gland is not an indication for tracheostomy but for laryngeal intubation.

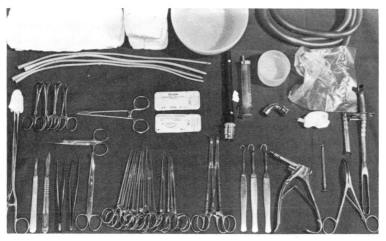

FIG. 18.5   Preparation for tracheostomy.

| | |
|---|---|
| Swabs and holder | 1 Nosworthy connection |
| Scalpels | 1 Catheter mount |
| 1 Toothed dissection forceps | Tape |
| 1 Non-toothed dissection forceps | Catgut, mersilk and needles |
| 8 Straight artery forceps | 1 Needle holder |
| 2 Curved artery forceps | 1 Stitch scissors |
| 2 Sawtellis forceps | 4 Towel clips |
| 1 Single hook | Assorted catheters |
| 2 Double hooks | Swabs |
| 1 Tracheal punch | Bowl saline |
| 1 Tracheal dilator | Pressure tubing |
| Selection of tracheostomy tubes | Syringe |

### THE TIME FOR OPERATION

The nurse must be familiar with the conditions in which a tracheostomy may be indicated, and once the possibility has arisen the instruments must be at hand and ready sterilised.

In a case of progressive respiratory obstruction a tracheostomy is usually indicated when the accessory muscles of respiration commence to contract, namely, the alae nasi and the sternomastoid. Recession of the epigastrium is also present. The patient is usually cyanosed, and the accompanying mental stress is very considerable.

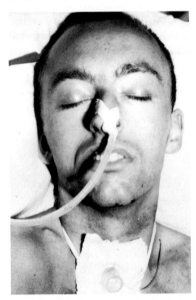

FIG. 18.6    Tracheostomy. General view.

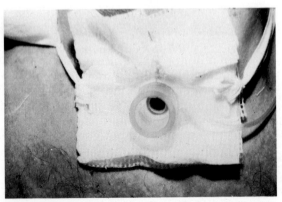

FIG. 18.7    More detailed view of tube in position in the same patient.

Artificial respiration will *not* be of the slightest use should the patient collapse, because he has not a free airway, and collapse due to respiratory obstruction is an indication for lightning speed in effecting an artificial opening.

## THE OPERATION

The instruments are shown in Fig. 18.5 but if the patient is collapsed and no instruments are at hand a penknife has, on occasion, been successfully used, and the nurse must bear in mind that of all instruments necessary in this grave emergency a knife is the most important. The patient's head must be kept well extended over a pillow or sandbag.

After the opening has been made in the trachea a tracheostomy tube, to which two tapes are attached, is inserted. The tapes must be tied immediately at the side of the patient's neck in a knot and bow. If they are tied at the back of the patient's neck they are uncomfortable to lie on, inaccessible and may be untied by mistake if the gown is also fastened by tapes. If a ventilator is to be used a cuffed plastic tube is essential.

## POSTOPERATIVE TREATMENT

The patient is exhausted and dozes off to sleep. He should be laid flat in bed, rolled from side to side hourly to promote drainage and exudate should be sucked from the tracheostomy tube. When he awakens he should be propped up and kept in this position for 48 hours. Metal tubes will require frequent removal and cleansing in a solution of sodium bicarbonate to ensure that they are clear. They should be shaken before reinsertion.

Deep breathing exercises are carried out under the direction of a physiotherapist. A suction machine must be available to enable the nurse to clear secretions from the airway, together with a supply of sterile Toronto catheters. Personnel should be trained in the methods used to avoid introducing infection into the trachea. Humidified oxygen may be administered via a tracheostomy mask or a T-piece such as the one shown in Fig. 18.4. A pair of tracheal dilators must be always at hand in case the tube is coughed or pulled out, and a pair of scissors to cut the tapes in case the outer tube becomes blocked. A spare correctly fitting tube should be available. Gentle handling is essential as the posterior wall of the trachea is very thin and easily eroded.

All these measures are designed to prevent pneumonia, which is a very likely complication.

Swallowing may be difficult but small amounts of fluid can usually be taken. If the patient is very thirsty fluids may be given parenterally.

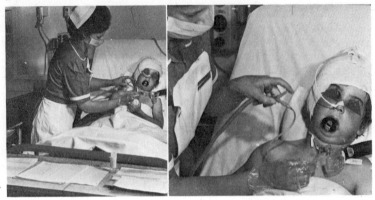

FIG. 18.8 Aftercare of tracheostomy. A, General background of intensive care. B, Suction through the tracheostomy.

If the case is one of carcinoma of the larynx a tracheostomy will be permanent, but in other cases the tube is removed when the cause of the obstruction has subsided. In children, removal of the tube may be followed by considerable fright because the voice is absent *unless the wound is completely covered.*

RULES FOR TRACHEOSTOMY MANAGEMENT
The following rules are essential:

1. Scrub the hands and wear a mask.
2. Use prepacked sterile disposable catheters.
3. Do not allow the catheter to touch *anything* before aspirating the trachea.
4. Discard the catheter after aspiration.
5. Replace the inner tube as required. A supply of autoclaved inner tubes should be available.
6. Clean the tracheostomy wound and renew dressing.
7. Keep the tracheostomy tube covered loosely with gauze.
8. Micro-organisms live everywhere and may kill if introduced into the bronchi. *Escherichia coli, Klebsiella bacilli* and *Pseudomonas* are the most common.
9. Always inflate the lungs after a suction session.

CARE OF A PATIENT WITH A TRACHEOSTOMY
The following articles should be kept at the bedside:

Tracheal dilator
Selection of sterile catheters, e.g. Toronto
Disposable gloves
Suction machine with half an inch of Savlon 0·5 per cent in the suction bottle

Bowl of Savlon 0·5 per cent

Brown wax bag

Small gallipot containing small amount of sterile normal saline to act as a lubricant. This sterile normal saline is removed from the container using a sterile syringe and needle.

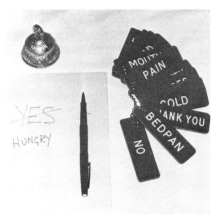

FIG. 18.9    On a table within reach of the patient should be a bell, a pencil, writing pad and communication cards.

The tracheostomy tube is held in position by tapes, which are tied at the side of the patient's neck.

The tube is sucked out whenever necessary, but at least at two-hourly intervals.

Disposable gloves are put on. The packet containing the catheter is cut at the wide end of the catheter, which is connected to the pressure tubing of the suction machine. The wrapper is removed.

The catheter is nipped in order to prevent suction, and dipped into the normal saline in order to lubricate it.

The tracheostomy tube is steadied and the catheter inserted not more than 4 inches. It is released to allow suction, turned, and slowly withdrawn while turning. Should it be necessary, the catheter can be reinserted once only.

When a Y-shaped connection is used, the side-arm can be opened or covered to prevent or allow suction.

After withdrawal the catheter is washed through with Savlon 0·5 per cent. It is disconnected and discarded into the brown wax bag. The pressure tubing is fixed to the handle of the suction machine using a bulldog clip. The gloves are removed and discarded into the brown wax bag.

CARE OF THE TUBE

A cuffed tube requires attention at intervals, e.g. 2-hourly or as otherwise instructed. The pharynx is sucked out especially if the patient is not swallowing. The tracheostomy tube is sucked out using another catheter. The cuff is released for 2 minutes and then reinflated.

The inner tube of a metal tube is removed, e.g. 2-hourly, and the outer tube sucked out. The inner tube is washed in sodium bicarbonate, and is sterilised in special Savlon or by boiling and reinserted.

*The wound* is cleaned as required, e.g. 4-hourly, using Savlon 0·5 per cent and the aseptic technique. A gauze swab may be placed under the tube if necessary.

*Emergency.* If the tube becomes dislodged and the patient is having difficulty in breathing, the tapes holding the tube are cut, the tracheal dilator inserted and held open to allow entry of air. Assistance is called for. The tracheostomy may require to be sucked out.


## OXYGEN THERAPY

Air contains about 20 per cent of oxygen. This is adequate to saturate the haemoglobin of the blood in a patient whose respiratory and circulatory systems are normal. In many surgical conditions the respiratory and cardiovascular systems have suffered from severe interference. The result is that the circulating haemoglobin is reduced in amount or is inadequately saturated with oxygen. For this reason the percentage of oxygen in the inspired air has to be increased.

The indication for use is hypoxia (deficient oxygen in the blood from any cause). The distress of respiratory failure is often really due to $CO_2$ retention, not to lack of oxygen.

### CAUSES OF HYPOXIA

1. **Respiratory obstruction.** This includes all conditions in which the normal exchange of gases in the lungs is impeded:

    (a) Laryngeal obstruction.
    (b) Laryngeal spasm.
    (c) Pneumonia.
    (d) Collapse of the lungs.
    (e) Pneumothorax.

2. **Acute circulatory failure and heart failure.** Stagnant anoxia.

3. **Diminished oxygen-carrying capacity.** Anaemia due to haemorrhage being the most important surgically.

4. **Increased oxygen consumption,** such as continuous hyperpyrexia—thyrotoxic crisis (p. 282) is surgically important.

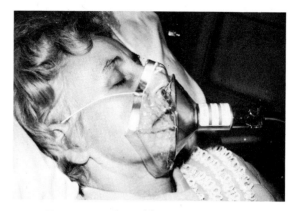

Fig. 18.10    Disposable oxygen Ventimask.

It is important to stress that the decreased respiratory movements which occur postoperatively may be due to:

(a) The effects of the anaesthetic not having worn off.
(b) Bandages being too tight and impeding respiratory movement. The patient whose chest is 'crushed' should nevertheless be tightly bandaged in order to stabilise the thoracic cage.
(c) Pain.

These may be indications for assisted respiration or analgesics rather than a supply of oxygen.

Oxygen is supplied in cylinders at a pressure of 2000 lb/per in² or possibly by a pipeline from a central depot. A reducing valve brings this pressure down to 5 lb per in² and a flowmeter is attached which measures the quantity of oxygen delivered in litres per minute.

Oxygen may be administered by:

1. A FACE PIECE—(a) the ordinary mask of an anaesthetic machine, (b) the polythene mask.
2. NASAL INHALATION—(a) nasal mask such as a Polymask, (b) nasal tube, Argyle's spectacles or a nasal catheter.
3. OXYGEN TENT—The oxygen tent has been largely abandoned. It is hot, septic and the concentration of oxygen is frequently inadequate.
4. INCUBATOR for newborn hypoxic cases.

*Method of administration*

Pure oxygen is administered until the patient shows the maximal improvement. The oxygen is then gradually reduced and the patient's condition is satisfactory only when he can inhale air alone without any deterioration. The usual rate of admin-

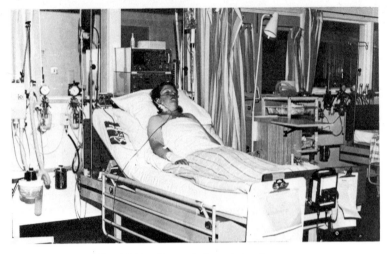

FIG. 18.11 General view—intensive care.

istration is 4 1 per minute. All oxygen should be moistened. The nose requires careful toilet if an indwelling catheter is being used and 0·1 per cent Hibitane in Xylocaine jelly is useful.

In patients such as chronic bronchitics who normally have a high blood carbon dioxide ($Pco_2$) and low blood oxygen ($Po_2$) care should be taken to limit oxygen flow to 4 litres of 24 per cent oxygen per min. to avoid total suppression of respiration or to use one of the special masks such as the Ventimask which restricts the inspired oxygen content to 24 or 28 per cent.

SPECIAL PRECAUTIONS TO BE TAKEN WITH OXYGEN THERAPY

There are no toxic changes in the fully formed tissues from up to a concentration of 70 per cent oxygen. Retrolental fibroplasia is a danger in premature infants. The most important danger is that of fire. This is increased by:

1. Greasing the valve.
2. Smoking, the use of a naked light or electric toys.
3. The use of spirit or ether for the treatment of the patient.
4. The production of static electricity—for example by too active bedmaking or nylon clothing.

Before connecting up the oxygen supply, grit should be blown out. When the oxygen cylinder is empty it should be removed and marked accordingly. If 'piped' oxygen is used the nurse must know where the cut-off valves are situated outside the room or ward in case of fire.

DETAILS OF ADMINISTRATION OF OXYGEN

The doctor ordering that oxygen shall be given to a patient, should indicate the means of administration and the rate of flow. The usual means are:

Argyle's spectacles
Ventimask
Edinburgh mask

In emergency, the nurse may give oxygen using the Argyle's spectacles with the rate of flow adjusted to 4 litres per minute.

The procedure is explained to the patient, and his co-operation obtained. The nostrils are cleaned using a wool swab held in sinus forceps and moistened in sodium bicarbonate solution. After use the swab is removed with dissecting forceps and discarded.

The nurse checks that oxygen is flowing from the piped supply. She fills the humidifier (nebuliser) with distilled water up to the level of the mark. The apparatus is connected and the flow of oxygen related to the prescribed rate. The spectacles or mask are placed in position. The patient is made comfortable. Observations are made on the effects of the oxygen on the patient's colour, breathing and general condition.

When oxygen is being administered intermittently, on the same patient, the spectacles or mask are stored in a clean paper bag attached to the locker, until next required.

The spectacles or mask and length of tubing are changed after 24 hours or more frequently as necessary. Being disposable they are discarded.

When the administration of oxygen is discontinued, the spectacles, mask and length of tubing are discarded. The humidifier is emptied, washed in Savlon 0·5 per cent, rinsed and dried, and placed back in position near the flow meter until required again.

When an oxygen cylinder is used, it is prepared and turned on outside the ward. The assembled apparatus consists of:

Cylinder with reducing valve, gauge and flow meter
Humidifier
Appropriate tubing
Appropriate means of administration.

HYPERBARIC OXYGEN THERAPY

A tiny amount of oxygen is dissolved in the blood plasma. This amount can be considerably increased if the patient is placed in a chamber and oxygen is administered at a pressure of 2 atm. This may be of value in saving a threatened limb. There is a specially devised bed which avoids the necessity

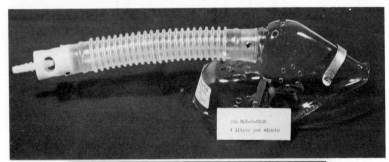

A

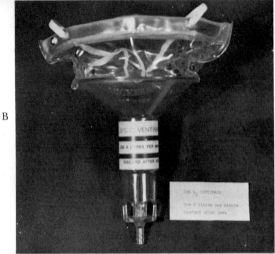

B

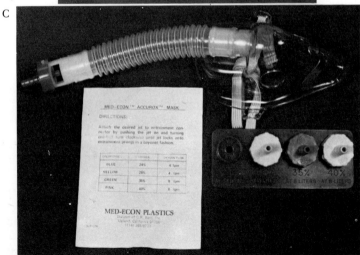

C

FIG. 18.12   Oxygen masks. A, Mix-O-Mask, 24 per cent. B, Ventimask. C, Mix-O-Mask variable.

of a pressure chamber. It has been used before megavoltage radiotherapy to increase the response of treatment. It is also used for patients in severe circulatory failure, for enhancing the chances of 'take' in extensive skin graft, combating carbon monoxide poisoning and in the treatment of gas gangrene.

## INTENSIVE CARE UNITS

An intensive care unit is one where there is the concentration of skill, equipment and staff required for the treatment or resuscitation of a seriously ill patient. The object is to maintain the highest level of medical and nursing care by day and by night. The essential features are:

### 1. STRUCTURE

Extensive floor space per patient is necessary and easy access all around the patient's bed should be provided. There should be good observation of the patient from a centrally placed panel. Exceptionally extensive electrical provisions are made for portable X-rays as well as for respirators, suction machines and monitoring apparatus. At the nurse's station are telephones and light indicators for night use, switches for the control of lighting and indicators relating to piped oxygen, suction and emergency electricity generation.

### 2. EQUIPMENT

This is necessarily on a lavish scale. The nurse cannot be expected to know how everything works but she should know what she may or may not do with it, whether it is working and what measures to take if it ceases to function. The most efficient suction machine will not function if the top of the reservoir is not fitted in an airtight manner! All the equipment necessary and already discussed in the sections on acute circulatory and respiratory failure must be available. A small laboratory near by is an essential.

Because of the ever-present danger of cross-infection, facilities for the total isolation of very clean from 'very dirty' patients are an essential feature of all modern intensive care units.

### 3. STAFF

To afford complete 24-hour coverage a three-shift system of duty is required with an average of five trained nurses and supporting nursing auxiliaries or ward orderly staff for each patient.

The types of condition for which patients are admitted vary enormously. They may be postoperative conditions, severe road accidents, coal-gas poisoning, frost-bite, myocardial infarction or cerebral thrombosis. Most will have some degree of respiratory, circulatory or metabolic disturbances. In addition to specialised procedures to counteract these conditions all patients require good basic nursing care. Careful records, attention to general and oral hygiene are as important as elsewhere in the hospital.

## CONTROL OF RESUSCITATIVE THERAPY

The control of resuscitative therapy, amongst which may be included oxygen, mechanical ventilation and the correction of acid base disturbances, is often achieved by reference to blood gas estimations. These are carried out on arterial blood taken into heparinised syringes. Specimens which cannot be examined at once should be refrigerated.

The normal values are:

pH      7·4
Standard Bicarbonate 25 mEq
$P_{CO_2}$    40 mmHg Base excess 0
$P_{O_2}$    100 mmHg

*Collection of specimens*
TAKING BLOOD FOR ESTIMATION OF BLOOD GASES
On a tray is placed:

A receiver
Heparin 5000 units per ml
Syringe 5 ml
Needle size 21 × $1\frac{1}{2}$
Wax carton of ice
Strapping
Red caps
Mediswabs
Packet of gauze swabs

A piece of strapping with the patient's name written on it is attached to the barrel of the syringe.

The doctor takes the blood from the patient's femoral artery. He removes the needle. He fixes a red cap to the nozzle of the syringe. He gently rotates the syringe. It is plunged into the wax carton of ice. It is taken immediately to the unit laboratory. The nurse maintains digital pressure on a gauze swab over the femoral artery puncture for at least 5 minutes.

# CHAPTER 19

# Burns and Scalds

Burns are caused by dry heat and scalds by moist heat. Burns are always more serious than scalds of the same extent. The clinical features and treatment are identical.

In practice it is necessary to decide whether or not the full thickness of the skin has been destroyed; if it has, skin grafting is necessary. The degree or depth of the burn is that of its deepest part. Modern classification recognises only three degrees:

Erythema (redness)
Destruction of the epidermis (superficial layer of the skin)
Burn of the full thickness of the skin

### CAUSES

1. Dry heat—flame.
2. Moist heat—scalds.
3. Chemicals.
4. Electricity.
5. X-rays and radium.
6. Friction is an occasional cause.

## CLINICAL FEATURES

The degree of general upset is proportional to the superficial extent of the damage rather than the depth of the burn.

1. Pain is usual, but is most marked in the more superficial burns because the sensory nerve endings in the skin are exposed. In deeper burns they have usually been destroyed.

2. Acute circulatory failure is always present if the burns are moderately extensive, and in more extensive burns it is profound.

*The treatment and nursing care of burns illness*

The care of the burnt area cannot be discussed in isolation from the general and metabolic changes which result from burning. These changes are complicated and not completely understood. They vary with the extent of the burns and the general physical condition of the patient. The institution of special units for the treatment of major burns has greatly improved the end results. The special features of burns illness are the prevention and treatment of:

1. Acute circulatory failure.
2. Infection.
3. Other metabolic changes.
4. The restoration of function and minimisation of deformity.

1. THE SUPERFICIAL EXTENT OF THE BURNT AREA is estimated on admission. The accompanying diagram from Wallace's 'Rules of Nine' is convenient. It is not often, of course, that the patient is burnt on the whole of the front of one arm or one leg so that another useful adjunct in the calculation is to assess an area covered by the surface of the patient's hand as 1 per cent. If the area exceeds 10 per cent in the child or 15 per cent in the adult the patient may die from circulatory collapse. Therefore burns of greater extent than this will require intravenous infusion.

2. DEPTH OF THE BURN. Superficial and partial skin thickness burns will heal if sepsis is excluded. Deeper burns will require grafting. In the occasional areas where there has been complete charring of the limb amputation may be necessary.

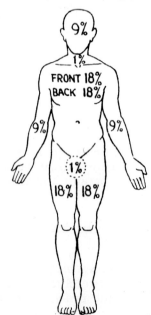

'RULES OF NINE'

SURFACE AREA AND FLUID
REPLACEMENT
I.V. FLUIDS FOR BURNS
OF 18 PER CENT OR OVER

ADULTS (18 years or over):
  1 bottle plasma  }  For each
  1 bottle saline   }  9 per cent.
CHILDREN (at 9 years):
  ½ bottle plasma  }  For each
  ½ bottle saline   }  9 per cent.

MAXIMUM NUMBER OF BOTTLES IN
48 HOURS:
  Adult, 12; child (9 years), 6.

  1 bottle = 540 ml.

FIG. 19.1  Wallace's 'Rules of Nine' for estimating fluid requirements in the first 48 hours after burns.

3. SITE. Certain additional measures may be necessary in certain sites. For example, tracheostomy will be indicated where the mouth or air passages have been severely burnt, or, occasionally for a deep burn of the neck. A dorsal slit or circumcision may have to be performed for certain burns in the genital area. Large burns of the trunk or burns involving wide areas on both aspects of the leg are particularly difficult to nurse, and a special bed for nursing the patient is of value.

4. AGE AND GENERAL CONDITION. The chances of a patient surviving severe burns will be greater in the previously fit and robust, than in the aged patient suffering from chronic illness. Epileptics form a notable percentage of patients who are accidentally burnt, because they fall on the fire during a fit.

### Management on admission

The patient should be admitted to a special resuscitation room and kept there until the danger of circulatory collapse has passed. He should be laid between sterile sheets and resuscitative measures are commenced at once by administering 500 ml of plasma (or plasma substitute) intravenously. In children an open infusion will normally be necessary and a nurse should have the necessary apparatus available. The first 500 ml may be given in a period of five minutes before any further observations have been made. Once the plasma is running the following observations are made and repeated at regular intervals:

1. The rate of the pulse.
2. Blood pressure.
3. Temperature.
4. The central venous pressure.

Blood is taken for estimation of:

(a) The haemoglobin level.
(b) State of the electrolytes.
(c) Haematocrit reading. This reading is an indication of haemo-concentration—that is to say an estimate of the amount of plasma lost and, therefore, a guide in determining loss of blood volume.

### Resuscitation

1. THE AMOUNT OF FLUID. The total amount of fluid to be given is calculated and half this quantity is given in eight hours and the remainder in 24 to 48 hours. The fluid loss each day may be as much as five litres from evaporation. If the urinary output is unsatisfactory Mannitol should be given at an early stage and if it is effective there will be a diuresis within an hour. If there is not, then its use should not be proceeded with.

2. TYPE OF FLUID. Plasma (or plasma substitute) is of the first importance. Normal saline is also given to maintain electrolyte balance and, if there has been red blood corpuscle destruction, some whole blood is usually given. Many give one half of the saline-plasma requirements as blood.

3. RATE OF INFUSION is determined by:

(a) Calculation of the total amount lost.
(b) Ensuring that urinary excretion is maintained (see below).
(c) Estimation of the central venous pressure.

4. SEDATIVES OR ANALGESICS are not always necessary, but if they are, they should be given intravenously.

5. STOPPING THE TRANSFUSION. This is never stopped before 24 hours and usually continued for 48 hours. The transfusion is continued until the blood tests show that stability has been achieved with very little fluid in the previous four hours, that is to say that the blood pressure, haematocrit and haemoglobin levels are maintained with the administration of not more than about 500 ml of fluid in this period.

*Maintenance of urinary excretion*

Special care is necessary to observe the volume of urinary secretion which may be diminished due to shock.

1. An indwelling catheter is inserted into the bladder and the amount of urine excreted hourly is measured. If it falls below 60 ml in the adult or 30 ml in the child the rate of the drip is increased.
2. If the patient is able, drinking is encouraged; if vomiting, nasogastric aspiration is necessary instead.
3. Urine is examined for the presence of normal and abnormal contents as well as for specific gravity.
4. The blood urea is estimated.

*Care of the burnt areas*

The principal object is the prevention of infection and covering the burnt area with skin as soon as possible. Superficial and partial skin thickness burns will heal if infection is excluded. Deeper burns require skin grafting. Special measures to be undertaken are:

1. BACTERIOLOGICAL. After admission swabs are taken from all burnt areas separately as a control and at regular intervals afterwards.

2. THE DANGER OF TETANUS in burns should not be overlooked and all burnt patients should be given tetanus antitoxin or given a booster dose of tetanus toxoid if appropriate.

3. MAINTENANCE OF ASEPSIS is very important and all in attendance must wear caps, masks, gowns and overshoes. Local

cleansing is not undertaken until the patient's condition is satisfactory and then consists of snipping away dead skin and cleansing with a mixture of Cetavlon and Hibitane known as Savlon 0·5 per cent. The surface is then dried with warm air or sterile towels. After this the burnt area may be treated by:

(a) *Exposure method.* The object of this method is to obtain and maintain a dry surface after cleansing with a detergent and drying with a hair drier if necessary.

Some surgeons advise that *no* antibiotic powder is used.

The sloughs are excised and grafting is performed as soon as possible in third-degree burns. The optimum time is 24 hours—if this is not possible the next time is 10 to 21 days.

(b) *Closed dressing principle.* The whole area is covered with tulle gras or melolin and secured with tapes to healthy skin. It is not redressed for six to eight days unless the dressing is wet with serum. Hyperpyrexia is due to the absorption of toxins but it should be remembered that when skin is destroyed the skin is less effective as an organ of heat loss and heavy dressings may be aggravating this condition. If infection occurs the appropriate antibiotic is administered. For fear of producing a generalised allergic reaction, antibiotic powders are not used locally.

*Burnt hand.* For burns of the hands the fingers are bandaged separately. Early grafting is advisable since tendons are often functioning and intact at the time of the burn, only to be destroyed by autolysis which is invariable beneath a third degree eschar. Obviously this is not possible if the patient's survival is in doubt and in such cases the hand may be enclosed in frequently changed plastic gloves soaked in a silicone.

Monafo has shown that if burns dressings were kept constantly moist with a 0·5 per cent solution of silver nitrate the heavy bacterial contamination from the air, so common when burns dressings are changed, would not arise.

4. SYSTEMIC ANTIBIOTIC THERAPY. This is usually confined to penicillin 0·5 megaunits b.d. Despite reports of penicillin sensitivity most surgeons treating burns advise the use of penicillin systemically and locally and alter it only on bacteriological evidence from the laboratory.

5. PRIMARY EXCISION AND SKIN GRAFTING. Localised full thickness burns may be excised as soon as the patient has been resuscitated.

6. SECONDARY SKIN GRAFTING is necessary in all full thickness burns and may be performed in a series of operations

depending on the extent of the area to be grafted. It is a particularly difficult decision in extensively burnt patients who are not doing well, but the consensus of opinion is that if one delays until the condition is ideal and the local area bacteriologically sterile many of these patients will have died. For these extensively burnt patients the following minimal standards are necessary:

(a) A normal blood haemoglobin reading. This can be achieved by blood transfusion.

(b) The absence of haemolytic streptococci. These are almost invariably sensitive to penicillin and can be killed in a few days. Grafting can be undertaken in the presence of staphylococci if the appropriate antibiotic is prescribed.

(c) A plasma protein reading of not below 55 g per l (5·5 g per cent).

7. In addition to these measures the burnt area is cleaned as much as possible:

(a) Eusol compresses followed by saline pads may be applied.

(b) Polymyxin cream may be used for cases heavily infected with *Ps. aeruginosa*. A 1 per cent solution of Framygen may be even more effective.

(c) Excision of sloughs in all deep burns is undertaken before separation occurs. The area is then covered with autografts or the viable cadaveric allografts with or without tissue typing. They are preserved in a skin bag in liquid nitrogen.

*Skin grafting*

Skin grafting will considerably reduce the time taken for a wound or burn to heal if there has been extensive skin loss. In addition, the scar will be more supple and the degree of contracture very much diminished.

PREPARATION OF THE DONOR AREA

Grafts may be taken in the form of thin sheets cut from the superficial layers of the skin (Thiersch graft), or large pedicle flaps (pedicle grafting). Pinch grafts have no place in modern plastic surgery since they leave a disfigured site and give an indifferent cosmetic result.

In cases for Thiersch grafting only the superficial cells (epidermis) of the skin are taken. In tube pedicle grafting the whole thickness of the skin is used. Antiseptics should not be applied to the donor area before grafting, since most antiseptics destroy the cells in the superficial layers of the skin. The limb or other area chosen is shaved, washed, and enclosed in a sterile towel.

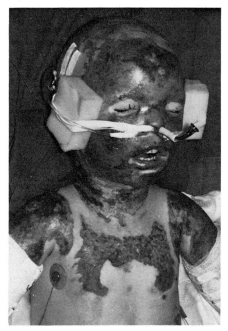

FIG. 19.2    Severely burnt child.

### PREPARATION OF THE RECIPIENT AREA

The wound is ready for grafting only when the granulations are healthy and sepsis has been almost eliminated. The granulating surface is healthy when it is smooth and does not bleed readily. As an additional precaution, a swab should be taken for bacteriological examination to determine the degree and nature of any infection which may be present. Antibiotics may be prescribed.

### CARE OF THE PATIENT AFTER SKIN GRAFTING

*The donor area* is always painful, and this may be minimised by the application of a soothing dressing, such as petroleum jelly gauze.

*The recipient area* is usually covered with tulle gras and a firm pressure bandage. The nurse must take the greatest care with the grafted area to see that it is not damaged while the patient is recovering from the anaesthetic. The dressing is usually left untouched for six to seven days, and in most cases the surgeon will prefer to perform the dressing himself. At the first dressing the old applications are floated off with sterile saline. In certain areas such as the perineum or buttocks the grafts themselves can be treated by exposure instead of dressings.

**SPECIAL COMPLICATIONS OF BURNS IN THE FIRST SEVEN DAYS**
Some additional special problems which may arise:

1. **Acute toxaemia.** This condition is not unlike the crisis which occurs in hyperthyroidism. The patient becomes excitable and later increasingly drowsy; the pulse increases in rate and diminishes in volume; the temperature rises to higher levels each day. The patient suffers from vomiting and diarrhoea. If the condition is unrelieved or fails to respond to treatment coma results.

*Treatment*
Continuous intravenous plasma transfusion and the administration of antibiotics are continued.

2. **Extensive local oedema.** This complication is not unusual, and is best overcome by a change in posture of the part so that the tissue drains by gravity. In the case of the hands, it is best overcome by suspension of the hands, adequately protected with dressings, from Balkan beams. Chymar, 10,000 units in 1 ml of normal saline twice daily for five days, given intramuscularly, is also effective.

3. **Loss of morale.** Morale is all-important to the immediate recovery. The physical weight of the dressings and the severe distress of the accident weigh heavily on many patients. Their dread of disfigurement is very great. The hair should be brushed and the patient should be encouraged to use cosmetics or anything which increases morale. This produces a sense of well-being and restores confidence.

It should not be forgotten that there may be deep psychological aspects in the relationship between parent and child following burns. Parents may feel a sense of guilt that their child has been burnt through some neglect on their part. In other patients the parents are aggrieved that the child has been burnt from its own fault.

4. **Metabolic changes.** There is a great loss of nitrogen and many other changes which are ill-understood. A high protein diet is essential to replace nitrogen. Complan (a food) is valuable in cases of burns, and vitamin C may be advisable in view of the large areas which have to be healed.

5. **Renal failure.** This may occur and the urine should be tested for albumin, which is a nitrogen loss and the volume measured each day, no matter how well the patient is progressing. A fluid balance chart should be kept.

6. **Pulmonary complications.** For example, pneumonia and bronchitis frequently occur, particularly in elderly patients. Pulmonary oedema, believed to be caused by unidentified toxins, may develop although the burning has not involved the respiratory tract.

7. **Liver failure and jaundice** may occur quite suddenly from toxaemia from tissue destruction or sepsis.

8. **Bone marrow suppression** may develop as a result of infection and cause anaemia.

9. **Contractures and deformities.** These are best overcome by early light splintage, active movements and early skin grafting.

10. **Gastrointestinal bleeding** from acute ulceration, the classical but rarest form being an acute duodenal ulcer (Curling's ulcer).

### CHEMICAL BURNS

Chemical burns are treated on lines similar to those described above, but those due to acid should be irrigated with sodium bicarbonate solution and those due to alkalis with 1 per cent acetic acid as soon as possible after infliction. With acid or alkaline burns of the mouth the following buffer solution may be used:

> Potassium dihydrogen phosphate (30 g)
> Disodium hydrogen phosphate (200 g)
> Aqua ad. 1 litre.

In addition to being used as a mouth wash it is suitable for irrigating the eyes.

The wide use of chemicals has led many firms to state how burns resulting from their products should be treated and burns centres throughout Great Britain can advise on treatment by telephone.

### X-RAY BURNS

X-ray burns require the application of an oily dressing. Patients who have worked as radiographers for some years are liable to develop squamous cell carcinoma (epithelioma) of the skin if the shield of the X-ray tube has been ineffective and X-rays are emitted.

On hair-bearing areas temporary depilation occurs after three weeks, or permanent alopecia (baldness) if the hair follicles are destroyed.

# CHAPTER 20

# Trauma

Higher speeds on the road with higher world population, higher buildings as well as more sophisticated industrial processes are some of the factors which have increased the incidence of disasters in which large numbers of people may be injured simultaneously. Most hospitals have contingency plans to deal with the work arising from a major disaster. A large hospital department receiving several accident and emergency patients every day will have the staff, facilities, and equipment to deal with all but the most overwhelming situation. In a major disaster it is essential, as far as possible, to distribute patients between neighbouring hospitals. On notification that a large number of casualties are to be expected contingency plans should be put into operation and will include summoning extra staff—nurses, surgeons, anaesthetists, radiologists and laboratory staff as well as stretcher bearers and ancillary staff.

## INITIAL SURVEY AND CLASSIFICATION

A rapid survey has to be made of the injured by the most experienced doctor present so that immediate treatment is given to those whose lives are threatened. However, the nurse in the accident department should cast her eyes frequently on patients whose injuries are apparently minor—who have not yet been formally and carefully examined or fully assessed. A small laceration may have penetrated deeply and signs of internal haemorrhage or perforation of an organ may become apparent only after arrival at hospital or after a first rapid assessment. Inevitably injury is not confined to the young or the fit, and some patients will be suffering from other pathology which may or may not have been diagnosed before the accident. The initial sorting will be into:

1. **Conditions which require immediate treatment**
   1. Severely injured but not immediately threatening life.
   2. Minor injuries.

**Life-threatening injuries** are:
   *Massive haemorrhage* amounting to near exsanguination. This is treated by blood replacement and, if possible, control of the

190

bleeding (Chapter 13). The only point to stress here is that if it is so overwhelming that there is no time for cross-matching group O Rh-negative blood is given immediately. If it is not available group O Rh-positive blood is used, but to give blood of other groups without cross-matching, however desperate the circumstances, is unjustified. Plasma or plasma substitutes are all that can be given.

The immediate requirements are:

(i) units of O −ve or, if not available, O +ve blood;
(ii) calcium chloride 1 gram every fourth unit of blood;
(iii) a solution of sodium bicarbonate 8·4 per cent should be given.

*Respiratory failure* (Chapter 18). A clear airway is essential.

*Cardiac arrest* will require the measures outlined in Chapter 15.

*Extensive burns* are infused with plasma on admission (Chapter 19).

*Profound shock* from whatever cause requires immediate treatment (Chapter 15).

*Coma.* When all possible urgent measures have been instituted an assessment has to be made of all their injuries and definitive treatment undertaken.

2. **Major injuries.** Major injuries although not immediately life-threatening may cost the patient his life; they include abdominal, chest and head injuries, multiple fractures and burns.

3. **Minor injuries.** Life-threatening, major or minor injuries all require careful assessment and formal documentation. The urine should be tested and if an anaesthetic, however short, is contemplated, steps must be taken to enquire that the stomach is empty or emptied by nasogastric suction if there is any doubt.

### ACCIDENTAL WOUNDS

There are three types of wound:

1. *Incised*, or clean-cut.
2. *Lacerated.* The tissues are jagged, torn and crushed.
3. *Punctured.* The skin wound is trivial, but the damage may be severe if a vital organ is punctured.

An abrasion is a wound in which only the superficial layers of the skin are damaged.

### MULTIPLE INJURIES

Multiple injuries may occur following a fall or a traffic accident, and open wounds may be only one aspect. The first essential in multiple injuries is to ensure that the patient has a free airway. If the patient is unconscious it is likely that he has a head injury, but if he is also in acute circulatory failure it is likely that he has other injuries as well. Injuries which may occur are:

1. Open wounds and lacerations.
2. Fractures of the limbs and spine—which includes the cervical, dorsal and lumbar spine.
3. Fractures of the skull. The facial bones, the jaw, maxilla and the nose should be examined.

**Acute circulatory failure.** This is considered in detail in Chapter 15. As good an estimate as possible of the amount of blood lost should be made. The blood loss may be to the exterior or into a body cavity. It is particularly important in multiple injuries to make due allowance for the amount of blood loss into the tissues around closed fractures. In the past, most patients with severe injuries have probably been inadequately transfused. A working rule is to allow, for every surface wound equal to the extent of the open hand, or, for a fracture or deep wound equal to the size of the closed fist, one unit of blood.

Resuscitation should be early and adequate.

**Infection.** A wound is clean, or non-infected, only when it is made under the aseptic conditions such as exist in an operating theatre. All other wounds, however clean they may appear to the naked eye, are potentially infected. The surface of the tissues which has been exposed is covered by a film of bacteria usually derived accidentally from the patient's clothing or from dust and soil. If this film could be removed by cutting a thin slice off the surface in one continuous piece, the conditions present in a clean wound would be almost exactly reproduced. Foreign bodies, of course, would also have to be removed. This procedure of removal of the superficial septic layer of a wound is known as excision. In practice it is impossible to follow this procedure literally, because in the superficial layer vital structures may be exposed, but as far as possible this is the aim.

After 12 hours infection may be well established, and excision of the wound will destroy the membrane formed by the white blood corpuscles which are protecting the deeper tissues. Therefore, if wounds are treated after 12 hours, it is usually better simply to remove obvious foreign bodies, and should pus develop make sure that drainage is adequate. The wound is left open and no sutures are introduced. Later, pocketing of pus may occur and further drainage may be necessary.

**Thrombosis.** Following severe injuries, older patients are particularly liable to thrombotic complications, some of which result in embolism. Controlled anticoagulant therapy has been shown to be of value in reducing them. It is commenced only *after* haemorrhage has been controlled.

## THE CARE OF THE WOUND

All patients who have sustained wounds, however trivial, must be given an intramuscular injection of tetanus antitoxin or tetanus toxoid or penicillin according to their immunity status (p. 71). Tiny punctured wounds are more likely to be a source of tetanic infection than large open wounds, because they are shut off from a free supply of oxygen.

Small incised wounds require only mild antiseptic dressings, such as flavine emulsion.

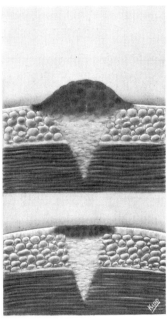

FIG. 20.1    Excessive granulations present an insurmountable barrier to the encroaching epithelium. Below: After cauterisation with silver nitrate.

*The general care of wounds*

The arrest of severe haemorrhage is the most urgent task. The methods of controlling haemorrhage are discussed in Chapter 13.

The resuscitation of the patient must be undertaken before any further measures are contemplated.

Following an accident a patient is liable to be very frightened and reassurance is very important. A permission form for operation should be signed. Before operation the wound is covered with a sterile towel.

*Preparation for immediate operation*

When the patient's general condition has improved, the bladder is emptied by the patient's own efforts if possible, and undressing is limited to a minimum if the condition has been critical. Atropine (0·6 mg) is injected hypodermically, and it is an advantage if the patient can be X-rayed before going to the theatre. Dentures must be removed.

*Operation*

The preoperative preparation of the skin will usually be undertaken by the surgeon after the patient has been anaesthetised. The skin is shaved and cleansed for a wide area beyond the wound. Superficial foreign bodies are usually removed. Excision of a thin margin of skin and the superficial layer of the wound is then carried out. After excision an antibacterial powder is usually insufflated. The skin is then loosely sutured. If suture is impossible because of loss of skin, a skin graft is performed. In late and infected wounds surgery is confined to ensuring that there is free drainage, but at the earliest possible date secondary suture or a skin graft is undertaken.

OPEN WOUNDS

Sometimes a wound is left open, dressed with petroleum jelly gauze, or insufflated with an antibiotic powder such as Polybactrin.

The edges of a wound must not be allowed to overlap. Unless raw edge is approximated to raw edge, healing is impossible. Similarly, if the edges of a wound are indrawn or sucked under due to loss of the tissue beneath, delay in healing will result.

*Complications* which can occur in a wound are:

Infection
Sloughing
Secondary haemorrhage (p. 110)
Severe pain, which is usually due to infection
A sinus or a fistula
The wound may gape, e.g. 'burst abdomen'
Haematoma (p. 125)
Sinking in of the edges.

*Immobilisation of wounds*

All wounds heal best when they are immobilised and covered. Daily dressings are not performed. However, the nurse must know when to suspect complications which necessitate inspection of the wound. The following are a guide that all may not be well:

1. The continued presence of pain.

2. Persistent rise of temperature.
3. Presence of toxaemia, indicated by the onset of vomiting, diarrhoea, loss of appetite and increasing pallor.
4. Increasing pulse rate.
5. Any symptom suggestive of tetanus (p. 70).
6. Any symptom suggestive of too tight a plaster or dressing, e.g. pain, tingling, or cyanosis of the tips of the fingers or toes.

## The healing of wounds

Healing by first intention is the aim in all wounds. The sutures are removed when the wound has healed, usually eight to 10 days later. When the sutures are about to be removed it may be noticed that there is some tension or swelling of the wound, due to a haematoma. If this is the case, the edges should be separated gently with sinus forceps and a small strip of rubber or plastic drain inserted for 48 hours.

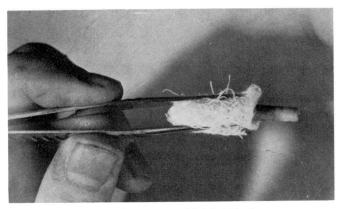

FIG. 20.2    Silver nitrate stick is held in forceps.

Gauze packing of the wound for haematoma or a subcutaneous collection of pus delays healing and blocks drainage. It should never be used. If the granulation tissue is excessive (proud flesh) and grows above the level of the skin, the exuberant patches should be burnt down by the careful application of a silver nitrate stick. The nurse must hold the stick in a pair of fine dressing forceps or special applicator and take care not to damage any portion of the patient's skin or her own hands. A wound which is large and septic may require irrigation with antiseptic lotions, such as eusol, Savlon (0·5 per cent) or hydrogen peroxide. The Entonox gas and oxygen machine may be used for producing analgesia when dressing a large infected wound. More usually omnopon 10 mg or Pethidine 50 mg is given intramuscularly half an hour previously. When an infected wound has become clean secondary suture of the skin may be performed or a skin graft may be possible.

*Chemotherapy*

Antibacterial drugs have revolutionised the healing of wounds and are used in almost all traumatic wounds. They may be prescribed locally or systemically.

Prolonged discharge from wounds and consequent loss of protein is liable to give rise to hypoproteinaemia and patients with wounds should have a diet rich in protein and vitamin C, which is an important constituent of the diet in effecting healing.

**Complications of wounds.** *Prevention of contracture* following a wound is a matter which requires constant attention. It is aided by proper splinting in the early stages and later by active movement. The prevention of oedema and swelling is also aided by movement once sepsis has been controlled. The rehabilitation of a patient who has been wounded is of considerable importance in helping him to overcome any dis-

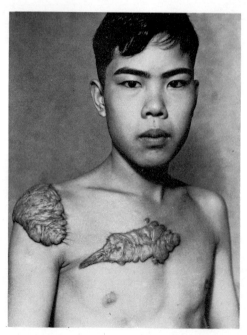

FIG. 20.3    Keloids. Extensive keloid scars following acid burns. Treatment by excision or radiation or the use of cortisone are all equally unsatisfactory.

ability, and often dispels any doubts he may have about his capacity to work. The nurse must supervise the movements. They are particularly important following wounds in the hand.

**Keloids.** A keloid is a condition of excessive thickening of a scar. It is particularly liable to develop after operations on tuberculous foci and following wounds in members of the coloured races.

*Treatment*

Excision is of no value. The use of 'Covermark', a tinted, opaque, non-irritant cream which is water and shower proof, may be advised. Cryotherapy or the local application of steroids (p. 216) may also be used to reduce these blemishes.

# CHAPTER 21

# Diseases of the Skin, Muscle and Tendon

Bed sores are an important complication which may develop from confining the patient to bed. In many cases they are preventable by skilled nursing, but in some cases no effort or skill can avoid their development, and the condition is frequently a terminal one.

*Causes and predisposing factors*

The root cause is long-continued pressure, and the pressure required need only be high enough to compress the blood vessel in conditions of hypotension resulting from shock or blood loss. Then otherwise tolerable pressure on the skin may cause a sore. Pressure causes discomfort, but in the debilitated and in paraplegics with a sensory loss, such discomfort may not be appreciated by the patient. The surface appearance of a pressure sore gives little indication of what may be its ultimate size.

**General**
(a) Emaciation due to malnutrition or disease.
(b) Senility.
(c) Diabetes, anaemia, and other severe constitutional disturbances.

**Local**
(a) Pressure. The patient's body weight renders movement difficult if he is obese. In a thin subject the bony prominences are exposed to greater pressure.
(b) Loss of skin sensation. This is usually due to a lesion of the spinal cord or the peripheral nerves.
(c) Incontinence is a potent source of bed sore formation, since the skin becomes moist and septic.
(d) Excessive sweating causes a moist skin.
(e) Friction such as too vigorous rubbing and the presence of foreign bodies—wrinkled sheets, breadcrumbs, etc.
(f) Impaired circulation, e.g. patients suffering from heart disease.
(g) Oedema.

THE PRESSURE AREAS

The pressure areas are those portions of the body on which the greatest weight is borne when the patient is recumbent, and it is at these sites that bed sores are liable to occur. They include the heels, buttocks, sacrum, scapular areas, elbows, the spinous processes of the vertebrae, and the occiput.

When the patient is lying on his side the whole skin area is liable to be affected, but more particularly the skin over the greater trochanter.

*The prevention of bed sores*

1. Pressure must be relieved by frequent change of posture, and the circulation revived by stimulation of the skin.

2. A carefully made bed, in which the sheets are pulled tight, smooth and freed from crumbs and wrinkles.

3. Sorbo or air rings and cushions are used if necessary, and the nurse should ensure that pressure is evenly distributed and that the patient is moved about in bed. Although frowned on by some authorities rubber rings are useful in the correct position.

4. The skin must be kept clean and dry.

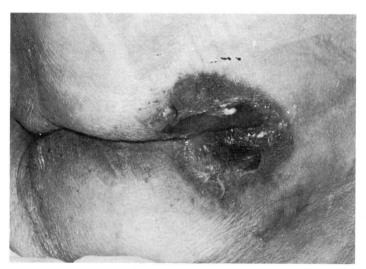

FIG. 21.1    Large bed sore.

All these objects are ensured by:

(a) Attention to the skin. The skin should be washed with soap and water, rinsed and carefully dried. The area is then stimulated by massage and/or a silicone preparation with powder, using a circular movement to assist circulation.

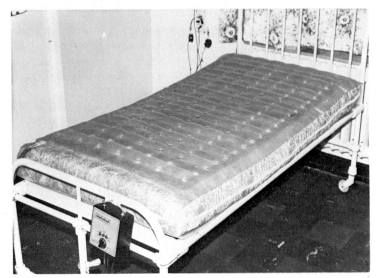

FIG. 21.2  The ripple bed.

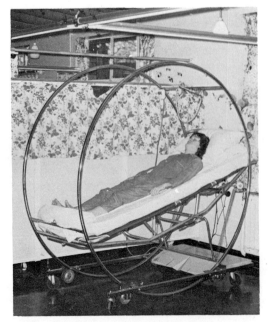

FIG. 21.3  A circo-electric bed.

Massage of the skin is still carried out with apparent success although in some patients soap and water may further dry the skin and may not be helpful. Silicone preparations are really only of use as a barrier against incontinence.

(b) The provision of a sorbo sheepskin or ripple mattress.

(c) Immediately incontinence occurs, the patient must be washed from the waist to the knees and dried thoroughly. All soiled bedclothes are changed and pressure areas massaged. Zinc and castor oil ointment or silicones form a waterproof covering for the skin. A Gibbon catheter is very useful to prevent bed-wetting in the incontinent patient. 'Inco pads' may be used. These are made of several thicknesses of soft paper which can be easily changed and are disposable. They are useful only in as much as they protect bed linen. If left in position too long they can also aggravate the skin by causing friction.

RIPPLE BED (Fig. 21.2) is a considerable advance in the treatment and prevention of bed sores. It has an alternating pressure-point pad used over the patient's ordinary mattress under the bottom sheet to provide regular, frequent automatic redistribution of the pressure areas. The pad consists of a Vinyl plastic pad with alternating sets of air cells running transversely across the width of the regular mattress, with an air pump which automatically controls the cycle. Single pads are now available and a new twin pulsator will operate two pads.

A CIRCO-ELECTRIC BED (Fig. 21.3) not only enables the patient to get out of bed unaided, but will change his position as often as desired even at intervals as short as 15 minutes or even less. It is controllable by the patient using an electric switch.

**Established bed sores.** When the lesion is still limited to an area of erythema of the skin, relief of pressure is most important. The patient's posture must be changed at least two-hourly, and on occasions the patient may be allowed to sit out of bed with considerable benefit. The doctor in charge of the case should always be asked if this is possible in a case of threatened bed sores. Moisture, friction and pressure are the three most important factors in causing and maintaining a bed sore.

The treatment prescribed above for the routine prevention of bed sores is continued to keep the circulation active in the skin around the bed sore. Cardinal rules in the treatment of bed sores are:

1. The relief of pressure.
2. Early debridement.
3. A high protein diet to make up for serum loss. If necessary a blood transfusion will replace serum loss and combat anaemia.
4. Excision and suture if suture is possible—if it is not, a skin graft is applied even over a bony prominence.

In some patients, particularly those in whom there has been complete transection of the spinal cord, the development of an ulcerated sore would appear to be inevitable, yet they almost never develop a bed sore when they are cared for in special spinal injury units.

If some part of the sore is healing by granulation, 1 per cent gentian violet or red lotion is of value. In the young subject who shows every sign of recovery from a long illness, and who has been unfortunate enough to develop a large bed sore as a complication, a further skin graft may be necessary to accelerate recovery. The most amazing fact about bed sores is their relative painlessness, and, curiously enough, the pain seems to diminish as ulceration deepens.

### ULCERATION

An ulcer is a breach of the surface. Important in maintaining the discontinuity of the epithelium and preventing healing are pathogenic bacteria, defective oxygenation as a result of venous or arterial disease, oedema from circulatory defects or infection, a defective nerve supply, and continued trauma.

### Types of ulcers
1. Inflammatory:
    (a) Non-specific, e.g. carbuncle which has pointed (p. 204).
    (b) Specific—tuberculosis, syphilis (p. 76), anthrax (p. 72).
2. Varicose (p. 237).
3. Bed sores (p. 198).
4. Trophic.
5. Malignant.
6. Rodent ulcer (p. 213).

The parts of an ulcer are:

> *The floor*—the portion which can be seen.
> *The edge*—side walls.
> *The base*, i.e. the portion that can be felt.

### COMPLICATIONS OF A SCAR

Wounds, ulcers, and burns which have involved the dermis leave a scar. Complications which may arise are:

1. Keloid formation (p. 197). This is very common after operations performed during pregnancy, following burns and after wounds in the Negro races.
2. Ulceration (from defective blood supply).
3. Contracture.
4. Neuroma (gives rise to pain).

5. Adherence to deep tissues.
6. Neoplastic changes.
7. Latent tetanus (p. 71).

## OTHER SURGICAL LESIONS OF THE SKIN AND SUBCUTANEOUS TISSUES

### INJURIES

**Bee and wasp stings.** The sting causes considerable pain. After removal of the sting by squeezing a compress of ammonia for a bee and vinegar for a wasp is applied.

**Dog bite** is treated with surgical toilet to the wound and the administration of tetanus toxoid and antibiotics. If the animal is suffering from hydrophobia (rabies), which is extremely rare in this country, the appropriate antitoxin must be obtained and administered as soon as possible to prevent the condition arising in the patient. The animal is isolated and kept alive to observe its behaviour before killing it when its central nervous system is examined for rabies.

**Foreign bodies.** Needles, splinters of metal and wood, and fragments of glass frequently become embedded in the tissues. If the end of the foreign body is protruding an X-ray is taken and the surgeon will advise if its removal is necessary. Most types of

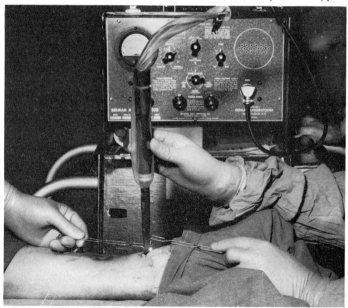

FIG. 21.4 Burman's metal locator. The electromagnetic metal detector based on the indications of a meter and a small loudspeaker operating simultaneously.

glass because of their lead content, are opaque to X-rays and therefore cast a shadow on the film because the component materials have a high atomic weight.

If it has been decided to remove the foreign body, the part is kept splinted and at rest and a further X-ray is taken immediately before the operation.

Removal of a foreign body in certain sites may cause greater damage than if it is left alone. Many foreign bodies cause no trouble and become surrounded by and embedded in fibrous tissue.

The Burman metal detector is an electromagnetic detecting device which will locate quickly and accurately metallic foreign bodies. Location is based on the indications of a meter and of a small loudspeaker operating simultaneously. The instrument, which is set to give sound of uniform pitch, remains unchanged until the probe approaches close to the metallic foreign body when the sound and meter reading both rise sharply. When used following an incision the probe is covered with a specially designed rubber jacket which can be sterilised by autoclaving or can be boiled. Non-responsive retractors supplied with the instrument are used for retraction.

## LOCALISED INFECTION OF THE SKIN

1. **Boils.** A boil is caused by infection of a hair follicle by the *Staphylococcus pyogenes*. The first symptom is a localised itching pimple which increases in size, and the surrounding area becomes indurated and painful. As pus forms on the surface a yellow discharge occurs. Later there is sloughing, which is replaced by granulation tissue as healing commences. Should resolution occur without suppuration, the condition is known as a 'blind boil'.

2. **Carbuncles.** A carbuncle is a gangrenous process of the subcutaneous tissues. It is due to infection of multiple hair follicles, and the commonest site is the back of the neck. Diabetics are particularly liable to develop carbuncles.

*Treatment*

If the patient is a diabetic the dosage of insulin will usually have to be increased and the co-operation of the physician sought. The best method of treatment of a boil or carbuncle is by administration of the appropriate antibiotic; resolution is usual and the acute stage is greatly shortened. If pus forms drainage will be necessary.

3. **Subcutaneous abscess** is a common condition. It is a frequent termination of cellulitis. The classical signs of acute inflammation are present.

*Treatment*
When pus is present drainage is necessary.

## TUMOURS OF THE SKIN
Papillomas and haemangiomas are fairly common.

**Malignant tumours** are:
1. Rodent ulcer (page 213)
2. Squamous-celled carcinoma (page 213)
3. Melanoma (page 213)

## SEPTIC FINGERS
Infection of a tendon sheath is responsible for the crippling disability which may be seen in many cases as the end result of a septic finger.

CAUSE. Septic pinpricks and cuts from glass are the usual causes.

*Symptoms*
1. Pain in the finger which is aggravated by movement.
2. The finger is swollen and throbbing.
3. Extension of the metacarpo-phalangeal joint is extremely painful.
4. Red lines on the arm (lymphangitis) and enlarged axillary lymphatic nodes (lymphadenitis).

General constitutional signs, flushed face, pyrexia, and loss of appetite, are present.

*Treatment*
1. Absolute rest. The arm should be kept supported in a sling.
2. Antibacterial therapy.
3. The patient should be encouraged to drink large quantities of fluid.

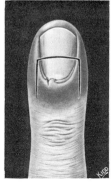

FIG. 21.5    Nail base removed for paronychia.

4. Incision and drainage followed by hypertonic sodium sulphate baths and active movement. Splinters or foreign bodies present will be removed at the same time.

Many surgeons require the application of a tourniquet to the arm when performing such operations. In addition, the general treatment of an acute infection is undertaken. Active movements of the fingers as soon as they are painless are very important.

*Paronychia* is the occurrence of infection around the nail bed. As soon as pus forms the bed is incised and the proximal half of the nail is removed to effect drainage (Fig. 21.5). The distal half is left covering the sensitive tissues. A new nail grows when the infection subsides and the portion of the old nail which has been left drops off. In a neglected case infection of the bone (the distal phalanx) develops.

*Pulp space infection.* The dense tissue of the finger tip is often infected by needle pricks. Unless early treatment is sought, necrosis of the underlying bone occurs.

*Diffuse infection of the spaces in the palm* may occur as a result of a tendon sheath infection or a subcutaneous abscess which has not been drained adequately.


## DISEASES OF MUSCLES AND TENDONS

Injuries are the most common affections of muscles and tendons. The muscles and tendons can function only when their contractions and movement are smooth and unhindered. Contusion or sprain results in swelling, which impedes their smooth action and gives rise to pain. Rupture of a tendon or muscle will result in complete loss of its function, since it is then attached only at one point.

*Treatment*

Rest, by splinting if necessary, is undertaken. The application of cooling lotions, such as lead and opium, relieves pain. When the pain has diminished, massage and active movements are commenced.

**Cut tendons.** Cut tendons commonly occur in the wrist area following wounds. Immediate suture is usually performed.

Rupture of a muscle or tendon may occur as a result of a violent strain and is commonly seen in athletes. Rupture of the soleus or a few fibres of the gastrocnemius is responsible for the severe cramping pain in athletes' calves after severe exertion. In certain cases osteoarthritis of the shoulder causes degeneration of the biceps tendon passing through the joint, and may result in complete rupture.

*Treatment*

Rest relieves the acute pain. If an important muscle or tendon has been torn, resuture may be undertaken, but in the presence of osteoarthritis such an operation would be contra-indicated.

**Infections.** Infections of the muscles are uncommon, apart from open wounds. Abscesses may occur as a complication of the administration of intramuscular injections, which should always be given on the outer side of the thigh. If an abscess develops, drainage is usually necessary.

**Chronic infections.** Tuberculosis is an occasional cause of chronic infection of the tendon sheaths, and when the condition occurs in front of the wrist it is sometimes known as a compound palmar ganglion.

**Ganglion.** A ganglion is a cyst on a tendon and the treatment is total excision. Sometimes crushing with a book is effective.

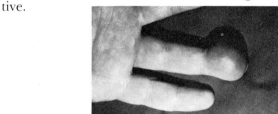

FIG. 21.6    Implantation dermoid of finger.

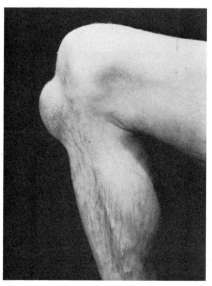

FIG. 21.7    Infrapatellar bursa.

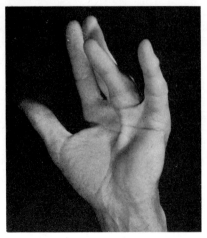

FIG. 21.8  Dupuytren's contracture.

**Tenosynovitis.** This is not uncommon from trauma and subsides with rest if necessary in an appropriate splint.

**Implantation dermoid cyst** (Fig. 21.6). May arise in the hand or fingers from pricks in which the superficial layers of the skin are carried into the deeper tissues.

### BURSAE

Bursae are small sacs containing serous fluid which 'oils' the tendons, etc., passing over bony prominences. The common sites are the elbow (olecranon) and the knee.

*Recurrent irritation* gives rise to enlargement, e.g. housemaid's knee. Infection may occur as a complication. An olecranon bursa is occasionally associated with a septic finger.

*Treatment*

Infected bursae are incised. An enlarged bursa is excised or aspiration may be advised and if it recurs excision undertaken.

### DUPUYTREN'S CONTRACTURE

This is a deformity resulting from contraction of the palmar fascia. Alcoholism and diabetes are contributing causes. The fascia in the palm, in the area corresponding to the ring finger, becomes a tight hard band. The finger is slightly drawn into the palm. Later, the little finger area is invaded. The index and middle fingers are not commonly involved. The fascia becomes adherent to the skin of the palm.

*Treatment*

No method of treatment is entirely satisfactory, and many patients find that the deformity causes little disability. The contracture should be stretched as frequently as possible to prevent an increase in deformity.

The operations which may be undertaken are:

1. Tenotomy to divide the band.
2. Excision of the fascia.

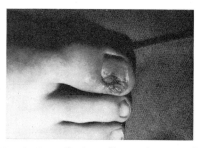

FIG. 21.9    Infection of ingrowing toenail.

### INGROWING TOE-NAILS

An ingrowing toe-nail is a condition associated with wearing badly fitting shoes. It is also caused by incorrect paring of the nails. Low-grade infection develops in the nail bed. Excision of the nail and its bed is undertaken.

### CORNS

Corns are due to the friction of badly fitting shoes. The central painful core consists of 'twisted' nerve fibres.

*Treatment*

Correction of the shoe fitting is essential. Locally, the corn may be painted with 10 per cent salicyclic acid in collodion, and a hot foot bath should be taken at night.

# CHAPTER 22

# New Growths

A tumour, or new growth, is a mass of cells similar to those of a body tissue, growing at the expense of the body and fulfilling no useful purpose. It is not true that tumour cells proliferate faster than normal cells. Further, it has become clear that a tumour is not a relatively stable mass of cells which increase in size and number as a result of a steady rate of cell division. It increases in size only when the rate of proliferation is higher than the rate of cell loss.

A new growth may be simple or malignant, and the difference is that unchecked a malignant growth will invariably kill the patient. Simple tumours are nonetheless important because, untreated, they may cause death by interfering with some vital function. A simple tumour of the meninges, for example, will cause cerebral compression and, unrelieved, the patient will die in a coma. A malignant growth is commonly known as a cancer.

THE CAUSE OF CANCER

The cause, or causes, of cancer are unknown, but there is, nonetheless, a vast amount of valuable information about the factors predisposing to its occurrence.

It is essential to realise that not all malignant growths are incurable, and year by year the number of cures is increasing. True, in some sites cancer is invariably fatal, but in others the results of treatment are highly successful.

PREDISPOSING FACTORS

1. *Heredity.* It is possible that there is a hereditary factor. Notable examples are the development of carcinoma of the colon in patients with familial polyposis and carcinoma of the oesophagus in the skin disease known as tylosis.

2. *Chronic irritation.* Chronic irritation is a definite predisposing factor in some cases. A squamous cell carcinoma (skin cancer) of the scrotum was common amongst chimney sweeps, and cancer of the lip was frequently associated with persistent smoking of an old-fashioned hot clay pipe. Excessive cigarette smoking is associated with the great increase in bronchial carcinoma. Constant irritation from coal-

tar products is responsible in some cases. *β-Naphthylamine* is a well-recognised bladder carcinogen.

Many pioneers of radiology lost their lives from skin cancer, the result of exposure to unprotected X-ray tubes.

3. *Chronic sepsis.* Carcinoma of the tongue is very frequently associated with long-standing syphilitic infection, and the condition hardly ever develops in a clean mouth.

In the pages which follow are described growths as they appear to the naked eye or under the microscope—that is, their morphological character. Malignant growths may well be due to the loss of essential cellular constituents or to faulty synthesis and logical treatment would lie in substitution or replacement therapy. The biochemical characterisation of cancer rather than a morphological one would then be logical. There is evidence that syndromes occur as a result of circulating hormones secreted by the primary tumour.

4. *Immunological aspects.* Tumours are not autonomous—that is to say they are not independent of all the normal constraints which contain tissue metabolism. It is known that spontaneous regression can occur and yet sudden reappearance may be made after a period of complete quiescence. It is of interest to note that circulating tumour cells often fail to establish metastases.

5. *Viruses* and alterations in the hormonal balance are other factors which predispose to malignant new growth. In experimental animals a condition indistinguishable from carcinoma of the breast can be produced by a virus.

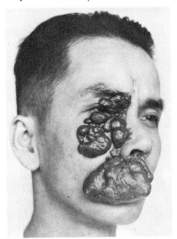

FIG. 22.1    From birth. Congenital naevus.
Naevi are frequently multiple, and superficial naevi may suggest a similar pathology in a deep-seated lesion. Spider naevi in a case of cirrhosis of the liver have a different cause.

SCREENING FOR THE EARLY DETECTION OF CANCER

This may take the form of:

*Exfoliative cytology*. Examples are:

1. Cervical smear for detection of carcinoma cervix (p. 619).
2. Screening of urine in rubber and dye workers who are liable to carcinoma of the bladder (p.476).

*Radiography* has been used for carcinoma of the breast but is not proven. More important in breast carcinoma is clinical examination of the breasts when smear screening is undertaken.

### SIMPLE NEW GROWTHS

Much confusion has arisen in following the terminology of tumour formation. The ending 'oma' simply means a new growth. A simple new growth is similar in substance to the tissue in which it arises and is named accordingly. Malignant new growths are named after the cells from which they arise.

Here we shall consider only the main types of simple new growths and the way in which they differ from malignant growths. Under the appropriate regions we shall consider their clinical features in detail.

| Type of growth | Tissue of origin |
|---|---|
| Lipoma | Fat |
| Neuroma | Nerve tissue |
| Chondroma | Cartilage |
| Myoma | Muscle |
| Osteoma | Bone |
| Fibroma | Fibrous tissue |
| Angioma (naevus) | Blood vessels |
| Myeloma | Bone marrow |
| Odontoma | Teeth |
| Adenoma | Gland |

A papilloma is a pedunculated tumour of the skin or of an epithelial lining. Some new growths are multiple. They have arisen separately and not from metastasis. Common multiple simple new growths are:

Lipomas
Neurofibromas
Naevi

CHARACTERISTICS OF SIMPLE NEW GROWTHS

1. The increase in size is slow. The tumour is limited by a capsule.
2. Spread into the neighbouring tissues does not occur. The tissue is pushed aside but not invaded.

3. They do not spread by the blood stream or by the lymphatic system.

4. They may cause symptoms as a result of their size or by pressure on the neighbouring tissues.

5. There is no tendency to recur after excision.

The usual treatment is excision or in suitable cases treatment by cryosurgery (p. 216).

## MALIGNANT NEW GROWTHS

The principal forms are:

1. **Those arising from the epithelial lined surfaces**

(a) *Squamous-celled carcinoma* (syn. epithelioma), which is a squamous-celled tumour growing from tissues covered by squamous cells, e.g. the tongue and skin.

(b) *Adenocarcinoma*, which is a glandular tissue tumour, e.g. breast, stomach, large intestine.

2. **Connective tissue tumours.** Sarcoma—this arises in bone (osteogenic sarcoma) or in fibrous tissues (fibrosarcoma).

3. **Pigment cells.** Melanoma arises in the pigmented layers of the skin and in the choroid of the eye. Simple pigmented moles may develop into malignant melanomas.

In between simple and malignant growths there is a number of borderline growths, the best recognised being a rodent ulcer of the skin. They are locally malignant in that they destroy tissue, but rarely spread to remote sites or into the lymphatic system.

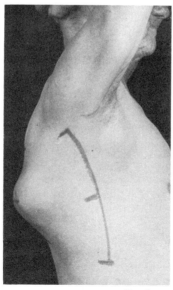

FIG. 22.2   Sarcoma of back.

Papillomas of the urinary tract, which were always known to become malignant if untreated, are now believed to be the first manifestation of carcinoma of the bladder.

## THE SPREAD OF MALIGNANT NEW GROWTHS

Malignant new growths may spread:

1. **Locally.** The growth increases in size and invades the neighbouring tissues.

2. **By metastasis** (i.e. by secondary growth formation).

(a) *By the lymphatic stream.* Carcinomas almost invariably metastasise or spread first by this route. The local lymphatic glands enlarge as spread progresses. Sarcomas invade the glands very late in their course.

(b) *By the blood stream.* The tumour may be widely disseminated to other tissues, and the deposit is also known as a metastasis or secondary new growth. This is a common method of spread of sarcomas, and this characteristic renders them rapidly fatal. Carcinomas have a lesser tendency to invade the blood stream in their earlier stages.

Secondary growths in bone are commonly the result of a primary growth in the breast, lung, prostate, kidney, and thyroid.

3. **By contact.** Tumours of the bladder have an evil reputation in this connection but the true explanation is probably that they are multicentric in origin.

4. **Transperitoneal implantation.** Cells shed from a growth of the stomach may fall on to the structures in the pelvis and give rise to secondary growths. The ovaries are the organs most frequently invaded by secondary growths in this way.

5. **Surgical implantation.** This is not a frequent occurrence, but is seen occasionally in the scar of an operation wound through which a new growth has been excised.

## CHARACTERISTICS OF MALIGNANT NEW GROWTHS

1. Untreated, the patient dies.

2. Increase in size is progressive. They have no limiting capsule.

3. Spread occurs to the other tissues as described above and gives rise to secondary growths.

4. Ulceration and infection are common, and many of the symptoms and signs are due to infection of the growth. Infection is particularly liable to result in secondary haemorrhage.

## SYMPTOMS AND SIGNS OF MALIGNANT NEW GROWTHS

The symptoms and signs described in this book, as we follow the course of new growths in each organ, are those of moderately advanced tumours. The early symptoms and signs are:

1. *A lump*—this should invariably be a cause for seeking medical advice.
2. *Bleeding*—from any part of the body. A few drops of blood lost even on only one occasion are important.
3. *Slight alteration in normal habits or functions*—to mention only a few: (a) increasing constipation; (b) difficulty with swallowing, walking, talking, or eating.
4. *Changes in metabolism.* Since some tumours such as those of the pancreas, the pituitary or the adrenal add to the function of these organs, a change in metabolism may be the first indication of tumour formation.

New growths in the early stages will be diagnosed only by careful clinical examination and painstaking investigation. When symptoms are marked the growth is usually well advanced.

BIOPSY. In cases of doubt, a small portion of the growth is removed and examined under the microscope. This procedure is often of great value in diagnosis, but is not without danger because more rapid spread of the growth may result. The recovery of malignant cells from the interior of organs or in secretion or excretion is sometimes of great value in diagnosis.

EXFOLIATIVE CYTOLOGY is the process by which cells recovered from natural secretions like the gastric juice or the urine are centrifuged, sectioned in a paraffin block and examined under a microscope. Scrapings from organs like the cervix of the uterus may be treated similarly, and the opinion of an experienced pathologist may be invaluable in the detection of cancer at a very early stage.

Biopsy and exfoliative cytology material will be examined by the pathologist. When a growth is malignant certain terms are used. Anaplastic means that cell division has been rapid. Another term used in this connection is undifferentiated which means that cells are very poorly formed and bear little or no resemblance to the cells from which they arose. They are more malignant than a growth in which the cells are well differentiated and more like the cells of origin. It can be compared to drawing a square with a pencil on paper. The normal accurate square is drawn with a ruler—normal cells—it takes time. Drawn more hurriedly without a ruler but joined together it will still resemble a square—well differentiated but not an accurate square. Drawn still more rapidly it may have only two sides and be unjoined—poorly differentiated and anaplastic —rapid and bad.

## TREATMENT

Many methods of treatment are attempted to eradicate the new growth. Radical surgery is justified only when there is a reasonable hope that the growth can be entirely extirpated. Hence, in the presence of secondary deposits beyond the regional lymphatic glands surgery is not usually undertaken.

*Radical treatment*

1. SURGICAL EXCISION consists of removal of the growth and the whole of the area between it and the lymphatic glands, together with the glands themselves. The results are best when the glands are not invaded.

2. RADIOTHERAPY. In certain sites, such as the tongue, where the mutilation of surgical excision is very great, this method is usually employed. In this particular growth it is quite as effective as operation. Radiations act by destruction of the cancer cells.

3. CRYOTHERAPY is the destruction of living tissue by cold. The fundamental premise of cryodestructive surgery is that the living cells are first injured and later die from the results of freezing. A machine circulates liquid nitrogen through a partially insulated probe. A cryolesion is produced around a central freezing point.

The majority of skin tumours, benign  and malignant, are best treated in this way. Postoperatively a slight haemorrhagic ooze may accompany the thawing process but ceases within a few hours. This may be followed by blister formation and subsequently by an eschar. This separates after several weeks and epithelialises.

*Palliative treatment*

1. RADIOTHERAPY is frequently of value in causing retrogression and, in the advanced case, may delay deterioration. In the presence of gross sepsis, however, it is not satisfactory, because the tumour is more resistant and infection may flare up. Radiotherapy is also a satisfactory method of relieving pain from secondary deposits in bone.

2. SURGERY. Palliative operations are frequently undertaken to relieve symptoms such as obstruction.

The duty of a doctor or nurse is to relieve suffering, and, although we may not be able to cure the patient of his disease, the treatment of his symptoms is all-important to him.

3. ADRENALECTOMY AND GONADECTOMY for carcinoma of the breast or prostate.

4. HORMONAL ANTIDOTES are still in the process of development. Prostatic cancer is treated with stilboestrol (5 mg t.d.s.) taken orally, and carcinoma of the breast in the male or elderly women by Ethinyl oestradiol 1 mg t.d.s.

5. CYTOTOXIC AGENTS also destroy bone marrow and the epithelium of the gastrointestinal tract—an effect which is put

to therapeutic use in the treatment of the leukaemias. The concentration of the drug at the tumour site is increased by:

(a) Injection into a malignant effusion.
(b) Injection into an artery supplying the tumour. (Regional perfusion.)
(c) Intravenous injection depending on the blood count.

Side-effects include leucopenia, diminution in platelets, alopecia, haematuria and nausea. The principal cytotoxic agents used clinically are methotrexate, cyclophosphamide and thiotepa.

Cytotoxic agents such as phenyl alanine mustard (PAM) for melanomas or nitrogen mustard for Hodgkin's disease are sometimes of value. They postpone death rather than cure the disease but methotrexate is usually a complete cure for chorion epithelioma. Other agents which are used are urethane for the leukaemias, and the folic acid antagonists, of which the most powerful is aminopterin, 1 mg daily. A short sharp dose of four drugs—quadruple therapy—may be used. One of the many group of drugs is:

Vinblastin
Prednisolone
Nitrogen mustard
Procarbazine.

*Local perfusion.* Nitrogen mustard or methotrexate destroy malignant tissue but also destroy blood-forming tissue. If the local concentration could be increased without the same high concentration escaping into the general circulation a better response could be anticipated. This is now possible by occluding the artery and vein supplying the part, cannulating the artery in a distal direction and joining the local circulation to an extracorporeal machine. The bone marrow may be removed to prevent damage from the nitrogen mustard, stored and later replaced.


## GENERAL NURSING CARE

The special treatment of new growths at their various sites is fully described in the chapters on systematic surgery, but we must consider briefly some general principles in the nursing care of patients suffering from malignant disease.

A nurse must never disclose to a patient that he is suffering from cancer. This does not mean that it can or should be always concealed, but this has to be considered carefully by all concerned in the treatment of the patient. Relatives should, of course, be informed, and if a severe operation or intensive radiotherapy is contemplated, the nature of the treatment and the risks should be explained to them simply and clearly. They form a useful link after the patient has left the hospital apparently cured, in encouraging him to return for examination for recurrences which may still be treatable.

The general body health must be improved as much as possible by good food, vitamins, and iron tonics. Blood transfusion is given if necessary. A tactful, cheerful nurse can do much to reduce mental trauma resulting from the necessary mutilation of operations for removal of new growths.

Special points of importance in the preoperative preparation are:

1. SEPSIS, IF PRESENT, MUST BE REDUCED OR ELIMINATED. An area of sepsis in a new growth encourages lymphatic drainage and spreads the growth. The mouth must be cleansed in a case of carcinoma of the tongue, and in cases of skin cancer an infected ulcer must be rendered as clean as possible by dressings. For growths of the colon, succinylsulphathiazole, (sulfasuxidine), phthalysulphathiazole or neomycin by mouth and enemas reduce bacterial contamination.

In the case of a patient suffering from carcinoma of the bladder, urinary antiseptics and bladder washouts are necessary if the urine is infected and render operation or radiotherapy very much safer. Antibiotics and the sulphonamide drugs will frequently be prescribed systemically to achieve the same object.

2. ADEQUATE REST FOR THE AFFECTED PART, and also for the body in general.


## RADIOTHERAPY

As the name implies, treatment by radiation includes radium, 'X-irradiation', and radioactive isotopes.

The aim of radiotherapy is either:

1. Radical to cure the disease.
2. Palliative to relieve a symptom such as the pain of a bony metastasis, dysphagia in carcinoma of the oesophagus or bleeding from a carcinoma of the uterus.

RADIUM

Radium emits several rays—alpha and beta particles, and gamma rays. Only gamma rays are used in the treatment of cancer.

The radium salt is enclosed in a platinum needle, the platinum absorbing the alpha and beta particles, which are highly damaging to the tissues.

*Application of radium*

Radium may be employed as:

1. INTERSTITIAL RADIUM. Needles are inserted into the growth and into the area surrounding it. They are left in position for a period of time calculated by the radiotherapist. The exact position of the needles is determined by the physicist.

2. SURFACE RADIUM. The needles are placed in a mould which is applied to the surface of the growth. The mould may be made of wax, sorbo, or dental stent.

3. RADON SEEDS. Radon is a gaseous emanation of radium. The seeds are radioactive for about nine days. This form of application is particularly suitable for sites such as the bladder, the parotid gland, the skin, and pharynx. The seeds do not require removal.

4. RADIUM BOMB. This is a machine rather like an X-ray machine. One or 10 g of radium is applied for a period of about two hours at frequent intervals.

5. INTRACAVITARY RADIUM, used in the natural body cavities, for example, in treating carcinoma of the cervix of the uterus.

RADIOTHERAPY (X-IRRADIATION)

Radiotherapy is of value when deep penetration is required and includes:

*Low or medium voltage* X-ray therapy used for superficial growths of the skin and for dermatological conditions.

*High voltage or deep X-ray* therapy used for the larger or more deeply seated malignant conditions.

*Supervoltage or megavoltage* therapy (over 1 million volts) is used in the treatment of deep-seated cancer and has the advan-

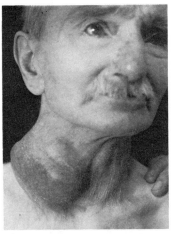

FIG. 22.3  Secondary malignant glands of neck.

tage that it does not produce the severe skin reactions or cause the same degree of constitutional upset so common with high-voltage X-ray therapy. Some growths are more sensitive to ir-radiation in a hyperbaric oxygen chamber.

RADIOACTIVE ISOTOPES

The radioactive isotope is a form of an element which be-haves chemically in the same way as its normal form, but be-cause of a different combination of particles within its nucleus, it is unstable and changes into a different element, releasing energy in the form of X-rays, gamma-rays, alpha and beta particles. The energy released enables them to be used in amounts small enough not to interfere with normal physio-logy and this is also the reason for their use in radiotherapy. They are used in three ways.

1. RESEARCH.

2. DIAGNOSIS. The most widely used is radioactive iodine, which is concentrated in thyroid tissue, and by using a Geiger counter, can outline the thyroid gland and show if any gland tissue lies retrosternally. Scans using special isotopes are now common to outline the kidney, the lungs, the bones, the liver and the pancreas.

3. TREATMENT. (a) Carcinoma of the thyroid—this some-times takes up radioactive iodine and the radioactivity concen-trated in the thyroid kills the carcinoma cells. Metastases from this tumour sometimes take up radioactive iodine. Radioac-tive iodine is also used to treat thyrotoxicosis.

(b) Multiple myelomatosis—radioactive phosophorus $^{32}P$ is injected intravenously and concentrates in bones.

(c) Caesium or cobalt is used as a beam in place of deep X-rays.

(d) Gold, injected into pleural and peritoneal fluid, com-monly abolishes the fluid, but does not cure the disease. It is a palliative treatment.

(e) Yttrium or preferably radioactive gold is implanted into the pituitary—this procedure has the same effect in breast car-cinoma as adrenalectomy, but can be used after adrenalec-tomy has failed.

All the substances actually injected into the body have a short life and the patient is not 'radioactive' for long. Also they are very local in their effects and other people can be in contact with them in safety.

Faeces and urine may need to be stored in protected con-tainers until any radioactivity in them has diminished to a minimal quantity. This usually takes only a few days; then the excreta can be emptied into the drains in the usual way.

*The mode of action of radiations.* The gamma rays or X-rays destroy cells which are about to divide. Cancer cells divide frequently, hence the more rapidly growing the tumour the more radiosensitive it is likely to be. Some damage to the skin and tissues is inevitable with radical radiotherapy, and this is known as a 'radiation reaction'.

*The care of the patient undergoing radium treatment*

Radical radiotherapy gives rise to general and local reactions.

GENERAL REACTION may consist of nausea and general malaise. From its effect on the blood system anaemia and leucopaenia may develop.

CARE OF THE RADIUM APPLICATION LOCALLY. The nurse must see that the radium does not slip out of place and must report any mishap at once. Loss of radium is prevented by keeping the patient in bed with a special sign, such as a large red 'R' hung over the bed to indicate that radium is being used. All dressings, etc. should be kept in a special bucket until the radium has been removed from the patient and the needles counted and found correct. All excreta are preserved while there is radium in her body and inspected before disposal.

PREPARATION OF THE SKIN. Only pure surgical spirit should be used for the preparation of the skin before the application or insertion of radium. Metallic substances which give off secondary radiations should not be used. These include pins, strapping, metallic chains, metallic lotions and ointments.

**Local reaction (radiation reaction)**

*On the intact skin* radium produces a painful erythema which, if severe, may lead to an indurated area of cellulitis. The stages are:

1. Erythema.
2. Dry desquamation.
3. Moist desquamation.

*On the surface of the growth,* for example, carcinoma of the tongue. Since the tissue is destroyed and some degree of infection is inevitably present, sloughing results.

Sepsis is controlled by antibiotics. The tongue is kept still by avoiding unnecessary speech and a pad and pencil should be provided. If a severe reaction develops a careful watch must be kept for secondary haemorrhage.

*Local disabilities induced by radiotherapy.* Damage which may occur from radiation includes:

1. Renal damage may develop following abdominal radiation and may induce acute or chronic nephritis followed about a year later by hypertension.
2. Osteoporosis may result in fracture after radiation of the cervical spine.

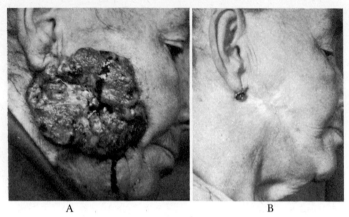

FIG. 22.4    Effect of radium. A, Squamous-celled carcinoma of cheek before treatment. B, Same case after treatment.

3. Radiation pneumonitis is a possible complication of radiotherapy to the breast.
4. Myelitis of the cervical spinal cord may arise from radiotherapy in the neck.
5. Damage to the rectum and sigmoid colon may occur after radiation to the cervix.
6. Fistula and perforation may occur from radiation necrosis.

All these local complications are diminished by improved techniques.

OCCUPATIONAL THERAPY AND REHABILITATION. The patient must be kept occupied while in hospital. Light work like rug making helps to pass away the time and take the patient's mind off his illness. The follow-up of patients suffering from cancer is important to the patient because recurrences are frequently treatable. It is also important to the hospital, so that the end results of treatment may be studied and correlated.

*Protection of the nursing staff*

Radium and X-rays are powerful poisons and sources of danger to the health of the nursing staff if adequate precautions are not taken. The nurse must not handle radium with the fingers. The nurse should not expose herself unnecessarily to radium, and the staff attending radium cases should be changed frequently and should wear small badges to indicate the level of radiation to which they have been exposed and should be tested regularly. A blood count should be performed every three months to detect early damage to the nurse's health.

## THE TREATMENT OF SYMPTOMS OF PATIENTS WHO ARE INOPERABLE

The treatment of inoperable cases is usually carried out away from an acute general hospital. It is nonetheless important from the nursing point of view; in fact, such patients call for the highest nursing skill.

1. GENERAL ATTITUDE TO THESE PATIENTS. Kindness, widespread human sympathy, and skill are called for in the highest degree in dealing with these patients in their misfortune. True, the end-result is death, but the good nurse must remember that her efforts and skill have not been wasted. Occasionally she will find that the patient who has been diagnosed as suffering from cancer lives on. The diagnosis has been mistaken, and an inflammatory lesion may have simulated a new growth. She will be abundantly rewarded when she finds that she has kept the patient in good spirits and fair health to enjoy, perhaps, many further years of useful life. A day will dawn when cancer will be as submissive to correct treatment as so many other hopeless diseases, which, in the past, have been brought into the field of certain cure.

2. ATTENTION TO PALLIATIVE MECHANISMS performed for the relief of symptoms, such as colostomy, must be scrupulously correct.

3. ATTENTION TO HYGIENE AND GENERAL NURSING, such as the care of pressure areas, must be faithfully observed.

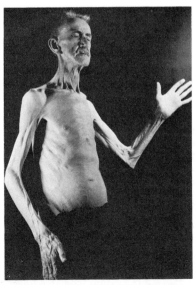

FIG. 22.5 Emaciation of the last stages of malignant disease.

4. THE RELIEF OF PAIN usually demands analgesic and narcotic drugs in ever-increasing doses, but the dosage should never be increased more than is absolutely necessary. Nerve section is sometimes necessary to relieve pain which is uncontrolled by morphia. For a pelvic growth intrathecal injections of absolute alcohol may be necessary. Radiotherapy is the most effective method of relieving pain due to secondary deposits in bone, but adrenalectomy may be undertaken if these are due to carcinoma of the breast. Anabolic hormones may relieve pain of secondary deposits in bone by preventing decalcification. They also delay metabolic breakdown in the body generally. Chlorpromazine (Largactil) reduces anxiety and is often useful.

5. LOCAL ATTENTION TO THE GROWTH. If the growth is on the surface, sepsis is usually very upsetting to the patient, but frequent dressings will render it less offensive. The use of a deodorant and antiseptic sprays will help to prevent a foul atmosphere in the room.

6. DIET. The diet should be varied, attractive, and, as far as possible, what the patient fancies.

7. OCCUPATIONAL THERAPY within the limits of the patient's strength should be encouraged.

8. The onset of symptoms suggestive of other diseases should be reported at once, since intercurrent disease may set in.

9. The patient should be allowed to do what pleases him, so far as is humanly possible.

10. Visitors should be encouraged. Scrupulous cleanliness, fresh air, clean bed and personal linen daily are most important. An attractive room with a quiet, happy atmosphere is ideal.

# CHAPTER 23

# Diseases of the Peripheral Arteries and Gangrene

The treatment of injuries has been fully considered in the chapter on haemorrhage.

Arteriosclerosis (hardening of the arteries) is a very common condition and is an important cause of senile gangrene. Much information about its nature and effect may be obtained by performing an arteriogram. In this procedure a radio-opaque solution is injected into the vessel to be examined and a series of radiographs is taken very rapidly because the blood flow in an artery carries it away quickly.

The needle for the intra-arterial injection is inserted into the artery percutaneously, or by a catheter inserted into the vessel after operative exposure.

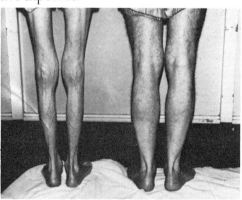

FIG. 23.1   Legs of old age showing absorption of the muscle mass due to the diminishing blood supply. Legs of youth showing good muscles.

## ANEURYSMS

An aneurysm is the bulging of a portion of a blood vessel wall. It may be due to damage by trauma, but more commonly it is due to atheroma. The condition is similar to the ballooning which may occur in the weakened wall of a rubber tyre, and sudden torrential haemorrhage will accompany a rupture of its wall. In the limbs and at the root of the neck ligation of the vessel is usually performed. The most common site, unfortunately, is the abdominal aorta, usually below the level of origin of the renal arteries, where ligation is not feasible but excision and grafting may be possible. Postoperatively the pulses in the arteries of the leg are carefully noted and the systemic blood pressure is recorded half-hourly. Anticoagulant therapy is prescribed by the surgeon.

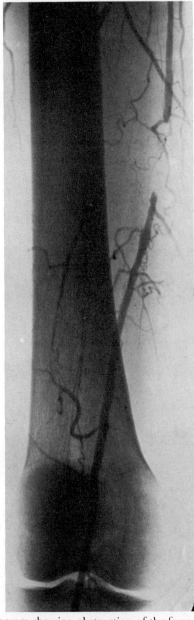

FIG. 23.2   Arteriogram showing obstruction of the femoral artery and path taken by the blood flow in collateral vessels.

## TUMOURS

Tumours of blood vessels are common. Many of these disappear spontaneously and a period of observation in infancy is always advisable before recommending active treatment. The capillary naevus, or haemangioma, is frequently seen in children and is treated if necessary by the application of carbon dioxide snow, or by excision. Cavernous haemangiomas are spongy tumours of veins, while pulsating tumours composed of arterioles are known as cirsoid aneurysms.

## PERIPHERAL ARTERIAL OBSTRUCTION

Vascular insufficiency is a common condition in the limbs and may be caused by pressure outside an artery, disease in the wall of the artery, blockage or partial blockage of the lumen. The changes may be sudden in onset or slow and progressive. The lesions which may give rise to this condition are many and varied and it is now usual to classify all these under the heading of—

### Vascular obliterative diseases

These may be sudden in onset due to an embolus or the ill effects of a ligature or tourniquet. The more gradual progressive form is usually due to arteriosclerosis.

*Symptoms and signs of arterial insufficiency*

1. CLAUDICATION. The patient complains of cramp-like pain, particularly in the calf, on walking.

2. REST PAIN is a symptom of very severe arterial occlusion. It is sometimes so severe that the patient is unable to sleep and hangs his foot over the end of the bed to get relief.

3. NUTRITIONAL CHANGES. The toes or finger-tips become insensitive, flaky and hard and the interdigital clefts become moist. There may be loss of hair and the muscles show wasting. If both legs are raised, the skin of the affected foot will blanch first. Recurrent infection may develop, and later, signs of frank gangrene, which may be wet or dry, will develop.

4. THE PULSES. In addition to palpating the pulses at the foot, the abdomen should be palpated for the presence of an aneurysm.

The gangrene will be dry if:

(a) The veins returning the blood to the heart are healthy, so that there is no water-logging (oedema of the part).

(b) The part is exposed to the air so that evaporation can occur.

(c) There is no infection.

Otherwise a wet gangrene will develop.

*Treatment of peripheral vascular insufficiency*

It should be made clear to the patient once this condition develops that his feet are now more precious than gold. The following measures are important and will delay the onset of gangrene:

1. AVOIDANCE OF INJURY

(a) The patient should not have a hot-water bottle in bed. He should wear loose bed-socks.

(b) During the day warm woollen, seamless socks should be worn and they should be inspected each day to see that there are no holes.

(c) His shoes should be of soft leather and lined with fur or wool.

(d) No garters or suspenders should be worn on the leg.

(e) Nail paring should be performed with great care and nails should be allowed to grow long so that there is no danger of injury to the nail bed (Fig. 23.3).

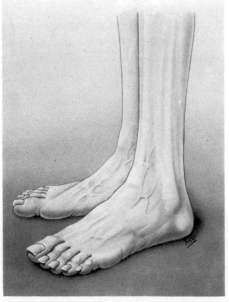

FIG. 23.3    Toe nails must not be cut short. Note the thin wasted limbs so characteristic of arterial insufficiency.

2. DIETETIC AND GENERAL MEASURES

(a) Tobacco must be avoided. This is probably the most important single factor in controlling the disease.

(b) Breathing exercises are of value because they aid the venous return.

(c) Walking should be continued but not to the extent of producing fatigue. The patient may increase his walking distance by learning to walk more slowly.

(d) Anaemia, however slight, is corrected and the blood should be examined at regular intervals to ensure that it is controlled. The volume of blood reaching the extremities is limited, therefore it is all the more important that its quality should not be impaired. In addition, the blood volume should be increased and Rheomacrodex is an excellent plasma expander—it dilates the vessels of the collateral circulation provided they are not affected by atheroma. It is administered intermittently over a period of 24 to 48 hours.

(e) The head of the bed should be raised not more than 20 cm to aid the flow of blood to the limbs.

(f) A diet which is nearly free of cholesterol and saturated fatty acids may be advised. This in practice usually means the avoidance of eggs and butter. It may be helpful in delaying the onset of vascular obliterative disease, but whether it has much effect on established disease is doubtful.

Drugs which cause vasodilatation are contraindicated because the usual cause is a localised patch of atheroma in a large vessel. They tend to dilate all the other vessels in the body, reduce blood pressure in the remaining patent vessels, and in effect reduce the volume of blood reaching the threatened part.

3. CONTROL OF INFECTION

There are infections to which all these points are susceptible. They may be fungoid or pyogenic. In all cases diabetes must be eliminated and if present must be standardised at once.

4. HYPERBARIC OXYGEN CHAMBER

Oxygen administered at two atmospheres for varying periods each day, or until recovery occurs, in acute cases will often save a limb. It increases the small quantity of oxygen which is dissolved in the plasma by more than sixteen times and in a diminishing circulation this may prove decisive in maintaining nutrition of the tissues.

5. SURGICAL MEASURES

These include sympathectomy and, in an occasional case where there is a localised block, the insertion of an arterial or plastic graft. In the upper third of the femoral artery localised blocks are treated by a femoro-popliteal bypass, using the saphenous vein on the same side. Another procedure is to core out the atheromatous lining—this is known as thrombo-endarterectomy. If a graft has been undertaken the patient has to be given anticoagulant therapy indefinitely.

If all these measures fail, gangrene develops, and gangrene always starts in the skin.

## GANGRENE

Gangrene is a condition of gross death of tissue. It may be massive in type, for example, the death of a whole limb; or it may be localised in form, for example, of the finger-tip, a bed sore, or carbuncle.

*Causes of gangrene*

1. LOSS OF BLOOD SUPPLY is the outstanding cause. This may be due to:
   (a) Embolism, or thrombosis, of an artery. Thrombosis formation is always slower than the effect from an embolus which is sudden and rapid.
   (b) Immobilisation of a limb in a plaster which is too tight.
   (c) Arteriosclerosis. The walls of the arteries are hardened and thickened and their lumen is diminished in calibre. A small patch of advancing atheroma readily obstructs a vessel in this condition.
   (d) Raynaud's disease—a disease which causes severe spasm of the small arteries.
   (e) Ergot poisoning, which produces spasm of the vessel with resultant diminution in the quantity of blood supplied to the area.
   (f) Thromboangiitis obliterans.
   (g) A tourniquet.
   (h) Thiopentone or similar drugs injected intra-arterially.
2. CHEMICAL OR PHYSICAL VIOLENCE
   (a) Carbolic acid burn.
   (b) Severe frost-bite.
   (c) Burns and scalds which may char the whole limb.
   (d) X-rays or radium.
3. INFECTION—*Gas gangrene* (p. 72).

Gangrene, apart from gas gangrene, can be of two types:

(a) *Moist.* The tissues are moist and infection spreads rapidly. Toxins are absorbed in the tissues which are still alive near to the gangrenous area. If the gangrene is moist, the area must be treated as a septic wound and amputation is usually undertaken as soon as the threat to life is apparent.
(b) *Dry.* This form is usually vascular in origin and the spread is slow. *So long as the part is kept dry*, the gangrenous portion may separate at a 'line of demarcation' where the blood supply is adequate.

The common clinical types of gangrene are:

Acute gangrene
Gas gangrene
Senile gangrene
Diabetic gangrene
Localised gangrene: (a) a carbuncle; (b) a bed sore
Raynaud's disease and thromboangiitis obliterans.

1. **Acute gangrene.** The commonest cause is the lodgement of an embolus at the bifurcation of the main vessel of the limb. The patient will probably be suffering from heart disease, and the heart itself is usually the origin of the clot.

*Symptoms and signs*

The patient suddenly develops severe cramp-like pain in the limb. The pain soon passes off, but the limb is insensitive and the patient is unable to move it. It is cold, pale at first and later blue in appearance and the local pulse is absent.

*Treatment*

Anticoagulant therapy is commenced at once. It may diminish the worst effects of the clot and prevent the common complication of a further embolus in another limb. As soon as possible the embolus is removed using a Fogarty's catheter. Postoperatively anticoagulant therapy is continued but, because of the risk of bleeding, this has to be carefully controlled. The peripheral pulses are palpated regularly to ensure the blood flow is satisfactory.

2. **Gas gangrene.** This condition has been fully discussed in Chapter 9.

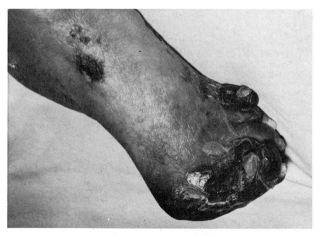

FIG. 23.4   Gangrene of feet.

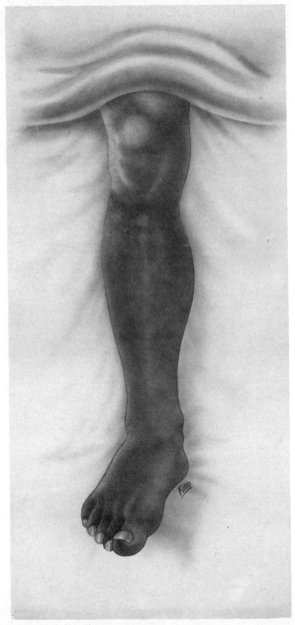

FIG. 23.5   Embolic gangrene.

3. **Senile gangrene.** This is an important condition, and will be seen with increasing frequency as our population ages. The patient is suffering from arteriosclerosis, which results in dim-

inution of the blood supply to the extremities. As a result a trivial injury, commonly a slip whilst paring the toe nails or corns, commences the gangrenous process. Pain is always severe if the limb is elevated.

CLINICAL FEATURES. The gangrenous part is cold and blue in the early stages. Later it is black, cold, insensitive and dry, unless infection has supervened.

*Treatment*

The principles of treatment are:

(a) To keep the limb cool so that its metabolism is diminished in a case of threatened gangrene. If the metabolic rate is low the limb can survive on the reduced quantity of oxygen available. The use of a fan may be desirable.

(b) To keep the affected part dry; this is often best achieved by exposing the part to the air without a dressing. The area is often mopped over with methylated spirit and any moist area is painted with gentian violet 1 per cent in spirit. Toes are kept separated with dental rolls. Pressure on the heel should be avoided and foam wedges and pads should be used.

(c) Removal of the sympathetic nerve chain results in vasodilatation of the collateral blood vessels and improves the blood supply of the skin in certain cases.

(d) Amputation of the limb at a point where the blood supply is adequate when the gangrene threatens the patient's life.

(e) Prevention of infection. Antibiotics may be prescribed, but may not be of value because they usually fail to reach the ischaemic part.

(f) To protect the limb Leonard (foam) pads are used.

NURSING CARE

These patients make great demands on the nurse's skill. Pressure is avoided around the gangrenous part. If the gangrene is dry, no dressing is applied and the limb is protected from the bedclothes by a bed cage. Since the blood supply is poor, the heel is very likely to ulcerate unless great care is taken to protect it from pressure. Heel rings are inadvisable because the heel still receives pressure from the inner circle of the ring. The patient should be nursed with the head of his bed elevated 20 cm.

Although vasodilators are contraindicated (p. 229) quinalbarbitone 90 mg is a barbiturate which may be given. It promotes vasodilatation which gives a sense of warmth and enables the patient to get ready for sleep. It also relieves pain, as does DF118 (dihydrocodeine).

4. **Diabetic gangrene.** Arteriosclerosis is a common condition in elderly diabetic subjects. Peripheral neuritis, which

renders the patient insensitive to pain and injury, is a common complication of diabetes mellitus; the result is that the patient may injure his tissues quite painlessly. Tissues saturated in sugar are an ideal medium for the proliferation of most bacteria, with the result that moist gangrene is an early complication.

*Treatment*

Gangrene is a very serious complication in a diabetic patient. The diabetes must be stabilised in co-operation with a physician. The septic area must be dressed, and as soon as the patient is fit amputation will usually be necessary.

5. **Localised gangrene** (p. 204).

6. **Raynaud's disease and thromboangiitis obliterans.** Division of the sympathetic chain which supplies the affected vessels is frequently undertaken to relieve pain and prevent the onset of gangrene.

In the case of the upper limb the operation is performed on the cervical portion of the chain. The skin over the neck, axilla, and back and front of the chest should be prepared. In affections of the lower limbs the lumbar sympathetic chain is divided and the area prepared is similar to that for an operation on the kidney.

The sympathetic nerves are sometimes temporarily anaesthetised with a local anaesthetic in the cervical region or a spinal anaesthetic in the lumbar region, to gauge what effect operation may have.

## AMPUTATIONS

An amputation may be indicated for:

1. **Trauma.** If the main vessels and nerves have been irreparably damaged or ruptured an amputation is necessary. Hopelessly mangled and lacerated tissues may also be an indication for amputation.

2. **Gangrene.**

3. **Malignant new growths.**

Seventy per cent of all amputations performed are on patients over 70 years of age.

All amputations for senile gangrene should have the skin prepared as described on p. 73, and all should have intramuscular penicillin for ten days from the moment of amputation. These measures are necessary to prevent gas gangrene in the amputation stump.

*Immediate after-treatment of an amputation includes:*

1. The treatment of acute circulatory failure.
2. The avoidance of injury to the stump.

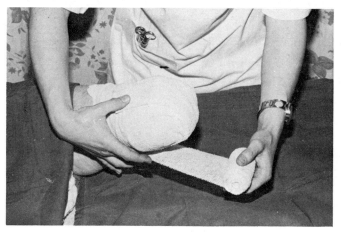

FIG. 23.6    Bandaging amputation stump.

3. The removal of a drainage tube, if one has been inserted, after 48 hours and the care of suction drainage if this has been used.
4. The removal of sutures about the tenth day.

## Complications

1. Reactionary haemorrhage in the first 12 hours.
2. Secondary haemorrhage (7–10 days). The presence of a small speck of blood on the dressing is the first warning of this complication and should be reported at once.
3. Infection, which may be associated with disease in the bone.
4. Phantom pains. The patient still complains of pain in the foot or hand which has been amputated, but in time this usually passes off.
5. Amputation neuroma—in which the cut nerve end forms into a small painful swelling.

*Care of the stump*

1. NO PILLOW should be placed behind the stump or flexion deformity will develop and make the fitting of an artificial limb more difficult.
2. THE BED is arranged so that the stump is in constant view in case haemorrhage should occur.
3. FROM THE FIRST DAY the stump must be wrapped in crêpe bandages or Flexoplast. It is now thought that the stump should be bulbous rather than conical for the modern prosthesis.
4. EXERCISE. The patient should be encouraged to put his joint through a full range of movements from the second day.

This is particularly important following mid-thigh amputation. The patient must turn on to the side opposite to the amputation and move the stump backwards (i.e. extension of the hip-joint). If this is not done when he is upright the stump will be pointing forwards.

5. AS SOON AS THE PATIENT is fit to be mobile out of bed he must be supplied with well-fitting crutches. Unless the crutches are of the correct size he will be liable to develop paralysis of the nerves of his arm from pressure on the nerves under the axilla.

6. MEASUREMENT OF THE CRUTCH. When held upright, the crutch should not reach higher than two fingers below the anterior axillary fold of the patient's armpit.

If for any reason the patient is in bed suffering from another illness and not wearing his artificial leg for more than two days, the stump should be bound. Otherwise it will swell and will not fit the artificial limb.

CHAPTER 24

# Varicose Veins

Varicosity of the superficial veins of the leg is a common condition. The great majority of cases are due to a primary defect in the valves of the veins themselves. A hereditary tendency is quite noticeable. Occasionally they develop as a result of an intra-abdominal new growth, or may, of course, be secondary to a previous deep vein thrombosis. Varicose veins which occur during pregnancy are produced by the relaxing effect of progesterone on the vein walls and the increased venous return from the uterus impeding the venous return from the lower limbs. If the foetus dies *in utero* the varicosities improve.

Untreated, the veins increase in size and extent and the skin, particularly in the neighbourhood of the internal malleolus of the ankle, becomes thin and pigmented. Later, ulceration may occur. A varicose ulcer incapacitates the patient greatly owing to its tendency to heal extremely slowly.

*Symptoms and signs*

Small varicose veins give rise to no symptoms, but some patients object to the slight cosmetic disfigurement. As they pro-

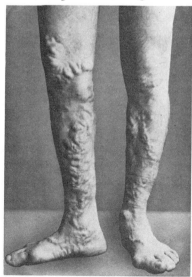

Fig. 24.1   Varicose veins.

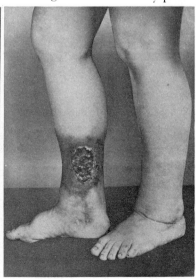

Fig. 24.2   Varicose ulcer.

gress, the veins are more prominent towards the end of the day and give rise to a feeling of heaviness in the legs. Inflammation and ulceration cause pain.

*Treatment*

Early cases are treated by injection, which effects obliteration in the blood vessel. A large variety of sclerosing solutions are available, and the surgeon will usually have his own preference.

By a combination of injecting all the communicating vessels and firm bandaging Fegan has treated quite large varicose veins without operation.

OPERATIVE TREATMENT

In cases where there is total incompetence of the veins, operation will usually be advised. This consists of ligation, always at the saphenous opening in the groin and usually along the course of the vein as well. *The skin of the whole leg, and also that of the suprapubic area and groin is prepared.* In the presence of enlarged glands in the groin, as a result of phlebitis, operation must be deferred until subsidence is complete, for fear that the wound may suppurate. As an alternative to ligation, excision or stripping of the vein may be performed. The vein and particularly the site of communicating veins between the superficial and deep veins are marked on the skin with a skin pencil or gentian violet paint. The limb must be firmly bound at the end of this operation to prevent widespread bruising. Whatever operation is performed, firm supportive bandages, blue line bandages, or elastic stockings should be worn for at least a month. A careful watch should be made for any allergic reactions to elastic stockings, adhesive pads or strappings. Any small venules which are then obvious have to be injected. Because of the increased risk of thrombosis postoperatively, a woman should cease taking contraceptive pills eight weeks before the operation.

### COMPLICATIONS OF VARICOSE VEINS
### AND THEIR TREATMENT

1. **Phlebitis.** Phlebitis or inflammation may follow slight trauma.

*Treatment*

The pain in the limb may be relieved by the application of lead and opium lotion, and an antibacterial drug may be administered systemically. Should suppuration occur, incision of the resulting abscess may be necessary. It is very rare for embolism to occur from a varicose vein. Alternatively the clot can be prevented spreading upwards by pads of adhesive sponge. The limb is then firmly bandaged from below upwards with Elastoplast and the patient is encouraged to walk about. In some cases anticoagulant therapy may be instituted. Rapid phlebitis extending towards the groin may require flush saphenofemoral ligation urgently.

2. **Haemorrhage** may be profuse if the vein is torn, and the first-aid treatment is to elevate the limb. Firm pressure and an antiseptic dressing are all that is necessary otherwise. If haemorrhage is excessive, however, hospital care is necessary and a blood transfusion may be advisable.

3. **Ulceration**
*Treatment*
The first and most important step in severe cases of ulceration is to confine the patient to bed and elevate the whole leg. If the ulcer is very septic it is cleansed by means of repeated dressings of eusol compresses. As healing occurs this may be replaced by petroleum jelly gauze. The patient is allowed to resume his normal work, and the limb must be encased in Elastoplast to give the necessary support to the veins. The bandage extends from the front of the foot to just below the knee. Discharge from the ulcer seeps through the Elastoplast, but the dressing is not changed for six or seven days.

Before its application the limb is shaved and a stirrup of 7·5 cm Elastoplast is applied.

The alternative method is to use a terracortril spray or Noxyflex applied daily through a window cut in an occlusive bandage now used with great effect. Aserbine cream or lotion used in a similar way is also effective.

If the foot becomes swollen the patient is confined to bed for 24 hours without a bandage. Before getting up the supportive bandage is again applied. This is important in all conditions in which the foot becomes oedematous on walking.

Later, surgical treatment of the veins in the form of Cockett's operation, which is a subfascial ligation of the perforating veins between the varicose veins and the deep veins, is undertaken. Occasionally a skin graft is necessary. Malignant change is a possible complication in an ulcer of long-standing.

# CHAPTER 25

# The Nature of Disease

Disease processes such as infection, haemorrhage, fluid loss and new growth have already been considered. Chapter 43 is devoted to severe congenital diseases in the newborn and in many subsequent chapters other significant congenital anomalies are described.

The causes of disease are of fundamental importance. The clinical picture as revealed by signs and symptoms has to be known if it is to be recognised and the correct treatment undertaken. Changes which result from disease have one or more of the following effects:

1. *Tissue destruction.* When it is gross it is known as gangrene or putrefaction; lesser degrees of destruction are termed necrosis.

2. *Obstruction* is a common cause or result of disease. Lesions occur in far dispersed sites in the body which have little or nothing in common aetiologically yet they share an identical, simple mechanical process. It is more likely to occur in the narrowest part of an organ or duct. Some of these sites are illustrated in Fig. 25.1.

Loss or diminution of blood supply is due to obstructive changes in the blood vessel walls or the valves of the heart. Solidification of normal contents in other channels results in stone formation in the biliary or urinary tract whilst the same process in the blood is called thrombosis. In addition to disease of the wall and obstruction of the lumen the whole organ may be compressed by pressure from without.

3. *Fluid leakage.* Fluid loss may be in a gross clinically perceptible form such as occurs in haemorrhage, perforation, ascites, burns, diarrhoea, vomiting or only in a more delicate physicochemical sense of change between the extracellular spaces and the blood.

4. *Degeneration.* The tissues wear out.

5. *Hormonal excess or inadequacy.*

In any illness an assessment has to be made of the nature of the changes produced.

## ANATOMICAL NARROWS

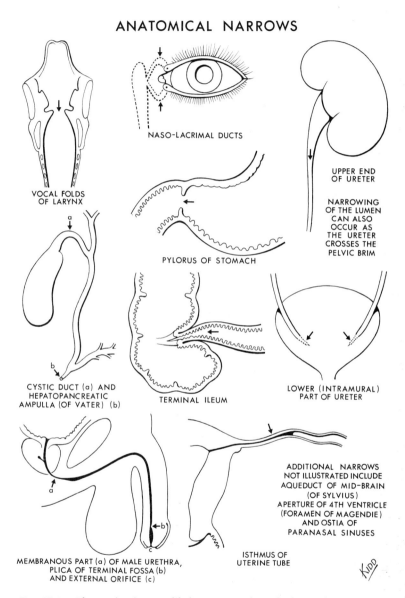

VOCAL FOLDS
OF LARYNX

NASO-LACRIMAL DUCTS

PYLORUS OF STOMACH

UPPER END
OF URETER

NARROWING
OF THE LUMEN
CAN ALSO
OCCUR AS
THE URETER
CROSSES THE
PELVIC BRIM

CYSTIC DUCT (a) AND
HEPATOPANCREATIC
AMPULLA (OF VATER) (b)

TERMINAL ILEUM

LOWER (INTRAMURAL)
PART OF URETER

MEMBRANOUS PART (a) OF MALE URETHRA,
PLICA OF TERMINAL FOSSA (b)
AND EXTERNAL ORIFICE (c)

ISTHMUS OF
UTERINE TUBE

ADDITIONAL NARROWS
NOT ILLUSTRATED INCLUDE
AQUEDUCT OF MID-BRAIN
(OF SYLVIUS)
APERTURE OF 4TH VENTRICLE
(FORAMEN OF MAGENDIE)
AND OSTIA OF
PARANASAL SINUSES

FIG. 25.1   Obstruction is more likely to occur where the lumen is narrowest.

## THE NATURE OF THE CHANGES PRODUCED

The following are a few examples of these processes:

(i) A small wound causes fluid leakage due to haemorrhage and fluid leakage occurs from the inflammatory
reaction in healing;

(ii) a 30 per cent burn causes fluid leakage and tissue destruction;

(iii) in a strangulated hernia containing a loop of small intestine the blood vessels to the bowel are obstructed
and the flow of intestinal contents along the lumen of
the intestine is prevented.

### THE DEGREE OR SEVERITY OF THE CHANGE

Taking the above examples—

(i) is usually completely trivial;

(ii) requires immediate and urgent treatment of the extensive fluid loss if the patient is to survive;

(iii) unless there is immediate surgical relief the patient will
die.

If the normal vital reactions (p. 243) of the body can restore
health no special treatment is required. If these reactions are
overwhelmed treatment is necessary.

Health is the preservation of a constant internal environment in the body. Small changes in this environment—the
'milieu intérieur' of Claude Bernard—produce reactions which
restore this state. Living cells apart from those of the skin are
provided with a fluid environment, with a constant hydrogen
ion concentration, osmotic pressure and temperature. Oxygen
and food are carried to the cells by the arterial blood which is
oxygenated in the lungs and waste products including carbon
dioxide removed by the venous blood and the lymphatic system to be eliminated by the lungs and the kidneys. The whole
process is regulated by the activities of the hormones and the
nervous system. Cannon named this restoration of a constant
environment 'homeostasis'.

Many diseases produce a state in which these reactions are
strained or severely threatened and unless efforts are successful in recreating conditions in which it is possible for the body
to readjust the patient will lose his life. Treatment must be
based on measures which logically assist these reactions and it
is very easy to aggravate the patient's condition by well mean-
ing but thoughtless action. For example, it is not so very long
ago that heat in the form of hot water bottles and radiant heat
cradles which appear so comforting in the management of the
shocked patient were used routinely. They forced dilatation of
the skin vessels which the physiological reaction was trying to

constrict to maintain the blood pressure as well as to retain fluid in the body and provide as much blood as possible to the vital centres within the brain (p. 136).

The measurement of the pulse, temperature and respiration are routine checks on the physiological state of the patient, but in serious conditions many more parameters of the body's activities have to be checked—the arterial blood pressure, the central venous pressure, the blood gases, the serum electrolytes, to mention only a few examples. Since the patient's condition is changing rapidly many tests have to be repeated at frequent intervals. In many cases a continuous check—monitoring—is essential. It is for this reason that a patient who requires such observation is nursed in an intensive care unit (p. 179).

Man has survived much injury and disease from Adam to the present day without the help of antibiotics, extensive resuscitative measures and all the other facilities of modern medicine, including the social services. It is but a few years ago that the pulse, arterial blood pressure, temperature, blood haemoglobin and the blood urea were the only physical and chemical measurements of his well-being. To understand what we are really trying to do to help the patient it is worth considering very briefly what vital reactions occur in the patient's body, all of which are designed for his survival. It is the study of these in depth that has enabled considerable progress to be made in the care of the patient.

VITAL REACTIONS

1. *Haemostasis* has been considered in detail on page 111. It is a natural reaction and, however large or small the haemorrhage, it is essential in controlling bleeding. Detailed study of its mechanism has enabled us to make good deficiencies of clotting factors as well as to prevent or disperse undesirable thrombus formation. Blood transfusion has saved the lives of patients whose blood loss has been too rapid and too great to be overcome by the body.

2. *The reaction to injury* explains how the body takes special precautions to conserve vital fluid and electrolytes when it is assaulted by injury, using the term 'injury' in the widest sense of physical trauma or bacterial invasion. The immediate changes are:

(a) Increased secretion of antidiuretic hormone by the pituitary. The result is that water is conserved in the body. The kidney secretes a highly concentrated urine of high specific gravity. The volume is small so that what fluid is lost as urine is used to the greatest advantage to remove the maximal quantity of waste products.

(b) *The adrenal glands* secrete large quantities of aldoste-

THE EFFECT OF A SEVERE HAEMORRHAGE

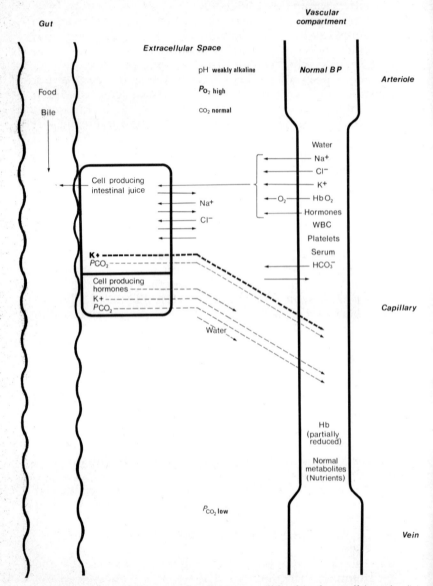

FIG. 25.2    Some of the normal exchanges at cell level in the small intestine in health (see text). K⁺ and Na⁺ pass freely across the cell membrane, $CO_2$ is excreted. Intestinal juice is produced and intestinal hormones are secreted and carried away in the venous blood.

FROM ANYWHERE IN THE BODY ON THE SAME CELLS

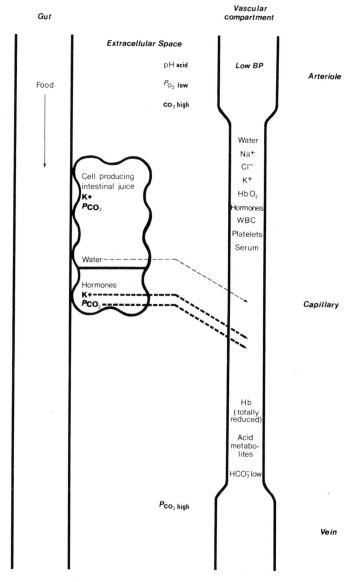

FIG. 25.3   The effect of a severe haemorrhage. The cell is denied oxygen and nourishment. Water is withdrawn from the extracellular space and ultimately from the cell. $CO_2$ first accumulates in excess in the cell in the extracellular space and in the venous blood.

rone which has the effect of retaining Na$^+$ in the body; K$^+$ is increased in quantity from the breakdown of protein tissue and an excess which is very toxic is freely excreted by the kidneys in larger quantities than normal. These changes are reversed when the body commences to rebuild—Na$^+$ is freely excreted and K$^+$ necessary for the building up of cells is retained.

There are many other reactions but the above are examples of the types of changes which occur.

3. *The inflammatory reaction* (p. 63) has already been discussed (p. 65) and the failure to occur may be fatal (p. 49).

4. *Physiological changes* in fluid loss, whether of whole blood, water, plasma or electrolytes (p. 49).

5. *Immunological reactions* generally so beneficial but a fuller understanding is necessary to treat and prevent organ rejection.

6. *Psychological reactions to disease* are important to the surgical nurse and the surgeon in the management of the patient and his disease.

All these vital reactions occur in and around a living cell in a fluid medium. The one essential is an adequate supply of blood and efficient venous drainage. Figure 25.2 illustrates in simplified diagrammatic form how the normal mechanism operates at the level of a single cell. For the purposes of illustration a single cell in the upper part of the small intestine secreting intestinal juice (succus entericus) is taken as an example and for the purposes of illustration only we shall assume that the adjoining cell secretes the hormone secretin which warns the pancreas that pancreatic juice should be secreted.

Figure 25.3 shows the changes which occur in the cell as a result of depletion of blood volume from haemorrhage anywhere in the body.

The junior nurse may well think—this is all very interesting, but has it any relevance to what she does at the bedside? Indeed it has. For example, it determines many nursing procedures.

1. THE POSITION OF THE PATIENT. It explains why pressure sores may develop and are kept active. The blood supply is compressed and the cell dies. If there is an excess of fluid in a limb from deficient venous drainage raising the limb will help increase the flow of fluid from the leg. When the femoral artery is blocked by an embolus the patient is nursed on the opposite side and not resting on his buttock, so compressing the little blood which could flow in from this area to the leg.

2. THE PREVENTION OF THROMBOSIS. It is obvious that the more dehydrated the patient the greater is the viscosity of the

blood (Fig. 25.3) and the more likely thrombi are to form. The risk of thrombosis is increased if the patient is immobilised or the blood platelets are increased as after splenectomy.

3. CORTICOSTEROID THERAPY by interfering with fluid exchange and causing water retention interferes with normal reactions. It also prevents the adrenal glands from functioning normally and in stress more corticosteroids have to be supplied or the patient will collapse since he is unable to react to injury.

6. THE POORER REACTION OF THE OLDER PATIENT is in large measure due to inadequate blood supply because the vessels are arteriosclerotic. Hormones, immune bodies, white blood corpuscles, and antibiotics are not so easily concentrated where they are required as they are in the younger patient with a better cardiovascular system.

5. ABNORMAL WHITE CELLS are ineffective in infection and the leukaemic patient is unable to deal with invading organisms. Shortage of white cells has a similar effect.

6. INADEQUATE RENAL OR PULMONARY FUNCTION results in a build-up of waste products.

The outstanding lesson that emerges from a study of the changes in disease at the cell level is that the shortest possible time that elapses from deprivation of blood and all the bad things it brings the better it is for health.

CHAPTER 26

# The Lymphatic System and the Spleen

## THE LYMPHATIC GLANDS

Lymph is a tissue fluid which drains by the lymphatic vessels to the lymphatic glands, and is conveyed to the blood stream by the thoracic duct and the right lymphatic duct. The glands (syn-nodes) form a meshwork and filter organisms or any particulate matter, with the result that inflammatory conditions of their substance are fairly common. The lymphatic system has a very important role in immunity.

### INFLAMMATORY CONDITIONS

**Acute lymphadenitis** (inflammation of glands). This is commonly due to an acute septic focus, such as a boil, tonsillitis, or a septic wound.

*Treatment*

The primary cause must be treated. Locally, a counter-irritant relieves pain, and in many cases the infection subsides without very much trouble. Occasionally suppuration occurs and incision and drainage may be necessary.

**Chronic lymphadenitis.** *Tuberculous.* This is now a comparatively rare condition. Resolution usually occurs with rest and antituberculous chemotherapy. If the glandular mass enlarges, excision of the glands is performed. A cold abscess may be aspirated or drainage may be performed and the gland removed by curettage. In the abdomen, tuberculous glands usually heal by calcification, and may give rise to symptoms on account of mechanical interference with the functions of the intestine. In the acute stage tuberculous peritonitis may arise as a result of dissemination in the peritoneal cavity.

*Syphilitic.* In primary syphilis the local lymphatic glands are always enlarged and painless. In secondary syphilis generalised enlargement of the lymphatic glands is the rule. The treatment is that of the causal condition (see p. 78).

**Hodgkin's disease.** Hodgkin's disease is a generalised enlargement of the lymphatic glands and of lymphatic tissue throughout the body. The glands are painless, discrete, and rubbery in consistency. Sooner or later the patient dies from mediastinal compression as the result of enlarged glands in the mediastinum or the thoracic cavity. The glands disappear with X-ray therapy 'like snow before the sun', only to recur at intervals. Nitrogen mustard therapy is used with good effect in most cases, or combined cytotoxic antimetabolite agents.

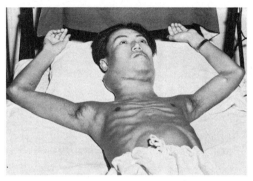

FIG. 26.1    A large mass of lymphadenomatous glands. (Hodgkin's disease.)

**New growths of the glands.** Primary new growths (lymphosarcomas) are rare, but secondary carcinomatous deposits in the lymphatic glands are very common indeed.

**Other causes of glandular enlargement.** In glandular fever and in several blood diseases, notably lymphatic leukaemia, the glands are enlarged. Removal of a single gland for pathological examination (biopsy) is frequently undertaken to determine the cause of the enlargement. The examination of a specimen of bone marrow obtained by puncture of the sternum is undertaken in some cases.

## THE LYMPHATIC VESSELS

1. *Lymphangitis* is common (p. 68).
2. *Lymphatic* obstruction may occur as a result of:

   (a) Invasion of the lymphatic channels by cancer cells (p. 214).
   (b) Invasion by certain organisms, or parasites, e.g. the condition of elephantiasis.
   (c) Surgical removal of regional nodes.

Conditions in which operative interference is possible are rare.

## THE SPLEEN

Closely allied to the lymphatic system is the spleen, and it is frequently enlarged in lymphatic tissue diseases. It is commonly

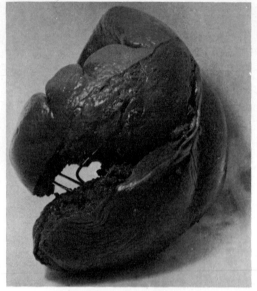

FIG. 26.2  Ruptured spleen.

enlarged in malaria. Removal of the spleen may be undertaken for:

1. Rupture.
2. Thrombocytopenic purpura in which steroid therapy has
   been tried without success.
3. Haemolytic jaundice.
4. Splenic anaemia and certain tropical diseases.

Rupture is the most common indication for splenectomy.
The spleen is torn in a crush injury of the left hypochondrium.
The patient complains of pain in the splenic area, and there
are signs of internal haemorrhage.

*Preparation for splenectomy*
The preparation is similar to that for any major abdominal
operation. A blood platelet count is almost always performed
before operation.
The spleen is situated in the left hypochondrium, and access
is difficult if the stomach is distended. For this reason a nasogastric tube is passed before the patient leaves the ward and
left in position during the operation and for 24 hours afterwards.

*Postoperative care*
Thrombosis is the only special complication to be feared,

and the measures described to prevent it (p. 129) should be energetically pursued.

Collapse or pneumonia of the lower lobe of the left lung is an occasional complication and may be prevented by deep-breathing exercises. Acute dilatation of the stomach is prevented by leaving the nasogastric tube in position and aspirating the stomach until it is emptying normally.

# CHAPTER 27

# Organ and Tissue Transplantation

The transplantation of living tissue in the form of skin, bone and the cornea has been possible for many years. The recent successful results of organ grafting are a beacon light to the possibilities of the future and careful examination of the associated difficulties and hazards provides guidance in the clinical management of these patients.

The aim of grafting or transplantation is that the tissues will survive and function. This it can do only if it is living when it is transplanted. Many tissues from such diverse sources as bone from a bone bank, kangaroo tendon from the kangaroo or catgut from the sheep are used in surgical practice in a dead or inert form. They form a supporting framework and may be absorbed. They have not been grafted and, therefore, do not live.

Certain terms are used to designate the origin of the (living) graft:

### Autograft

The tissue is taken from and grafted into another position in the same individual. When the blood supply has been re-established the graft functions normally for the life-time of the individual. This procedure has been possible for a long time and a well-known example is skin grafting in a patient

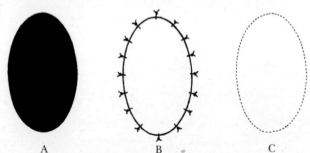

A                    B                    C

Fig. 27.1   Autograft. Skin defect (A) is closed by autograft of skin (B) and remains healed when the graft has 'taken' (C).

who has been burnt. Healthy undamaged skin is taken from one area to cover the burnt areas.

## HOMOGRAFT (ALLOGRAFT)

The graft is donated by another individual of the same species (in this case from one human being to another). It may survive for a time, but sooner or later it is destroyed. The process which destroys it is an immunological mechanism known as the homograft reaction.

The main problem in homograft transplantation, apart from the exercise of uncommon surgical skill, is to find a method of suppressing or diminishing the immune reaction between the host (the patient) and the graft. Discovery of a safe

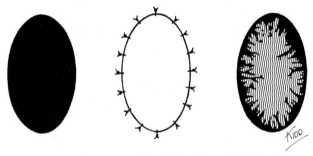

FIG. 27.2    Homograft reaction. Skin defect (A) is closed by homograft of skin (B) and gradually withers away (C) owing to the homograft reaction.

method of controlling the homograft reaction would enable spectacular surgical advances to be made and transplantation of the heart, the lungs, the kidneys and the liver may well then be regular surgical procedures.

## HETEROGRAFT (XENOGRAFT)

The tissue is grafted from a different species.

## THE NATURE OF THE HOMOGRAFT REACTION

There are two types of reaction:

1. The host develops cellular and humoral antibodies which react with antigens from the grafted organ.
2. The development of antibodies by the grafted organ against the antigens of the host. When severe the graft kills the host—this is known as Runt's disease.

The first reaction destroys the graft. Its survival time is dependent on the closeness of the genetic relationship between the donor and the host. Thus in twins who are genetically identical, grafts of tissue or even organs such as the kidney will survive for a life-time because the graft is, in fact, genetically an autograft. In closely related individuals there may be long survival of the homograft, but breakdown is unavoidable in the long run.

The transplantation antigens which provoke the reaction are present in nucleated cells of the body and it seems almost certain that it is the lymphocytes that invade the graft and in some way destroy it. Serological identification of the strongest antigens could lead to radical improvement in the selection of donors.

Homografts of the cornea survive as they cannot provoke or respond to a state of immunity because they have neither blood-vessels nor lymphatics.

## Modification of the homograft reaction

The successful survival of a homograft depends on modification or suppression of the homograft reaction. So far it has proved impossible to suppress it. The following measures are taken:

1. CLOSE GENETIC RELATIONSHIP increases the possibility of graft tolerance. As relationship becomes more remote the difficulties of the procedure multiply.

2. BLOOD COMPATIBILITY between the recipient and the donor in the ABO and Rh systems must be constant.

3. TISSUE TYPING of donor and recipient. HLA antigen is present on the cell surface.

4. ANTILYMPHOCYTIC SERUM.

5. IMMUNOSUPPRESSIVE DRUGS include azathioprine and Cortisone. Achromycin C is used in the control of rejection upsets. Drugs suppress the production of antibodies against rejection.

6. IRRADIATION. Whole-body irradiation has been abandoned but small doses of local irradiation of the donor organ may diminish the severity of the rejection reaction.

## Clinical application

Kidney transplants are now reasonably successful with careful tissue typing and computerised national and international kidney banks. The young patient with irreversible chronic renal disease is particularly suitable. Partial suppression of the rejection reaction is caused by uraemia which is of course incidental and an indication for the operation. More recently cadaver grafts have been used. The kidney differs however from other organs in that haemodialysis can again be used if the graft has failed. Almost every organ in the body, apart from the brain, has now been transplanted, with dismal results.

## ETHICAL PROBLEMS

The relatives or friends of a dying uraemic patient will offer to donate one of their kidneys, no matter how small the chance of success. The surgeon must balance the chance of success against the risk to the healthy donor, as the patient himself has nothing to lose. Much controversy has arisen about the moment of death in patients with irrecoverable head injuries whose organs may be suitable for transplantation.

## NURSING MANAGEMENT

The main problem is to prevent infection and, despite every care, many patients have developed significant infection. The principles of preventing surgical infection are applicable, but the special hazard is that these patients are particularly susceptible to infection owing to the use of immunosuppressive drugs.

In detail, the following special measures are necessary.

1. ISOLATION. A four-roomed suite in which the ward containing a single bed is air-conditioned, communicates with an anteroom and this in turn leads to a changing room and the sister's office.

Theatre gowning is essential for all attention on the patient. The walls and floors of the suite are washed with a solution of Hycolin 1 : 60. The room should contain an electric kettle for making hot drinks. A field telephone connects the patient to the sister's office and visits of doctors and nurses must be kept to the minimum.

2. BACTERIOLOGICAL CONTROL. Swabs are taken from the floor of the ward to limit infection. All medical and nursing staff who, in any case, are limited to the smallest possible number must have nasal, throat and skin swabs taken. The patient is also swabbed and homo-transplantation delayed if any pathogenic organisms are isolated.

3. SPECIAL PREOPERATIVE MEASURES include the supply of autoclaved pyjamas and bed linen.

4. POSTOPERATIVE CARE. Special measures are taken to prevent infection and include the supply of food which has been sterilised by gamma-ray irradiation in sealed packets of double-wrapped nylon on aluminium foil plates. Crockery and cutlery are also supplied wrapped and sterilised. The outside of bottles of blood or bottles of other fluids is sterilised by immersion in a solution of 1 : 60 Hycolin for five minutes. These measures are necessary for four to six weeks until the leucocyte and platelet counts begin to rise. Systemic antibiotics are used if infection occurs.

**Complications.** In addition to the ordinary hazards of a major surgical operation, the following complications are particularly liable to occur:

1. *Infection*. Measures to prevent it have been discussed above.

2. Infective hepatitis (p. 385).

3. *Haemorrhage* from deficiency of platelets following methods to suppress the homograft reaction, has been particularly troublesome.

4. *Failure* (rejection) of the homograft.

## SPARE-PART SURGERY

In addition to whole organ replacement, 'spare parts', some very functional, some only cosmetic, are widely used in surgery. As bioengineering develops, considerable developments are certain to emerge. Examples in practice are:

*External spare parts*. Limbs. Hearing aids. Eyes. Spectacles. Teeth. Wigs.

*Internal spare parts*. Artificial joints. Ring prostheses. Arteries. Dacron prostheses. Heart valves. Spitz-Holter valve.

*Artificial nerve*. Cardiac pacemaker (p. 325).

*Circulation*. Heart-lung machine (p. 323).

*Renal clearance*. Haemodialysis (artificial kidney) (p. 452).

*The blood*. Whole blood and special components.

*Tissues*. Skin. Bone. Cartilage.

# CHAPTER 28

# The Mouth, the Face and the Tongue

A patient suffering from a surgical lesion of the face or lip usually seeks medical advice in the early stages of the disability. The mildest lesion of the face is usually of some concern even to the most self-effacing individual, and facial disease or deformity can depress the morale of a patient out of all proportion to the size or severity of the lesion. Unsightly scars or naevi will effect profound changes in the attitude and outlook of the patient. They may affect his whole life, and the importance of the work of the plastic surgeon is very considerable.

## WOUNDS

Wounds of the face, because of the abundant blood supply to the part, heal rapidly, and for the same reason gas gangrene is almost unknown in this area. Thorough cleansing and the removal of grit is important, as failure to do this results in an ugly discoloured scar. Sepsis is rare. The fine stitches inserted should be removed on the third or fourth day to avoid permanent stitch marks. Dressings are unnecessary and the wound may be left exposed.

A depressed fracture of the malar bone is not uncommon, and early elevation is undertaken so that the cheek prominence is restored.

## INFLAMMATORY CONDITIONS

1. **Cellulitis and carbuncle.** The lips may be affected. Infection of the upper lip, once regarded as a most dangerous condition, is now easily resolved by the use of antibiotics.

2. **Chancre of the lip.** A primary syphilitic lesion (chancre) may appear on the lip. The glands in the neck are enlarged.

3. **Chronic inflammatory conditions.** Chronic inflammatory conditions are not common. The rhagades of congenital syphilis may be seen as healed scars in the adult. Chronic thickening with fissure formation may occur as a result of syphilis, and the treatment is that of the causal disease.

4. **Cysts of the face.** Sebaceous cysts are common, particularly on the nose and around the ears. They are due to block-

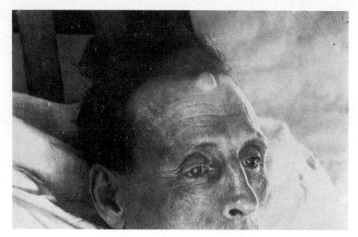

FIG. 28.1　Sebaceous cyst of scalp.

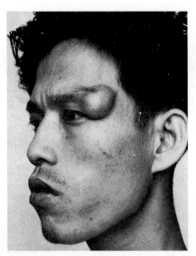

FIG. 28.2　External angular dermoid cyst. The overlying skin is freely movable.

age of the duct of a sebaceous gland. The pent-up secretion of sebum is responsible for the swelling, and the lining of the cyst is the stretched sebaceous gland. The treatment is excision.

Dermoid cysts may form at the line of fusion of the skull and face and may be found at the root of the nose or over the external angular process of the orbit. Since they may have an intracranial connection, excision is usually not undertaken until the age of 14 years, when skull fissures are solidly fused.

# NEW GROWTHS OF THE FACE AND LIPS

## SIMPLE TUMOURS

Simple tumours, particularly naevi, may be disfiguring. They are usually treated by destruction with carbon dioxide snow, by surgical excision or by radiotherapy if they do not regress spontaneously. The best method is probably by cryosurgery (p. 216).

## BASAL-CELL CARCINOMA
### (Syn. **Rodent ulcer**)

A rodent ulcer usually occurs on the upper part of the face, and is frequently situated dangerously near to the eye. It is locally malignant and, untreated, will erode the bones of the face and skull until a septic meningitis kills the patient. Its progress is very slow at first.

CLINICAL FEATURES. In the early stages there is a tiny yellow ulcer with a rolled edge. Later, diffuse sepsis may render the whole area raw and purulent.

TREATMENT. Radium to the surface, excision or cryodestruction are effective. In late cases the eyeball may have to be removed.

## SQUAMOUS-CELL CARCINOMA
### (Syn. **Epithelioma**)

Cancer is commoner on the lower than the upper lip, and used to be frequently associated with a long-standing habit of smoking a hot clay pipe.

CLINICAL FEATURES. The growth appears as a hard nodule which later becomes either papilliferous and watery in appearance, or it assumes the characteristics of a typical malignant ulcer. The base is fixed and the edge is hard and everted. The lymphatic glands underneath the chin and the lower jaw enlarge as spread occurs. Untreated, the tumour erodes the lower jaw.

TREATMENT. Surgical excision, radiotherapy or, better, cryosurgery may be used. The glands are treated by subsequent block dissection.

## CLEFT LIP AND CLEFT PALATE

Cleft lip and cleft palate are congenital deformities due to the failure of fusion of the various tissues forming the lips and the palate. Cortisone intoxication, virus infections such as rubella, oxygen and vitamin deficiency, as well as radiation damage during foetal life, are now known to be causal factors. Cleft lip almost invariably affects the upper lip, and may involve one or both sides. It may occur alone or in association with a cleft pa-

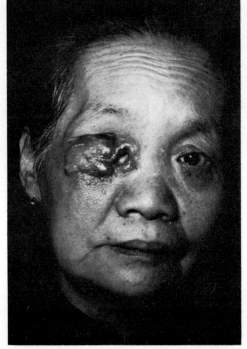

FIG. 28.3    Rodent ulcer.

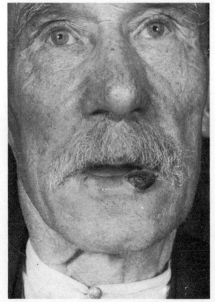

FIG. 28.4    Squamous-cell carcinoma of lower lip.

late. In all cases there is some deformity of the face and nose. A cleft palate may involve the hard and the soft palate or only a portion of the soft palate. The disability of these lesions may be summarised as follows:

1. There is obvious cosmetic deformity.
2. Feeding is rendered difficult, and undernourishment may result unless very special care is taken.
3. Nasal catarrh and respiratory infections are common because the mouth and the nose communicate.
4. The speech is seriously impaired.

*Treatment*

A cleft lip is repaired as soon as possible. The edges are freshened and sutured together under a general anaesthetic.

The orthodontist by making a plate for the newborn baby with the cleft palate can aid the baby to suck. Furthermore modification of the plate can mould the cleft into correct alignment before surgical closure is undertaken. This has given vastly superior cosmetic results; in particular, deformity of the nose is very much reduced.

The repair of a cleft palate is undertaken in the first year or two of life. The soft palate must be repaired if good speech is to be attained. The hard palate may be united by suture, or the cleft may be blocked with an obturator (a dental plate similar to that on which artificial teeth are set).

PREOPERATIVE CARE OF A CASE OF CLEFT LIP

The infant must be trained to take food from a special spoon (Fig. 28.5) or dropper, and his reaction to this form of

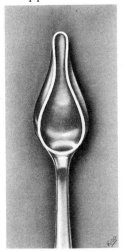

FIG. 28.5   Spoon adapted for feeding infant with cleft lip or cleft palate.

feeding must be satisfactory before operation is contemplated. Sucking with a soft teat is preferable if a dental plate can be fitted. He should be gaining weight. The blood haemoglobin should be not less than 80 per cent. The mouth must be gently rinsed or swabbed very carefully with glycothymolin or other suitable mouthwash, and swabbed with sodium bicarbonate solution to remove the mucus. Preoperatively, systemic antibiotics will usually be prescribed to counteract any infection which may develop.

Swabs of the nose and throat should be taken before operation and the child should be in hospital for at least a week.

### POSTOPERATIVE CARE OF CLEFT LIP

1. Antibiotics will be continued postoperatively. The wound is left exposed. The mouth and nose must be carefully and frequently cleansed so as to avoid infection. The sutures are removed on the fifth day after operation or earlier as the surgeon directs.

A Logan's bow may be applied for fourteen days to keep the lip in the normal pouting position.

2. The arms are splinted lightly to prevent the infant 'picking' the dressing.

3. Feeding must be as careful as before operation.

4. Rest is essential. Crying must be reduced to a minimum, since it tends to stretch the suture line. Sedatives, such as chloral hydrate, are prescribed at frequent intervals for four or five days after the operation.

### PREOPERATIVE CARE OF CLEFT PALATE

The child's general condition must be satisfactory before operation is performed and sepsis must be eliminated. The mother can be assured of a good cosmetic result. Removal of the tonsils may be advised but this practice is avoided if possible as removal of the tonsils and adenoids tends to impair effective palatopharyngeal closure.

### POSTOPERATIVE CARE OF CLEFT PALATE

1. The arms should be splinted to prevent the child injuring the suture line in the mouth. The patient is propped upright in bed. Atropine (0·3 mg) is administered to diminish salivation for two or three days.

2. Feeding is carefully carried out. Since the mouth is now smaller than previously, and also very tender, there may be considerable difficulty in feeding. The diet should consist of milk, jelly, blancmange, fruit juice, and soup. Rusks, vegetables, and toast are avoided lest the sutures line in the mouth should be injured.

3. The mouth is cleansed with several spoonfuls of sterile water before and after every feed.

4. The stitches do not require removal, since catgut is usually employed and will dissolve spontaneously. Wire sutures, if inserted, will be removed by the surgeon.

5. Rest is secured, as described in the postoperative care of a cleft lip.

Continual supervision and further operations to correct associated deformity are necessary until adult life.

A long convalescence is necessary, and the child must be under the care of a speech therapist as soon as possible after operation.

## THE MOUTH AND THE TONGUE

The most serious disease inside the mouth is a carcinoma originating in the buccal mucosa or in the mucous membrane of the tongue. The condition is frequently associated with chronic irritation, and is rarely seen inside a clean mouth.

### GLOSSITIS
#### (Inflammation of the tongue)

(a) **Acute.** This may be due to a sting from a wasp, or it may occur as a result of acute streptococcal infection. Certain anaemias and blood diseases, particularly the leukaemias, may be predisposing factors in the occurrence of extensive glossitis.

Acute glossitis is not a common condition, but when it does arise it is extremely urgent, since a swollen tongue may fill the mouth and the nasopharynx, causing death from asphyxia.

TREATMENT. Ice packs should be applied to the tongue. In the event of respiratory distress appearing, the nurse should hook the tongue forward at once by means of tongue forceps. In all cases preparations should be made for an urgent tracheostomy, should this be necessary.

(b) **Subacute glossitis.** Subacute glossitis, due to antibiotics causing vitamin $B_2$ deficiency, is probably the commonest form of all, but it may result from the use of cytotoxic drugs.

(c) **Chronic.** Chronic glossitis is usually syphilitic in origin. In the early stages the surface of the tongue is red, firm, and fissured. Later it is white and cracked in appearance (leukoplakia). The condition is a pre-cancerous one, and a growth may develop in one of the fissured clefts.

TREATMENT. The affected area will usually be excised and sent for microscopical examination. Antisyphilitic treatment is given (p. 78). Jagged teeth, septic roots, or other sources of local irritation are removed. In some cases cryosurgery is performed.

## CYSTS IN THE MOUTH

1. Simple mucous cysts are not uncommon.

2. A ranula is a cystic swelling of the floor of the mouth.

3. A dermoid cyst may protrude into the floor of the mouth.

Excision is the usual treatment.

## ULCERATION OF THE TONGUE

Ulceration of the tongue may be:

1. **A dental ulcer.** A dental ulcer is always situated on the side of the tongue in the neighbourhood of a jagged tooth.

2. **Tuberculous ulcer.** A tuberculous ulcer is usually associated with advanced pulmonary tuberculosis. It is always extremely painful. The application of 20 per cent chromic acid paint to the ulcer aids in its cure, but in intractable cases a local anaesthetic, in the form of orthocaine powder, is dabbed on to the surface to enable the patient to partake of nourishment in comparative comfort. Happily the condition is now very rare.

3. **Syphilitic ulceration.** Syphilitic ulceration is painless, and the ulcer has a typical punched-out appearance.

4. **Malignant ulcers.** These are discussed below.

5. **Aphthous ulcers.** Aphthous ulcers are characterised by the development of single or multiple erosive lesions in the oral mucosa surrounded by an area of oedema and hyperaemia. They vary in size from 2 to 10 mm and may be episodic. In women, characteristically they occur premenstrually. The aetiology is unknown, but oestrogen therapy is effective in healing most patients with premenstrual aphthous ulcer as well as in some in whom the ulcer is not related to the menstrual cycle. Stilboestrol 3 mg daily is a suitable dosage.

# NEW GROWTHS OF THE TONGUE

## SIMPLE NEW GROWTHS

1. Papilloma.

2. Angioma.

The patient feels the nodule. In the case of angiomas slight haemorrhage is usually present. These growths are excised with a diathermy knife.

## MALIGNANT NEW GROWTHS

Carcinoma is the most common growth of the tongue, and its incidence has been reduced by routine dental care. Leukoplakia is a predisposing factor of which syphilis is one aetiological cause (but a diminishing one).

*Symptoms and signs*

The patient is usually about 60 years of age, and the teeth and gums are almost invariably septic. Pain may be present in the tongue or referred to the ear, so that the patient complains of earache.

**Haemorrhage.** Small haemorrhages are common once ulceration has occurred. A massive fatal secondary haemorrhage is a not unusual termination.

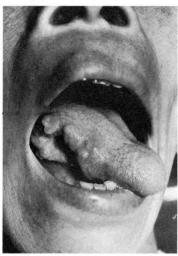

FIG. 28.6   Squamous-cell carcinoma of the tongue.

**Ulceration.** Ulceration has usually occurred by the time the patient seeks advice. It takes the form of a sloughing ulcer with a firm, indurated base and a large everted edge. As the disease advances the patient may be unable to protrude the tongue from his mouth. Salivation is excessive as a result of irritation, and the exudation of pus which results from secondary infection of the growth. Secondary deposits occur in the lymphatic glands in the neck.

COURSE OF THE DISEASE. Untreated, death occurs from:

1. Broncho-pneumonia, which results from the inhalation of the infection in the growth.
2. Secondary haemorrhage.
3. Starvation and exhaustion as a result of pain, and extension of the growth into the tissues of the neck and mouth.

*Treatment*

DENTAL TREATMENT

Dental treatment must be undertaken before any surgical treatment can be attempted.

## SURGICAL TREATMENT

Excision of the tongue is rarely performed today, but in passing it is interesting to note how remarkably well successful cases of excision can speak after the operation. Nonetheless, it is an extremely mutilating procedure. If this is contemplated the external carotid artery on the same side as the growth is usually tied before the operation, and the skin of the neck should be prepared.

## RADIOTHERAPY

Interstitial radium is the treatment of choice usually applied to the primary growth, but radiotherapy has given disappointing results in the treatment of the glandular field.

The glands are almost always treated by what is known as a 'block dissection' of the neck. This is usually undertaken after the primary growth has been treated by radium or excision. For this operation the skin is prepared from about 15 cm below the clavicle up to the hair-line.

### Nursing care

The patient with radium in the mouth requires very special care. *The threads of the needles* must be securely fixed on the face with strapping and regularly inspected and counted to ensure that a radium needle has not been swallowed. All excreta are inspected before disposal. Frequent bland mouthwashes must be given, and a fluid diet, as rich as possible in protein and other nutrients, must be provided. Meat soups, eggs, milk, jellies and fruit juice to which glucose has been added can all be taken.

He should be nursed upright in bed and provided with:

1. A bowl into which saliva can drain.
2. Gauze swabs or disposable tissues to wipe his lips. The bowl for salivation and the swabs should be checked in case they contain a radium needle.
3. A pencil and paper to communicate his wishes.

*Pain* is usually severe, and morphia may be necessary for its relief. Earache, although not due to an organic cause in the ear, may be treated by the instillation of phenol drops (5 per cent) into the ear and a cotton-wool plug. They act as a counter-irritant at the site to which pain is referred.

*The radium reaction* is frequently severe, and secondary haemorrhage is most liable to occur two or three days after the radium has been removed. Its risk is minimised by frequent cleansing of the mouth and encouraging the patient to wash out the mouth as often as possible. Chemotherapy may be prescribed to control infection. Should bleeding occur, the nurse must pull the patient's tongue well forward with the tongue forceps. This frequently controls the haemorrhage temporarily. If this is not successful, the common carotid artery pressure point at the root of the neck must be compressed at once and medical aid summoned without delay.

## THE SALIVARY GLANDS

The normal healthy mouth, apart from cleansing of the teeth, does not require mouthwashes. The mouth of the patient who is toxic, dehydrated or forbidden to take fluid becomes dry and more septic than usual. He has little stimulus to excite salivation. The result is that infection creeps up the ducts down which saliva normally flows profusely, and an inflammatory condition develops in the gland. It is for this reason that moistening of the mouth, and mouthwashes, are so important in preventing infection in the conditions just mentioned. Even better than moistening the mouth is to stimulate the flow of saliva, and this can be achieved by giving the patient chewing gum or barley sugar.

### ACUTE SIALADENITIS
#### (Acute inflammation of a salivary gland)

This is due to the conditions which we have mentioned above, and is common only in the parotid glands.

*Symptoms and signs*

The face is tender and swollen over the affected parotid gland. The patient complains of difficulty in opening his mouth.

*Treatment*

The prevention and treatment have already been indicated, namely, mouthwashes, chewing gum and drinking plenty of fluids, if they are allowed. Should suppuration develop, incision will be necessary.

### ACUTE NON-SUPPURATIVE PAROTITIS
#### (Mumps)

This is a virus infection and an entirely separate condition. Both parotid glands are usually swollen. Orchitis and very rarely pancreatitis may occur as complications.

### CHRONIC SIALADENITIS AND SALIVARY CALCULI

The secretion from the parotid gland is thin and serous; that from the submandibular gland is thick and mucoid. As a result of obstruction or stricture of the duct, a low-grade chronic inflammation may arise in a gland. In some cases a calculus forms and blocks the duct. Because of the thicker secretion, 95 per cent of calculi are formed in the submandibular gland.

### Symptoms and signs

The patient complains of a swelling in the submandibular region which increases in size at meal times and diminishes in the periods between meals. The enlarged gland can be palpated. A radiograph is taken to prove the presence of a calculus.

### Treatment

Treatment may consist of:

1. Removal of the calculus.
2. Dilatation of Wharton's duct with lacrimal probes.
3. Excision of the gland.

A calculus in Wharton's duct is removed from inside the mouth. No special local preoperative preparation is necessary. Postoperatively, these patients may be sent from the theatre with a small swab in the mouth, which is attached outside to a pair of Spencer Wells forceps. The patient is usually coughing by the time he leaves the theatre, and the swab can be removed shortly afterwards. It is unusual for severe haemorrhage to develop. Stitches in the mouth are usually of catgut and do not require removal.

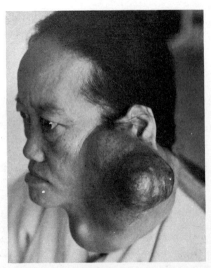

Fig. 28.7  Mixed salivary (parotid) tumour. This is an extreme example, but despite its size there is no facial paralysis and the lesion was benign.

Dilatation of Wharton's duct is usually undertaken for strictures; dabbing the surface with local anaesthetic may suffice, or no anaesthetic may be necessary. The preparation for an excision of the gland is similar to that for excision of the lymphatic glands of the neck.

### PAROTID TUMOURS

1. Mixed parotid tumour—75 per cent are benign. The superficial lobe of the parotid gland is excised.

2. Carcinoma—usually involvement of the facial nerve occurs. It is treated by total removal of the parotid.

3. Some rarer tumours, such as adenolymphoma, may occur.

## THE TEETH AND THE JAWS

In the first or deciduous dentition there are 20 teeth which erupt at intervals from about six months to 2 years of age. The permanent teeth, which number 32, follow the deciduous teeth and commence to erupt at the age of 6 years. They continue their eruption until the age of 12, when only the third molar (wisdom) teeth are unerupted. Their eruption occurs in the late teens. The roots take three years to develop completely after the teeth have commenced to erupt.

Each tooth forms a firm joint with the jaw, being held in its socket in the alveolar bone by a fibrous ligament, the periodontal ligament, which is attached to the tooth root and to the bone.

### ABSCESSES ARISING FROM THE TEETH

An abscess arising from a tooth may be the cause of infection at remote sites in the body. Infection arising from teeth may be of two types:

Open

Closed

1. *Open sepsis.* Open sepsis occurs almost invariably from infection of the gum margins and from decayed teeth and roots. It is commonly caused initially by the deposits of calculus (tartar) which irritate and inflame the gum margins. It is known as open sepsis because the infected material drains into the mouth. The pus forms in the pocket between the gum margin and the root of the tooth and drains into the mouth producing halitosis (bad breath). Infection may spread to the sinuses, tonsils and stomach. Open oral sepsis predisposes to chest infections after general anaesthesia.

2. *Closed sepsis.* Closed sepsis is considerably more important than the open type. Infection almost invariably com-

mences as dental caries (decay) and if this is untreated it spreads and infects the pulp of the tooth, from which it is but a short step to the jaw and the venous blood stream, through which it is passed around the body. Such bacterial spread (bacteraemia) is dangerous in patients suffering from congenital or rheumatic heart disease because it can lead to bacterial endocarditis.

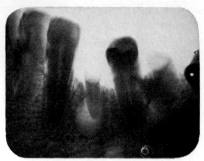

FIG. 28.8A    Root abscess $\overline{|4}$

## Dental abscess

1. *Acute*. An acute dental abscess (alveolar abscess) arises from an infected tooth. The onset is heralded by acute pain, increasing in severity. Swelling is not marked at this stage.

About the third day there is characteristically a sudden remission of the pain as the inflamed, congested tooth pulp dies. Soon the infected material escapes through the root end and produces inflammation of the periodontal ligament. This makes the tooth tender to touch and to bite on, and pain returns in the jaw. With the pus tracking through the periosteum into the soft tissues, a generalised swelling occurs. The patient feels unwell, looks ill and the temperature, which should not be taken in the mouth, is elevated.

Treatment consists of extraction of the offending tooth. This will usually provide sufficient drainage, but in the presence of extensive facial swelling with pus, external drainage may be necessary in addition. Antibiotics will be used in severe cases. Nursing treatment, apart from vigorous hot mouthwashes, is on the general lines of an acute toxic condition.

2. *Chronic*. A chronic abscess may follow an acute abscess which has pointed in the mouth, leaving a sinus which has failed to heal. More commonly they are chronic from the beginning, caused by low grade infection from the dead pulp of a tooth over a prolonged period.

## ODONTOMES

Odontomes are cysts or tumours arising from the cells from

which teeth are formed. Excision and removal of the epithelial elements is undertaken, together with malformed dental hard tissues—i.e. masses composed of enamel, dentine and cementum in differing proportions.

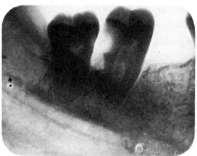
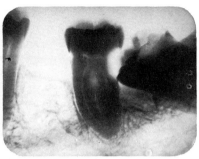

FIG. 28.8B Dental caries in first molar tooth.

FIG. 28.8C Impacted third molar (wisdom tooth). Caries in adjacent molar.

## DENTAL CARIES

Dental caries is a very common disease in civilised peoples and its treatment is a matter for the dental surgeon. It is the progressive destruction of the enamel and dentine of a tooth by acids produced by oral bacteria. The bacteria (which are part of the normal flora of the mouth) convert carbohydrates such as sugar and starch to acid—e.g. lactic acid, which can slowly dissolve the hard tooth tissues. The dental plaque, a film lying on uncleaned teeth, is the site where bacteria act to produce the acid. It follows that in simple terms, caries can be controlled by (a) reduction of the amount of sugar in the diet, and particularly by cutting down the duration of time it is present in the mouth; (b) removal of dental plaque by brushing between the teeth conscientiously; (c) making tooth structure more resistant to acid attack by applying fluoride gels to the teeth or, better still, incorporating fluoride in the developing tooth through the intake of fluoridated drinking water. The addition of minute quantities of fluorine (as sodium fluoride) to water supplies where this element is naturally lacking significantly reduces the incidence of dental caries.

A nurse should never advise a patient to have his teeth extracted, however bad they may appear—only to seek dental advice. Conservative treatment may well be possible.

## HAEMORRHAGE FOLLOWING THE EXTRACTION OF TEETH

As we would expect, this may be primary, reactionary or secondary. Reactionary, or intermediate haemorrhage, occurring a few hours after extraction is by far the most common and is probably caused by excessive vigorous rinsing of the mouth or by licking the clot and dislodging it.

*Treatment*

The head is raised on pillows and the mouth cleaned and examined with a good light. A pressure pack is placed over the bleeding socket. A gauze swab soaked in hot water and wrung out is placed over the socket and the patient is instructed to bite on it. 'Surgicel' gauze may be packed into the socket before applying the pressure pack. If this fails, the gum will probably have to be sutured, usually after giving a local anaesthetic. Make sure the patient does not suffer from a constitutional bleeding disorder—e.g. purpura, haemophilia or is on anticoagulants. Reassurance is important and 15 mg morphia may be useful to reduce apprehension and agitation.

### FRACTURES OF THE JAW

Almost all fractures of the jaw are caused by violence—e.g. the car accident victim or the boxer. Pathological fractures occasionally occur as a complication of osteomyelitis or as a complication of a large dental cyst or neoplasm.

The immediate treatment is to ensure a free airway. The muscular control of the tongue, because of its dependence on an intact lower jaw, may be lost in a fracture and if the patient is laid flat on his back there is a considerable risk of the tongue falling back, causing asphyxia. This may be prevented by placing a suture through the tongue, by tongue forceps, or by nursing the patient lying on the face until either the mandible has been immobilised in a forward position or the patient's control of the tongue has returned.

All patients suffering from a fracture of the jaw are transported in the prone position.

*Treatment of fractures of the mandible*

The aims of treatment are reduction of the fracture, its immobilisation and prevention of infection. It may be immobilised by:

1. Gunning splints (in the edentulous patient).
2. Eyelet wiring.
3. Cast metal splints.

The teeth are fixed together either by wires or metal cap/splints to ensure correct relationship upper to lower. If they occlude correctly then the bone, of necessity, must be in correct alignment. Maintaining the teeth in occlusion may be necessary for six to eight weeks. The mouth is syringed with sodium bicarbonate 1:60 using a Higginson's syringe, and as soon as possible the patient is encouraged to clean his teeth with a small toothbrush and paste. Food, which has to be in liquid form, may be introduced by a catheter and funnel, or by flexible straw. Meals should be small and given frequently.

### ACTINOMYCOSIS

This is an example of chronic infection due to a fungus which may occur in the jaw. Classically, an extensive brawny swelling develops and in the later stages multiple sinuses which discharge sulphur granules are present. An alternative form simulates an acute dental abscess, but healing is delayed. Infection usually arises following a dental extraction or any lesion involving a breach of the oral mucous membrane. The organisms are present in normal mouths, but can occasionally enter the tissues and produce a persistent infection.

Treatment consists of the administration of penicillin (1 megaunit daily) for three months, or tetracycline for a slightly shorter period. Surgery is confined to providing free drainage from the abscess.

### TUMOURS OF THE JAW

**Simple tumours.** Simple tumours are usually osteomata. They are not very common. Simple tumours of the mouth such as fibromas are often seen, particularly if an irritant factor such as an ill-fitting denture is present.

**Malignant tumours.** These may be—

1. *Sarcoma.* A sarcoma may develop in the upper or lower jaw.

2. *Carcinoma.* A carcinomatous growth may arise in the lining of the maxillary antrum. It extends in all directions, upwards towards the eye, inwards to block the nostril, downwards eroding the hard palate, and forwards into the muscles and skin of the face.

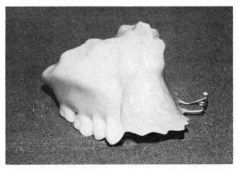

FIG. 28.8D    Dental obturator to repair palatal defect.

*Treatment*

Radiotherapy and surgery are usually combined in the treatment, the affected half of the upper jaw being removed. The dental surgeon will make an appliance to repair the loss of tissue.

# THE NECK

## WOUNDS

Wounds in this area bleed freely, and deep wounds may open massive blood vessels, like the carotid artery or internal jugular vein. A further danger of a wound in this area is damage to the larynx or trachea with resulting respiratory obstruction. Tracheostomy may be necessary.

## SWELLINGS IN THE NECK

Swellings in the neck are common. They are:

1. Lymphatic glandular swellings (p. 248).
2. Goitre (Chap. 29).
3. Sebaceous cyst (p. 258).
4. Thyroglossal cyst, which arises in the midline above the prominence of the thyroid cartilage. It arises on a vestigial tract running from the tongue to the thyroid. Excision is the usual treatment.
5. A branchial cyst, which arises high in the neck near the angle of the lower jaw. It is a developmental abnormality. Excision is usually performed and it may be quite an extensive operation.
6. Cystic hygroma is a condition of dilatation of the lymphatic vessels. It occurs in children and frequently becomes mildly infected. Infection sometimes results in recession. Excision is the usual treatment.
7. Ludwig's angina, which is a dangerous condition of cellulitis of the floor of the mouth.

Rapid swelling appears even before pyrexia. Tracheostomy instruments should always be ready in case of respiratory obstruction. The patient should be kept very still as heart failure may cause sudden death.

# CHAPTER 29

# The Endocrine Glands

## DISEASES OF THE THYROID GLAND

The endocrines or ductless glands secrete hormones into the blood stream. The glands whose secretion is essential in conditions of stress are connected by very short veins to the general circulation so that the concentration of their hormones in the blood can be increased very rapidly. Normal functioning of all the glands is necessary for the maintenance of good health. In this chapter much space is devoted to the thyroid gland because its lesions are surgically more significant. This emphasis may well change as knowledge increases and many lesions which we now treat as diseases of the thyroid are already recognised to be only a manifestation of imbalance originating elsewhere in the endocrine system.

A goitre is an enlargement of the thyroid gland. The thyroid gland is an endocrine gland situated at the root of the neck in front of and at the sides of the trachea and oesophagus. The diseases to which it is subject are unusual in that they do not

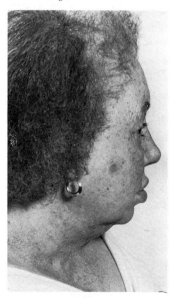

FIG. 29.1   Myxoedema showing thin hair and dry skin.

conform to the pattern of those to which we are accustomed elsewhere.

The thyroid secretes three hormones:

Thyroxine
Tri-iodothyronine
Calcitonin.

The first two hormones, of which thyroxine accounts for 90 per cent, are essential for normal growth in infancy and for the maintenance of a balanced metabolism in adult life. If iodine is deficient in the diet, or if the demands of the body for thyroxine are temporarily in excess of the gland's capacity to produce it, the gland substance may enlarge in an attempt to compensate. Later, the enlargement may subside evenly and smoothly, but frequently it is so large or retrogression so patchy that the patient is left with an irregular nodular goitre. The absence of the gland, or the failure to produce sufficient thyroxine, results in cretinism in infants and myxoedema in adults. The whole tempo of the activities of the body is depressed in these conditions. On the other hand, an excessive amount of secretion results in the condition known as thyrotoxicosis, with the result that the whole pace of the patient's activities is accelerated.

A thyrotropic hormone (thyroid stimulating) in the pituitary regulates the production of thyroxine which is manufactured in the secretory cells of the vesicles of the thyroid. Iodine is taken up from the blood and when the hormone is released into the blood stream it combines with the plasma proteins. This is known as the protein-bound iodine (PBI). An increase is a manifestation of excessive thyroid secretion and a diminution occurs in myxoedema but it is now more usual to estimate the level of thyroxine in the serum.

Secondarily, as a result of enlargement, symptoms due to pressure on the neighbouring organs may occur.

Calcitonin—a serum calcium-lowering hormone which inhibits bone destruction is now known to be secreted in the thyroid—in addition to thyroxine.

## SIMPLE ENLARGEMENTS OF THE THYROID

Simple or non-toxic enlargement of the thyroid is fairly common. The gland usually enlarges in the neck, but occasionally the enlargement occurs behind the upper portion of the sternum (retrosternal goitre).

*Causes*

During periods of special stress, such as puberty, the calls for thyroxine are greater, and a diffuse enlargement of the gland may occur. It is physiological in origin, and the colloid goitre of puberty requires no special surgical intervention.

Since iodinised salt has been used, endemic goitres with a definite geographical distribution have almost disappeared.

The simple enlargement may subside if not excessive, or subsidence may occur in one portion of the gland and not in another. This process results in the production of nodules in the gland. They may be single (adenoma) or multiple, known as nodular goitre.

*Symptoms and signs*

The most obvious and frequently the only complaint is the goitre itself. A goitre always moves on swallowing. Surgical interference is indicated if the patient complains of:

1. Pressure symptoms, which may be:
   (a) Dysphagia (difficulty in swallowing).
   (b) Dyspnoea (difficulty in breathing—the trachea, which is normally round in shape, is so compressed on both sides that it may be 'scabbard' in shape).
   (c) Hoarseness due to pressure on the recurrent laryngeal nerves.
2. Cosmetic disfigurement.
3. Symptoms suggestive of toxic or malignant changes.

Radiography of the trachea and chest is usually ordered to determine the degree (if any) of the deformity of the trachea resulting from pressure.

*Treatment*

Surgical operation consists of partial thyroidectomy. The after-care is similar to that of toxic goitre (p. 281), but antithyroid drugs are unnecessary.

## Complications of a simple goitre
1. The onset of toxic symptoms.
2. The occurrence of haemorrhage into an adenoma with the sudden onset of severe dyspnoea.
3. Malignancy.

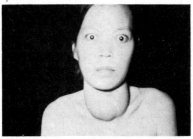

FIG. 29.2    Simple (non-toxic) goitre.

## THYROTOXICOSIS

Toxic goitre is a condition in which the secretion of thyroxine is excessive in quantity, and the disease is commoner in women.

The disease may commence in a gland which was previously normal, or it may develop in a thyroid already subject to simple enlargement. The former is described as primary thyrotoxicosis or Graves' disease and the latter as secondary thyrotoxicosis. The main distinction is that the patient is usually older in the secondary type and the heart muscle is less fit to withstand being driven so much faster. The other clinical distinction is that the eye signs, particularly exophthalmos, are nearly always present in Graves' disease.

*Symptoms and signs*

The onset of toxic symptoms may follow a severe mental shock or anxiety. The thyroid gland may be very large, or there may be almost no enlargement at all. The severity of the symptoms bears no relationship to the size of the goitre. The symptoms are those of an accelerated metabolism. The body is being driven even faster.

GENERAL SYMPTOMS

1. The skin is moist and vascular. Sweating may be profuse, and cold weather is preferred to a warm sunny day.

2. The eyes are protruding (exophthalmos), staring, and have a frightened look. This is common in Graves' disease but unusual in secondary thyrotoxicosis in the older patient.

3. Loss of weight is marked but the appetite is good.

4. Tremors of the fingers are present.

5. Mentally, the patient is hyperexcitable, nervous, and difficult to get on with. Frequently the patient with a toxic goitre will insist on leaving hospital in the midst of treatment.

6. Diarrhoea and vomiting may be present, and are due to overactivity of the intestinal tract.

CARDIOVASCULAR SYMPTOMS

The heart rate is always increased and palpitation is a common complaint. The systolic blood pressure is raised and the diastolic pressure lowered, with the result that the pulse pressure is increased and the pulse is full and bounding.

Later, irregularity of the heart beat occurs, usually in the form of atrial fibrillation, and unrelieved, the patient dies of cardiac failure, which is usually associated with acute mania.

RADIOIODINE TRACER studies may be necessary to reveal thyroid overactivity in atypical cases. The blood PBI (p. 276) and serum thyroxin level are raised and the blood cholesterol level lowered.

*Treatment*

1. Mild cases may be treated medically by sedatives and prolonged rest which will include rearrangement of the patient's life. Carbimazole (Neo-Mercazole) (10 mg t.d.s.) or other antithyroid drug may be given until the patient's weight is rising and then reduced to smaller doses. Agranulocytosis is now comparatively rare but should always be considered as a possible complication of this drug. The disadvantage of all antithyroid drugs is that in the presence of moderate enlargement they increase the size of the gland. Radioactive iodine is being used with increasing frequency.

2. For severe cases and for moderate cases where the patient must lead his normal life and earn his living, subtotal thyroidectomy or radioactive iodine therapy gives the best chances of permanent cure.

Radioiodine is contraindicated in:

(a) Patients under 40 years of age for fear of causing carcinomatous change in the thyroid.
(b) Pregnancy.

It is specially indicated in:

(a) Recurrent thyrotoxicosis where a second operation carries a much higher risk of damage to the recurrent laryngeal nerves.
(b) In patients with concurrent medical disease which precludes safe operative intervention.

*The nursing care of a case of thyroidectomy for thyrotoxicosis*

All patients require a period of medical treatment before operation can be undertaken.

The operation is performed when the heart rate settles down to about 80 to 85 per minute—in fact when the patient is in a euthyroid state, that is a condition of normal thyroid function. The patient is now feeling better, less excitable and gaining weight. This is confirmed by a normal serum thyroxine reading.

The patient is admitted to hospital 48 hours before operation to check the sleeping pulse rate, which will be normal if the patient is euthyroid.

DRUGS which are used in the preoperative stage are:

(a) Carbimazole (Neo-Mercazole) is given for several weeks before admission but its administration is stopped ten days before the operation. Some surgeons continue antithyroid drugs up to the day of operation.

(b) Lugol's iodine (0·3 to 0·9 ml  t.d.s.) in milk is given. It has a remarkable effect in causing the complete subsidence of most of the symptoms of the disease for a brief period, and when its effect is at its maximum, usually after 10 to 14 days, operation is performed.

(c) Propanolol (120/160 mg daily in divided doses) may be used as the only preoperative preparation for thyroidectomy.

(d) Sedatives quieten the patient and ensure sound sleep. Phenobarbitone (30 mg t.d.s.) is usually sufficient.

(e) Digitalis is given if atrial fibrillation is present. This is given in the form of digoxin (0·25 mg) sufficiently frequently to control the fibrillation.

OBSERVATIONS:

(a) The sleeping pulse rate is the most important guide of progress.
(b) The *heart rate* must be counted if the patient is fibrillating (Fig. 29.3).

*Immediate preoperative care*

1. THE ANAESTHETIC. An ordinary general anaesthetic is given. Morphia and atropine are usually prescribed preoperatively.

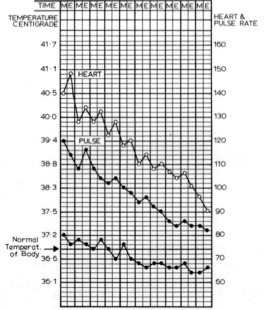

FIG. 29.3  The pulse and heart rate must be recorded in atrial fibrillation. (*The uppermost graph is the heart rate.*)

2. PREPARATION OF THE SKIN. The neck, the upper half of the chest area, the axillae, and the upper arms must be shaved and washed with 2 per cent hexachlorophane soap.

THE OPERATION. Up to nine-tenths of the gland is removed at operation. The wound is closed and drained through a tube brought out through a separate stab incision.

*The postoperative care*

1. POSITION IN BED

If a general anaesthetic has been administered, the patient is laid in the left lateral position until recovery takes place, and is then propped up, supported by a back-rest.

2. TREATMENT IMMEDIATELY ON RETURN FROM THE THEATRE

(a) Digoxin (0·25 mg) may be given subcutaneously, especially if the patient was fibrillating before the operation.

(b) The respirations are frequently shallow and slow. A careful watch is necessary, and oxygen administered if required.

(c) The patient should swallow a little fluid as soon as possible, as it serves to clean the mouth and reduce the tendency to infection. The patient should speak only in a whisper so as to decrease the pain in the neck.

(d) The bedclothing should not be too heavy, and frequent cold sponging is important as sweating is invariable. A room which is too warm must be cooled by a fan.

3. DURING THE NIGHT

(a) *Haemorrrhage.* A careful watch must be kept for excessive

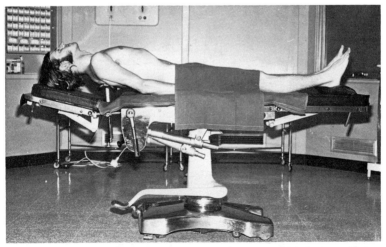

FIG. 29.4   Position for thyroid operation. Note shoulder support.

bleeding. It is important to remember that the site to look for haemorrhage is at the *back* of the dressing.

(b) *Drugs* to encourage sleep are prescribed and given before the patient is too lively.

CARE OF THE TUBE. The tube is removed not later than 48 hours after the operation and the stitches should be removed on the fourth or fifth day. If Michel's clips have been used, alternate clips should be removed on the third day and the remainder on the fourth day. After the fifth day a collodion dressing is all that is necessary. If serum collects in the wound aspiration may be necessary.

OBSERVATIONS. Two-hourly temperature and hourly pulse recordings must be made for two to three days.

### Complications and their treatment

*Haemorrhage.* Some bleeding is usual, but excessive haemorrhage must be notified at once. Severe haemorrhage will cause bulging of the wound and severe dyspnoea due to formation of a haematoma. Reopening of the wound may be necessary.

*Tetany.* Removal or trauma of the parathyroid glands may result in tetany. The patient complains of a tingling and numbness of the face, lips and hands, and twitching of the muscles. Most cases subside spontaneously, but calcium gluconate usually gives rapid relief. The blood calcium is estimated. More remotely a high dosage of vitamin D or AT10 (a synthetic steroid) increases calcium absorption from the intestine.

Apart from tetany, it is advisable to estimate the blood calcium three months after thyroidectomy. It has been shown that latent parathyroid deficiency may give rise to such distressing conditions as bilateral cataracts.

*Respiratory complications.* Soreness of the throat and neck are almost invariable complaints, and are soothed by giving the patient blackcurrant pastilles to suck. Pneumonia and bronchitis may occur.

*Hoarseness.* Hoarseness is usually due to the trauma of the operation, and clears up rapidly. Occasionally it is caused by damage to the recurrent laryngeal nerve and this will be seen when a laryngoscope is passed and the vocal cords are not moving. In cases where both nerves have been damaged, the paralysed vocal cords lie almost in apposition so that the space between them is negligible. The result is that the patient has acute respiratory distress and tracheostomy must be performed without delay.

*Thyrotoxic crisis* is an alarming condition which may cause death very shortly after the operation. In the first six to 24 hours after return from the theatre the patient may develop all the signs of a toxic goitre in an extremely acute form. With modern antithyroid drugs it is now extremely rare.

TREATMENT requires hypothermia, large doses of hypnotics, oxygen and intravenous fluid replacement and sodium iodide intravenously, and propanolol.

*Myxoedema* may occur as a remote complication in about 10 per cent of patients but not all show deposition of mucopolysaccharide substance which gives the typical 'solid' appearance in this condition.

*Recurrent thyrotoxicosis.*

### *Instruction to the patient on leaving hospital*

Two or three months are necessary to gain the full benefit from the operation. Weight increases and, three months later, most patients are fit to lead a normal life. The patient can be reassured that a necklace will adequately conceal the scar. Many patients now feel the cold and must wear warmer clothing.

### EXOPHTHALMOS

The cause is not understood but is thought to be due to excessive secretion of anterior pituitary hormone. It usually occurs as a complication of hyperthyroidism although occasionally it occurs in euthyroid patients. If untreated the exophthalmos, in progressive cases, leads to corneal ulceration and ophthalmoplegia.

### *Treatment*

1. Hyperthyroidism is controlled.
2. Diotroxin, which resembles the thyroid hormones, is administered to damp down the anterior pituitary secretion.
3. The patient wears spectacles with broad side pieces to prevent the exposed cornea from outdoor dust.
4. In the early stages radiotherapy to the orbits in small doses (600 rad) may produce dramatic results.

If improvement does not occur with the above measures, tarsorrhaphy is performed.

Finally, orbital decompression is carried out in an effort to prevent ophthalmoplegia in advanced resistant cases.

### RADIOACTIVE ISOTOPES

Radioactive iodine is now used in the diagnosis and treatment of thyroid gland diseases. This material disintegrates with the emission of energy in the form of gamma rays which can be detected by Geiger counters. In diagnosis, a small (tracer) dose is given orally or intravenously and the amount in the thyroid and in the urine measured. A high thyroid uptake with low urinary excretion is indicative of hyperthyroidism, whilst a low thyroid uptake and high urinary excretion suggests hypothyroidism. Treatment by this means can be given by a large dose and is used at present for those in whom surgery is contraindicated and medical treatment not suitable. In thyroid cancer about 10 per cent of patients take up sufficient radioiodine in the gland and its metastases to be treatable by this method.

Certain thyroid carcinomas are under the influence of the anterior pituitary gland and by the administration of thyroid hormone the growth may be suppressed.

### NEW GROWTHS OF THE THYROID

An adenoma is the commonest new growth. Many malignant neoplasms arise in a pre-existing adenoma and have a particular tendency to metastasise in bone. Spread locally is into the trachea, oesophagus, skin and veins of the neck. In only a few cases are radioactive isotopes of value. Radical surgery may be performed if the disease is not too extensive and some types of tumour are slow growing and have a good prognosis.

### INFLAMMATIONS

1. **An acute abscess.** This may develop in the gland, and is usually secondary to some other acute infection, such as pneumonia or influenza. Incision and drainage may be necessary.

2. **Chronic inflammation.** Tuberculous and syphilitic infections may occur. A diffuse iron hardness of the gland sometimes occurs and is known as Riedel's thyroiditis. Its main importance lies in its tendency to resemble carcinoma.

A rare but interesting type of chronic inflammation of the thyroid gland is Hashimoto's thyroiditis which is thought to

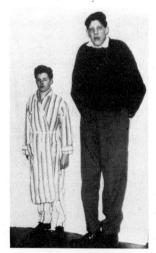

FIG. 29.5   Gigantism.

be an auto-immune disease. In this condition the body reacts to some of its constituent proteins.

## DISEASES OF THE PARATHYROIDS

The parathyroid glands control calcium metabolism. Disease may arise from:

1. *Excess of parathormone* which decalcifies the bones and produces a skeletal condition known as osteitis fibrosa cystica. Ultimately the excessive calcium in the blood causes renal failure. The disease is usually associated with an adenoma of one parathyroid gland.

Intermittent excessive secretion of parathormone may be associated with renal stone formation. Careful calcium balance studies may be necessary to detect this abnormality.

2. *Lack of parathormone* results in great irritability of the nerves, causing spasm and twitching. Known as tetany, it may be caused by conditions other than lack of parathormone, for example, excessive vomiting or hyperventilation (usually of hysterical origin).

## DISEASES OF THE PITUITARY GLAND

Affections of the pituitary gland are many, and complicated. Those of surgical significance are:

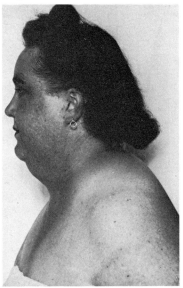

FIG. 29.6  Cushing's syndrome in the adult, showing buffalo hump, acne, hirsutes, plethoric appearance.

## TUMOURS

Space-occupying lesions affect the skull and after eroding the sella turcica press on the optic chiasma. Tumours, or hyperplasia produce acromegaly or Cushing's disease. In infancy hyperpituitarism may cause gigantism. Excision or destruction of the pituitary by radiation may be carried out to decrease oestrogen production in advanced carcinoma of the breast.

## DISEASES OF THE ADRENAL GLANDS

Tumours may occur in the cortex or the medulla. Tumours of the medulla include phaeochromocytomas which cause hypertension. Tumours or hyperplasia of the cortex may produce Cushing's disease, or Conn's syndrome or virilism.

Secondary tumours or any lesion producing destruction of the adrenal cortex causes Addison's disease. The adrenals are most frequently operated on to decrease oestrogen production in advanced carcinoma of the breast (p. 298). Both adrenals are removed and cortisone replacement therapy commenced.

**The gonads.** Anomalies of the testes and ovaries produce a large variety of constitutional disease if the internal secretions are diminished. Examples are Klinefelter's and Turner's syndrome.

# CHAPTER 30

# Diseases of the Breast

The breast is the common site for carcinoma in women. Simple or non-malignant masses are also common, and are broadly known as fibro-adenosis.

Fibroadenosis is a condition of residual thickening of certain portions of the breast, due to a failure of hormonic balance. Its importance lies in the differentiation from a new growth. Acute inflammation terminating in the formation of an abscess may complicate lactation, but is unusual at other times.

## GENERAL SYMPTOMS AND SIGNS OF BREAST DISEASE

Apart from an acute inflammation, the early symptoms are few and unobtrusive.

1. *A lump in the breast* is frequently the only complaint, and the general physical upset is slight.

2. *Pain* is unusual and, when present, is only a 'prickling sensation' which occurs before menstruation. It is unfortunate that growths are usually painless in the early stages, because of all symptoms pain is the one which compels a patient to seek advice.

3. *A discharge from the nipple is not uncommon.* It may be:

(a) *Blood.* This is diagnostic of a duct papilloma or a duct carcinoma.

(b) *A clear, thin discharge* may result from a cyst of the breast.

(c) *A milky discharge* may occur for some time after lactation.

(d) *A green or brownish discharge* is seen occasionally as a result of fibroadenosis.

A discharge from the breast should be tested for the presence of haemoglobin. In a patient under 40 years a breast in which no lump can be palpated but in which there is a discharge from the nipple containing blood, is treated by careful observation. In a patient over 40, a simple mastectomy may be advised.

## CONGENITAL ABNORMALITIES

Congenital abnormalities, apart from retraction of the nipple, are uncommon. An accessory nipple or breast is the most interesting.

An accessory nipple is a small red nodule usually much smaller than the adult nipple and situated in the same longitudinal line as the nipple. It may be noticed by the nurse when washing the patient, who may be either a man or a woman.

An accessory breast is usually unilateral, and the patient complains of swelling of the lower chest or abdominal wall in the same longitudinal line as the breast. The swelling usually appears at puberty and may or may not possess a nipple. The treatment usually advised is excision, because of the cosmetic asymmetry and inconvenience. Injuries to the breast may take the form of an haematoma or fat necrosis. Fat necrosis gives rise to a very firm swelling which may be mistaken for a carcinoma.

### INFECTION OF THE BREAST

*Acute mastitis.* This is not uncommon during lactation, when cracks or fissures are likely to develop in the nipple and areolar regions. Acute lactational mastitis also develops in an area of milk engorgement due to a blocked lactiferous duct. A breast engorged with milk is an excellent medium for the proliferation of organisms usually staphylococci or more rarely streptococci.

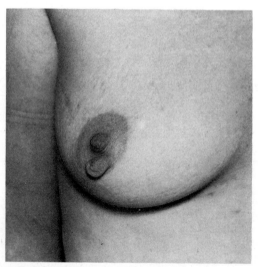

FIG. 30.1   Accessory nipple.

*Symptoms and signs*

The affected portion of the breast is painful, tender, warm and indurated. The patient feels ill and the general signs of inflammation may be present. As pus develops, throbbing pain occurs and the patient is pale and tired from lack of rest and toxic absorption.

*Treatment and nursing care*

PREVENTION

*Breast abscess* is best prevented by careful preparation of the nipple in the last two months of pregnancy and the institution of scrupulous hygiene during lactation. The nipples should be massaged with a good toilet soap and water. Rolling the nipples between the fingers may get them accustomed to the friction of sucking. Any suitable ointment may be applied twice weekly but is not really necessary.

TREATMENT OF ESTABLISHED INFECTION

1. IN THE EARLY STAGES before suppuration has occurred the administration of celbenin is likely to be of most value since most organisms are resistant to penicillin. The infant should be weaned from the affected breast, which should be elevated and supported. A sedative is usually prescribed to promote sleep. The infant, of course, is fed at the other breast. The practice of manual expression of milk from the breast if excessive milk production occurs whilst breast feeding avoids galactocoele formation.

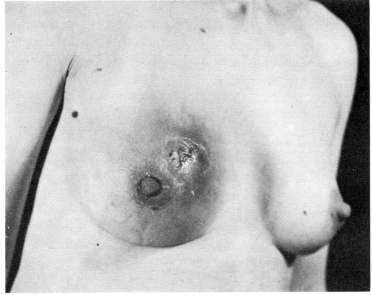

FIG. 30.2    Breast abscess.

2. DRAINAGE is necessary as soon as pus forms, and a tube is usually inserted. At this stage weaning is inevitable from both breasts, and stilboestrol 5 mg b.d. for three days and 5 mg once daily for a further three days is given. This programme of stilboestrol administration diminishes the risk of vaginal bleeding on withdrawal. Stilboestrol, however, increases the risk of venous thrombosis and for this reason some surgeons advise that it be withheld and a sample diuretic prescribed.

ANTIBIOMA. Occasionally an acute mastitis treated with antibiotics forms an encysted abscess, the pus is buried beneath a thick firm wall and a month later the patient is worried because she has a large lump in her breast. Simple incision and drainage are all that is necessary.

AFTERCARE

The tube should be removed about the fifth or sixth day, according to the amount of drainage, and the wounds dressed with eusol compresses.

Later, when the granulating surfaces are clean, Savlon (1 : 200) may be used until healing has been completed.

*Complications of incision.* Haemorrhage is the only serious complication. It is not common, but is sometimes severe. Firm pressure with a bandage is usually sufficient to control it.

**Chronic inflammation of the breast**. Chronic inflammation is rare. A tuberculous abscess is seen very occasionally.

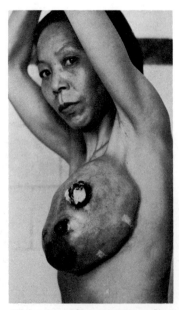

FIG. 30.3　Giant fibroadenoma of breast.

# FIBROADENOSIS AND SIMPLE TUMOURS

The breasts enlarge and develop their adult characteristics at puberty, due to hormonal influences generated in the pituitary, the ovary, and possibly in the thyroid gland. During each menstrual cycle, some slight enlargement of the breasts occurs, to be followed by retrogression until the next cycle, unless pregnancy ensues.

During pregnancy the breasts enlarge, produce milk after parturition, and, later, retrogress when the child has been weaned. Normally this periodic enlargement and retrogression occurs evenly throughout the whole of both breasts. Occasionally, however, due either to the excessive enlargement of one segment or the failure of another to subside evenly, irregularity may occur in the breast substance, with the result that the patient complains of a lump, which is usually painful in the days immediately before menstruation. These lumps, or masses, are known as fibroadenosis. They may take several different forms, which we shall consider presently, but the important fact to remember is that they are essentially the same, however much their clinical forms may vary.

## FORMS OF FIBROADENOSIS

1. **Generalised.** The whole of one or both breasts may be hard and irregular.

2. **Fibroadenosis.** May be limited to one segment or quadrant of one or both breasts.

3. **Cystic type.** Cyst formation is a predominant feature.

*Symptoms and signs of fibroadenosis*

1. The mass is always mobile in the breast tissue.

2. The lump is not felt as easily with the flat of the hand as between the finger and thumb.

3. The nipple is not retracted.

4. Pre-menstrual pain in the breast is not uncommon.

5. The consistency is usually firm and rubbery and not iron-hard in nature.

6. The lymphatic glands in the axilla are not grossly enlarged and are never hard and fixed.

*Treatment*

The local mass is usually excised and examined under the microscope so that the diagnosis can be confirmed with certainty, and nothing reassures the patient more. The cavity in the breast is almost obliterated, but a small drain may be brought out through a separate stab incision, and the main wound in the skin is closed. The drain is removed in 24 to 48

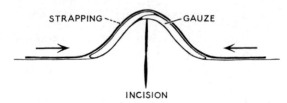

FIG. 30.4 Diagrammatic cross-section of wound (incision) showing correct method of applying strapping over gauze to pull edges together as indicated by arrows.

hours. To prevent separation of the wound and consequent broadening of the skin scar the sides of the incision must be supported by gauze and strapping or Elastoplast drawn up from the sides so that the wound is not flattened (Fig. 30.4).

Simple mastectomy is almost never advised today for fibro-adenosis.

### TRUE SIMPLE TUMOURS OF THE BREAST

These lesions include:

1. **Fibroadenoma.**
2. **Cystadenoma.** Occurs in slightly older women and grows to a larger size than a fibroadenoma.
3. **Duct papilloma.** This is a benign tumour which arises in one of the terminal lactiferous ducts. It causes a blood-stained discharge from the nipple. As these tumours are liable to develop into duct carcinoma, excision is advisable.

## CARCINOMA OF THE BREAST

Every woman who discovers a lump in her breast has a not unnatural dread that it is a carcinoma. Unfortunately, this dread too often results in concealment of her condition until it is too late, yet the breast remains one of the most favourable sites for the treatment of a new growth. The earlier treatment is instituted, the greater the chances of cure.

### VARIETIES OF CARCINOMA OF THE BREAST

1. **Scirrhous carcinoma.** This is the commonest form. It is hard in consistency.
2. **Encephaloid carcinoma.** Encephaloid carcinoma is a softer growth and spreads more rapidly than the scirrhous type.
3. **Duct carcinoma.** The rarest growth. It is characterised by bleeding from the nipple and is occasionally associated with an eczematous-like condition of the nipple and areola (Paget's disease). It is a favourable growth to treat.
4. **Acute carcinomatosis of lactation.** Fortunately rare. The

patient develops a growth while lactating, and the great vascularity of the breast at this time causes rapid spread.

*The spread of carcinoma of the breast*

1. LOCALLY, spread occurs by increase in the size of the growth, invasion of the skin overlying the growth and invasion of the pectoral muscles of the chest wall.

2. LYMPHATIC SPREAD occurs to the axillary lymphatic glands and later to the supraclavicular group. Spread to the lymphatic glands in the chest may occur early in growths of the inner segments of the breast.

3. SPREAD BY THE BLOOD STREAM may result in invasion of the bones, particularly the vertebrae. The liver may also be invaded by this route.

CLINICAL STAGING OF CARCINOMA OF THE BREAST

*Stage 1.* A small growth with no localised spread.

*Stage 2.* Evidence of local extension such as a skin attachment but no enlargement of the glands.

*Stage 3.* In addition the glands are enlarged.

*Stage 4.* Disseminated spread.

Although clinically a growth may be stage 1, undetected secondary deposits may already be well established and the disease is in fact already well advanced.

*Symptoms and signs*

1. A painless, hard, irregular mass in the breast is the usual complaint. It has been noticed as a rule while washing, or as a result of a trivial knock. It is easily felt with the flat of the hand. There is usually some elevation of the breast. With a lump in the breast, as in vaginal bleeding, the greatest service a nurse can do is to refer the patient immediately to her doctor.

2. Attachment to the skin and the deeper structures, namely, the pectoral muscles and the ribs, occurs as the growth extends.

3. Recent retraction of the nipple may be present. This sign is diagnostic.

4. A coarsening of the skin, known as *peau d'orange*, may be present, due to blockage of the subcutaneous lymphatic vessels.

5. Ulceration and fungation occur in late and untreated cases.

6. The lymphatic glands in the axilla may be enlarged and hard.

7. Mammography is sometimes of value.

8. Frozen microscopic section as soon as the lump has been

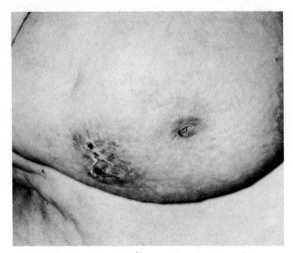

FIG. 30.5    Carcinoma of breast showing *peau d'orange*.

removed is the only certain method of diagnosis in the very earliest cases.

9. Early detection should be increased if the breasts of every patient who has a cervical smear are palpated for swellings.

10. Thermography with an infra-red detector reveals increased vascularity and is an occasional help in diagnosis.

*Treatment*

The measures considered below are widely practised and the best form of treatment for each patient has to be carefully considered. Recently some surgeons are of the opinion that the course of carcinoma of the breast is uninfluenced by treatment while others believe that local excision of the swelling or simple mastectomy without removal of the axillary glands has much to recommend it, the theory being that the glands, if they are uninvolved, are a protection to the patient.

1. BONE SCANNING may be undertaken before deciding the appropriate method of treatment.

2. RADICAL MASTECTOMY (i.e., removal of the breast, a large area of skin over the breast, the pectoral muscles and fascia, together with axillary fat and lymphatic glands in one continuous piece).

3. RADIOTHERAPY is usually used to supplement a simple or radical removal or to delay the growth in inoperable cases. Some surgeons advise radiotherapy alone or followed by simple mastectomy.

4. SIMPLE MASTECTOMY is the most commonly practised operation followed by radiotherapy only if the glands are invaded. It is also performed if it is possible in late cases to reduce fun-

gation and sepsis, which are particularly distressing to the patient.

5. HORMONE THERAPY is sometimes unexpectedly dramatic in its effect. It consists of oestrogens for the post-menopausal woman and androgens in the pre-menopausal patient to alter the prevailing internal hormonal environment. It is used for recurrent carcinoma.

6. BILATERAL ADRENALECTOMY (p. 298).

7. CHEMOTHERAPY. Thiotepa (an intramuscular nitrogen mustard preparation), 15 mg twice or thrice weekly for a maximum of 300 mg, has given good immediate results. Methotrexate may be given intravenously or intra-arterially. Quadruple therapy (p.217) may be given.

Regular white cell counts are performed to avoid agranulocytosis.

## Nursing care of a case of radical mastectomy
### PREOPERATIVE CARE

X-rays to exclude secondary deposits in the chest, the ribs and the spine will usually have been taken before admission. Anaemia is corrected by a blood transfusion.

Operation is not undertaken until the patient is free from any acute respiratory infection.

### PREPARATION OF THE SKIN

1. LOCAL. Both axillae are shaved, the affected one because it comes into the incision, and the opposite one because the bandages pass around it. The area of both breasts, the arms to the wrists, and the abdomen to below the umbilicus, are washed with 2 per cent hexachlorophane soap.

2. THE THIGH. The ipsilateral thigh should be shaved and washed so that it is ready as a donor area should a skin graft be required. It must *not* be painted with antiseptics which kill the superficial cells from which the graft is cut.

### THE OPERATION

The prepared area is generously towelled off.

THE CARE OF THE ARM DURING THE OPERATION. The arm is held by a nurse until the patient is towelled for operation. It is held abducted, one of the nurse's hands holding the patient's wrist and the other hand resting on the table to protect the patient's radial nerve on the lower third of the humerus. The nurse must be careful not to over-abduct the arm for fear of causing damage to the large nerve-trunks. It is then fixed on a suitably padded side arm of the operating table.

POSTOPERATIVE CARE

The patient is laid on her side on return to bed. A blood transfusion may be running. When recovery from the anaesthetic has taken place, the patient is propped up and a pillow is placed at the bottom of the bed, so that she can push against it with her feet.

The patient gets out of bed next day.

*Haemorrhage and care of the drainage tube.* A tube is invariably inserted, and in the first 24 hours oozing of blood and serum always occurs. A careful watch must be kept for haemorrhage, and the dressing can be repacked if it becomes saturated. The bandage must be firmly secured. Any excessive haemorrhage should, of course, be reported at once. The tube is rotated and eased a little after 24 hours and removed after 48 to 72 hours. Some surgeons prefer suction drainage of the axilla and the tube is attached to a suction machine or Redivac drain.

*Pain* is relieved by morphia (15 mg), which is usually prescribed on the night following the operation.

CARE OF THE WOUND. After removal of the tube the stab wound is covered with a mild antiseptic, such as flavine.

The edges of the wound should be inspected for undue tension during dressing, and stitches are released if necessary. Ballooning of the flaps may occur, and air and serum are evacuated by aspiration or the gentle insertion of sinus forceps. The flaps themselves must be observed for sloughing, and, should it occur, eusol is an excellent dressing for aiding the separation of sloughs.

THE SUTURES are removed as follows: alternate sutures are removed on the tenth day and the remainder on the twelfth day.

If a bare area has been grafted great care must be taken to

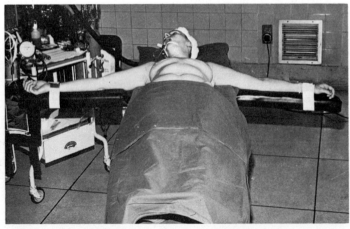

FIG. 30.6   Position for operations on the breast.

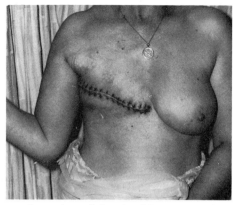

FIG. 30.7  External rotation of the shoulder joint is the only movement which it is important to recover in the first week following mastectomy. If this is full, abduction will also be full.

'float off' with sterile saline the innermost dressing, which is usually a small flap of tulle gras.

CARE OF THE ARM. It is important to commence arm movements on the second day after operation, but it is unwise to insist on much abduction for four or five days. The wound is disturbed and serum oozing increases. The patient must be encouraged to externally rotate the shoulder joint gently, and by the tenth day should have no trouble in touching the back of her head with her hand. If she has full external rotation at once she will have no difficulty in achieving full abduction. This is important, since her greatest disability will be in fastening her clothes at the back and doing her hair.

DIET. The patient should drink large quantities of fluids as soon as post-anaesthetic nausea has ceased. The nurse must remember that in the early days the patient will require some assistance with drinks and food because of the disability of the arm. Her locker or bed-table should be placed on the side opposite to that on which the operation was performed.

## Complications

1. *Respiratory complications* are not uncommon, since respiration may be impaired by the trauma of the operation and the restriction of chest movements caused by the firm bandaging. Deep-breathing exercises assist in preventing respiratory complications.

2. *Sloughing of the flaps.* Should extensive sloughing occur, skin grafting must be undertaken later, when the area has granulated cleanly. Sloughs must be removed and sepsis reduced to a minimum as soon as possible. Eusol compresses are valuable before and just after the sloughs have separated, followed by hypertonic saline compresses.

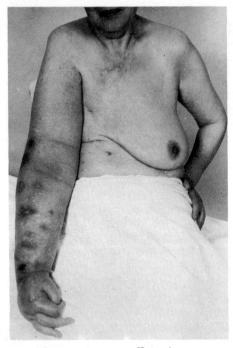

FIG. 30.8   Heavy oedematous arm, sufficiently severe to dislocate the shoulder.

3. *Oedema of the arm* may occur immediately if ligation of the axillary vein has had to be performed. More remotely, it may be due to lymphatic obstruction, constriction of the axillary vein from fibrosis or to recurrence of the growth and is a most distressing symptom. Elevation of the arm at night may control moderate swelling.

4. *Thrombosis* of the axillary vein may occur occasionally.

ADVICE TO THE PATIENT ON LEAVING HOSPITAL

The patient may be referred for a course of radiotherapy when the wound is soundly healed, six to eight weeks later. In some cases subsequent removal of the ovaries may be advised. She should report back to the operating surgeon at regular intervals.

*Cosmetic deformity.* This is easily concealed by a TruLife prosthesis attached to the patient's clothing.

*Adrenalectomy for disseminated carcinoma of the breast*

Bilateral removal of the adrenals may be indicated in disseminated carcinoma of the breast or prostate when it is beyond other methods of control. Other indications for bilateral removal of the adrenals are selected cases of Cushing's syndrome.

PREOPERATIVE MANAGEMENT

Patients selected for adrenalectomy are always at an advanced stage of the disease. Their general condition must be carefully assessed. The extent of the malignancy must also be mapped out carefully. A low blood count must be corrected by transfusions. Hydrocortisone is given by intramuscular injection of 100 mg one hour before operation. Both adrenal glands are usually excised at one operation but if it is decided to remove one at a time the opposite is removed 10 days later. Because of danger of delay in healing and trauma on the table to a healing wound, the stitches from the first wound are not removed until the second operation has been completed. Pethidine, 50 to 100 mg, is preferable to morphia because of the danger of liver damage from secondary deposits.

The striking benefit of adrenalectomy is the immediate relief of pain in most cases of secondary deposits in bone. After eighteen months to two years most patients relapse.

POSTOPERATIVE CARE

Following operation hydrocortisone is given in 100 mg doses, intramuscularly six-hourly, for one day. Close observation of the blood pressure is essential, and if the patient becomes hypotensive the dosage and/or frequency of hydrocortisone must be increased. This is reduced to two doses of 100 mg on the next day after operation and continued orally as cortisone acetate in 25 mg doses six-hourly for two days. On the fourth day cortisone is reduced to 75 mg and from the sixth day most patients are maintained on a dose of 50 mg a day. It is explained to the patient that the adrenal glands, which produce a substance called cortisone, essential to life, have been removed. Cortisone must be taken in tablet form for the rest of the patient's life. The patient should take a normal diet with plenty of salt. A few patients require in addition fludrocortisone (a minerocorticoid) 0.1 mg daily. If she is not feeling well or gets tired, she should return at once. If she vomits, cortisone can be given by injection. If she goes abroad, she must make sure that she can get a maintenance dose of cortisone or she will die. It is essential that patients should carry 'steroid cards' to the effect that they are on maintenance cortisone therapy.

When adrenalectomy is performed for carcinoma of the breast the ovaries are also removed so that no oestrin-producing tissue remains in the body. The patient who has had only one adrenal removed requires replacement therapy—the other adrenal may be functionless from secondary deposits.

*Hypophysectomy*

As an alternative to adrenalectomy removal or destruction of the pituitary may be advised.

PREPARATION

The patient is admitted a week before operation and the urinary excretion of 17-ketosteroids estimated. The uptake of radioactive iodine is estimated for subsequent assessment of thyroid function.

Six days before operation cortisone, 50 mg by mouth, rising to 400 mg on the day of operation, is administered. Half of this is given by mouth and the other half by intramuscular injection.

Pleural or ascitic collections are aspirated.

The usual preparation for craniotomy (p. 520) is undertaken for a transfrontal approach. An alternative approach either for excision or for the implant of yttrium-90 is transphenoidally.

POSTOPERATIVE CARE

The pituitary controls all the other ductless glands so that removal causes widespread effects and the postoperative care reflects some of the methods of dealing with this upset. Consciousness is quickly regained: 350 mg of cortisone is given and gradually reduced to 50 mg daily.

The wound heals uneventfully: 300 mg of DOCA may be implanted beneath the sheath of the rectus muscle in the abdominal wall before discharge from hospital.

**Special dangers**
1. Lassitude.
2. Anorexia.
3. Low blood pressure.
4. Danger of infection.
5. Electrolyte imbalance—salt depletion, retention of potassium and a rise in blood urea.

Salt capsules, 4 g daily, may be given if the blood pressure is low. If the blood pressure is raised salt is forbidden.

**Occasional complications**
1. *Fits.* The risk may be diminished by administering phenobarbitone, 30 mg daily.
2. *Diabetes insipidus.* Forty mg of post-pituitary snuff, once to three times daily, may be advised.
3. *Hypothyroidism.* Thyroxine may be given but is to be avoided if possible on account of the danger of stimulating the neoplasm.

After adrenalectomy or hypophysectomy vomiting is a most important *symptom* and is usually due to lack of cortisone.

THE SURGICAL SIGNIFICANCE OF CORTICOSTEROIDS

The adrenal glands secrete adrenaline and noradrenaline from the medulla and hydrocortisone (Cortisol), aldosterone and some other androgens and oestrogens from the cortex. Hydrocortisone is the natural hormone and can now be made synthetically. Cortisone, prednisolone and a number of other substances are synthetic compounds with similar properties. Hydrocortisone output of the adrenals is under the control of the adrenocorticotrophic hormone (ACTH) secreted by the pituitary. ACTH output is governed by the amount of hydrocortisone in the blood. Aldosterone is the main hormone responsible for maintaining electrolyte balance and is not controlled by the pituitary.

Patients who have been on corticosteroids for any length of time usually have a medically induced adrenal insufficiency due to the suppressive action of the administered steroids on the pituitary gland.

The dose of cortisone should be increased before, during and immediately after operation to cover the increased demands made by anaesthesia and surgical intervention. Failure to observe this principle may lead to death of the patient from acute adrenal insufficiency.

Corticosteroids may be used as:

1. Replacement therapy, e.g. Addison's disease, hypopituitarism, and after bilateral adrenalectomy.

2. Therapeutically. Apart from adrenal insufficiency, cortisone is widely used in the group of diseases known as the collagenoses: notably rheumatoid arthritis, scleroderma, periarteritis nodosa, and lupus erythematosus. In addition it may be used in such diseases as iritis, thrombocytopenic purpura, and status asthmaticus.

Corticosteroids given in a dose beyond what is normally required for the maintenance of life causes the body to: (1) retain sodium salts, (2) excrete potassium salts. If more than 50 mg is used potassium chloride (3 g daily) should be given to make good the increased excretion of potassium salts. In addition a low salt diet is necessary. The patient who has undergone bilateral adrenalectomy, on the other hand, should take a normal salt diet because her replacement dosage of cortisone is equal to the normal secretion of the hormone.

Many patients receiving corticosteroid therapy may come for urgent surgical intervention and the dosage of steroids has to be increased before and after operation.

There are many complications of cortisone which may be of surgical importance. The commonest are:

1. Reactivation of a latent pulmonary tuberculous focus.
2. Bleeding from a peptic ulcer.
3. Development of silent fulminating infections, for example, appendicitis.
4. Rapid development of cardiac failure.

5. Oedema including 'moon'-shaped face usually due to overdosage.

Other complications include thrombosis, osteoporosis, psychosis, and skin reactions such as acne and mild hirsutism.

## DISEASES OF THE MALE BREAST

Since the male breast is a vestigial organ, disease is uncommon.

*Fibroadenosis* is the most common simple lesion and is frequently due to pressure from braces. The treatment is excision. Gynaecomastia, which may be very painful, is sometimes seen as a complication of stilboestrol therapy for carcinoma of the prostate. At puberty, and sometimes in the newborn infant, enlargement of the breast occurs.

*Carcinoma of the male breast* occurs occasionally, accounting for 1 per cent of all breast cancer. The symptoms and signs are the same as in women, but because there is almost no breast tissue for the growth to invade, fixation to and invasion of the underlying muscle and ribs occur very early.

CHAPTER 31

# Diseases of the Lungs and Thorax

Surgery of the chest has shared in full measure in the advances in chemotherapy, blood transfusion and anaesthesia. It has also benefited by an increased understanding of the physiology of respiration, and operations inside the thoracic cavity are as common as surgical operations elsewhere in the body.

## INJURIES TO THE THORAX

1. **Fractured ribs.** Fracture of the ribs is a common condition caused by a crushing injury. The pain over the affected rib is severe and is aggravated by respiration. If the underlying lung has been torn, air may escape into the subcutaneous tissues and give rise to a swollen crepitant condition known as surgical emphysema, or into the pleural cavity, giving rise to pneumothorax. A double fracture of the ribs is more dangerous because paradoxical respiration may occur in the flail section of the chest, producing a shift of the mediastinum. A firm pad and bandage are necessary for seven to ten days. If a pad does not control it then a tracheostomy is performed and the patient is connected to a mechanical respirator. Operation to wire the ribs together may be necessary.

In older patients, pneumonia is very liable to follow even a moderately severe injury, and this complication is more likely if the patient is kept at rest in bed.

*Treatment*

The main objects of treatment are the relief of pain and the prevention of pulmonary complications.

For the first 24 hours the patient is usually kept in bed. An accurate estimate must be formed of the extent of the damage to the underlying lung. Laceration of a blood vessel or laceration of the lung may cause an effusion of blood into the pleural cavity. This is known as a haemothorax.

Since fractures of the ribs unite easily without any particular treatment, every effort must be made to relieve the pain and encourage the patient to move about. Strapping is the usual method of treatment, but the injection of a few millilitres of 2 per cent novocain into the fracture will usually effect complete relief.

2. **Haemothorax.** Haemothorax is a collection of blood in the pleural cavity. It may follow a fracture of the ribs or a penetrating wound of the chest. The symptoms are those of pleural irritation, viz., pain, which is worse on breathing, followed by relief as bleeding increases. If the bleeding is profuse, dyspnoea and the signs of internal haemorrhage will be present. The presence of a considerable quantity of blood in the pleural cavity causes further outpouring of fluid from the pleura due to the irritant effect of blood. In many cases the collection of blood absorbs spontaneously; in others aspiration or evacuation by open operation may be necessary.

3. **Penetrating wounds of the chest.** If a 'sucking' wound (i.e., a wound in which air is sucked in and out of the wound in the chest wall) is present it must be covered with a small pad of sterile petroleum jelly gauze as a first-aid measure. After acute circulatory collapse has been treated the wound is excised, foreign bodies are removed and the wound is closed. The complications are:

(a) *Pyothorax.*
(b) *A persistent sinus.*
(c) *Lung abscess.*

## ACUTE INFECTIONS OF THE CHEST

### PYOTHORAX

A pyothorax (or empyema) is a collection of pus in the pleural cavity, which compresses the lung and displaces the heart.

The commonest cause is infection of the pleural cavity secondary to an attack of pneumonia but it may follow a wound in the chest, perforation of the oesophagus or spread from a subphrenic abscess.

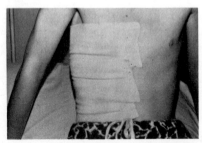

FIG. 31.1   Strapping for fracture of one or more ribs.

*Clinical features*

Examination reveals the presence of fluid in the chest of the patient who is obviously toxic. The diagnosis is confirmed by aspiration of pus from the pleural cavity.

BACTERIOLOGY

Whilst almost any organisms may be responsible for the infection, the commonest causal organisms are:

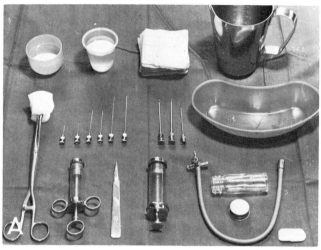

FIG. 31.2A   A tray for chest aspiration:

| | |
|---|---|
| Sponge-holding forceps | Cannulas |
| Labat syringe | Three-way connection and |
| Martin's syringe | tubing |
| Infiltrating needles | Specimen bottle |
| Aspirating needle | Swabs |

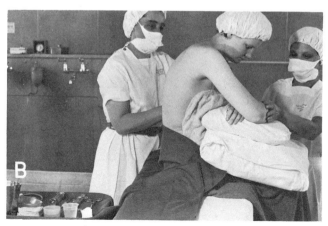

FIG. 31.2B   Good positioning for chest aspiration.

1. The staphylococcus.
2. The haemolytic streptococcus.

*Treatment and nursing care*

GENERAL TREATMENT

POSITION IN BED. If dyspnoea is present, the patient usually prefers to sit up supported by a back rest. He must be allowed to assume whatever position he finds most comfortable.

LOCAL TREATMENT

ASPIRATION. This is essentially for diagnosis and determination of antibiotic sensitivity. Neomycin 1 g is inserted after the first aspiration before sensitivity is known. Then when the report returns the appropriate antibiotic is injected after repeated aspiration. This usually clears up the condition. If not, intercostal closed drainage for seven to ten days is undertaken. Later still, if the condition has not resolved, rib resection and open drainage are undertaken.

PROCEDURE FOR CHEST ASPIRATION. (a) A basic trolley is prepared, additional items on the bottom shelf are:

Gown, mask, gloves
Local anaesthetic, syringe and needles
Green towels
Iodine
Set of aspirating needles
Three-way tap
No. 5 drainage tube
30 or 50 ml syringes
Measure jug
Artery forceps

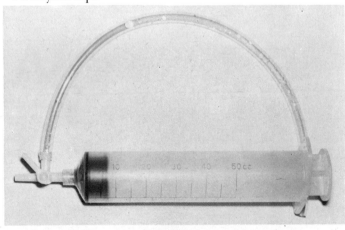

FIG. 31.3   Three-way tap and syringe and tubing.

Specimen tubes
Sealing agent, e.g. Nobecutane, 'stamp dressing'.

(b) The nature of the procedure is explained to the patient and his co-operation is obtained. Privacy is ensured. (c) The doctor prepares himself. The trolley is taken to the bedside. The pyjama coat is removed and the patient made comfortable and supported in the sitting position either leaning forwards or backwards as the doctor requires. (d) The nurse opens the outer wrappings of the basic dressing pack, opens other packets as required, and assists the doctor to assemble the apparatus. The doctor performs the procedure, assisted by the nurse. (e) The nurse observes the patient's general condition, in particular noting his colour and pulse. Any changes and any tendency to cough are reported to the doctor. She gives help and reassurance as appropriate. (f) On completion of the procedure, the doctor withdraws the needle and seals the wound. The patient is dressed and made comfortable. Observations are continued on his general condition, colour and breathing. (g) The trolley is covered and removed. The fluid is measured, the amount recorded, the necessary specimen taken and the re-

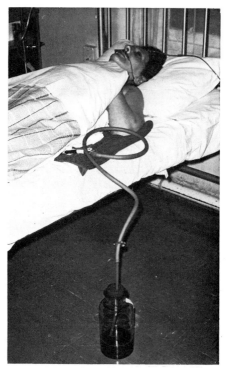

FIG. 31.4   Closed drainage of the chest.

mainder discarded. The aspirating needles are rinsed in cold water, placed in the appropriate container, and returned to the C.S.S.D. Any specimens are sent to the laboratory.

DRAINAGE. Drainage consists of the insertion of a large tube into the lowest part of the pleural cavity, usually after resection of about 5 cm of a rib. The wound is closed around the tube. If the tube is allowed to drain on to the dressings the drainage is described as 'open'. On the other hand, if the tube is connected to a bottle half-full of an antiseptic lotion, outside the bed and completely shut off from the atmosphere, the arrangement is known as 'closed' or underwater seal drainage.

CARE OF THE TUBE. Pyothorax may require prolonged drainage, but the original tube is left in place for two days and then changed. The reinsertion of the tube may be difficult but a laminaria tent inserted into the sinus for 12 hours dilates it painlessly and a tube of the original size may then be inserted. Drainage is continued until the abscess cavity is completely obliterated. The diameter of the tube should not be reduced but the length can be shortened as required. Persistent pain suggests that the tube has been incorrectly reinserted.

Radiographs and sinograms are invaluable in gauging progress.

The tube is secured to a very large pad of Gamgee by means of a large sterile safety-pin, or sutured to the chest wall. The tube should be surrounded by an antiseptic dressing such as proflavine.

MEASUREMENT OF THE QUANTITY OF DISCHARGE. In the closed drainage method the amount of pus discharged each day is

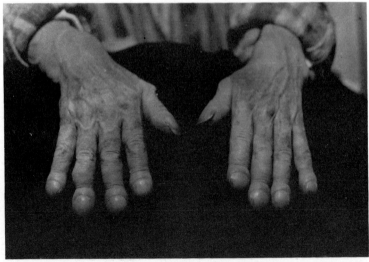

FIG. 31.5   Clubbing of the fingers.

measured, and a chart should be kept.

BREATHING EXERCISES. Selective breathing exercises under the care of a skilled physiotherapist are essential.

**Chronic pyothorax.** An acute pyothorax may become chronic. The discharge of pus continues, the cavity remains unobliterated, and the general health of the patient deteriorates. Clubbing of the finger-tips and amyloid disease may develop as a result of the existence of prolonged suppuration.

*Treatment*

1. Obvious faults such as inadequate drainage, the neglect of respiratory exercises or the presence of a foreign body are corrected and treatment continued as for an acute pyothorax.

2. If the visceral pleura is fibrosed the lung cannot expand. The cavity must be excised or obliterated by the approximation of the chest wall to the lung, which is achieved by an operation known as thoracoplasty (p. 312). If the underlying lung is diseased by tuberculosis or a neoplasm, resection of the lung may be necessary.

### LUNG ABSCESS

An acute abscess may develop in the lung as a result of the aspiration of septic material from the throat or vomitus, as a result of intestinal obstruction. This is particularly liable to occur as a result of anaesthesia, or following an operation on the teeth, the mouth, or the throat. The failure of a patch of pneumonia to resolve or the presence of a foreign body in the bronchus are not uncommon causes.

The patient is ill and may complain of a cough. Sweating, wasting, loss of appetite, and persistent high temperature are usual. The sputum is profuse, purulent, and foul if the abscess is draining into the bronchi, but if, as is usually the case, the abscess is walled off, sputum is not copious.

The abscess may burst into a bronchus and the pus will be coughed up. This may result in healing, but occasionally the rupture results in such an outpouring of pus that it runs into all the bronchi of both lungs, with the result that profuse dissemination of the infection occurs, if the patient is not fatally overwhelmed at once.

*Treatment*

The vast majority heal with treatment by postural drainage and chemotherapy. Lobectomy is the usual treatment for an abscess which fails to resolve with medical treatment. Very rarely external drainage may be necessary.

### BRONCHIECTASIS

Bronchiectasis is a condition in which the smaller bronchi and bronchioles are enlarged, stretched, and have lost their elasticity. There will usually have been a history of pneumonia, a severe attack of measles or whooping cough, associated with severe chest complications. With the use of antibiotics and improved social conditions any severe form of bronchiectasis has now become rare.

## Symptoms and signs

Cough with profuse purulent sputum, which is sometimes foul. It is more copious in the morning and may vary with

A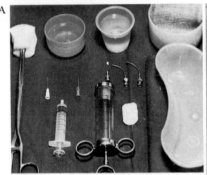

B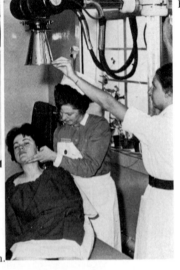

FIG. 31.6A  Tray for bronchogram:
   Sponge-holding forceps
   5-ml Disposable syringe
   Labat syringe and intercricoid needle
   Swabs.

FIG. 31.6B  Positioning for bronchogram.

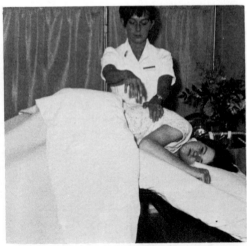

FIG. 31.7   Postural drainage for 'pre-bronchogram'.

change in posture. It is occasionally bloodstained. Intermittent attacks of pneumonia and pleurisy may occur.

This diagnosis is confirmed by a bronchogram.

*Treatment*

Removal of the affected area is the treatment of choice, and this takes the form of excision of one lobe of the lung (lobectomy) or of the whole of one lung (pneumonectomy).

PREOPERATIVE CARE

In addition to the general preoperative care of thoracic surgical patients, postural drainage is essential in cases of bronchiectasis.

1. GENERAL MEASURES. The patient must have plenty of rest, but is not kept in bed all day. Fresh air and sun tone up his body, and a verandah if available is a very suitable place to carry out preoperative treatment.

The patient must be kept interested, and an occupational therapist will be able to suggest some light, interesting work to occupy his mind. This preoperative stage may last from one to two months.

2. DRAINAGE OF THE CAVITIES. This is achieved by the use of postural drainage. This consists of placing the patient's body in such a position that pus will drain by gravity from any cavity in the lung into the bronchi and so may be coughed up. For example, a cavity in the right lower lobe would be drained by laying the patient on his left side and raising the foot of the bed. For this purpose a Nelson bed or one improvised on its principles is generally used. The exact position is determined by the site of the disease, and the surgeon will give precise instructions. Postural drainage should be undertaken every four hours.

*The surgical treatment of pulmonary tuberculosis*

The extended use of streptomycin, PAS and INAH now enables most cases of pulmonary tuberculosis to be cured by medical treatment alone.

In some cases, however, the damage to the lung has been so great before the diagnosis is made and the medical treatment started, that although the tuberculous infection has been sterilised, the changes in the lung are such that removal of the affected area is indicated. Again, some patients' organisms become resistant to the drugs before they are all killed, and surgical treatment may be required to eradicate the infection. Some patients, too, will remain apparently healed for long periods of time and then break down again, and surgical extirpation of the lesion may be required.

Thoracoplasty is an operation undertaken to collapse the lung by approximating the chest wall to the affected lung by the resection of a number of ribs on the affected side, usually five or seven, rarely ten. It is associated with extrapleural stripping of the apex of the lung to assist any cavities to collapse.

The operation is usually performed in stages, since it is a severe undertaking. The patient is usually under 55 years of age and the disease is preferably unilateral.

PREOPERATIVE CARE requires prolonged sanatorium treatment so that the patient is as fit as possible.

POSTOPERATIVE CARE is similar, in general, to that of a case of lobectomy.

The following additional points are of importance:

1. A firm many-tailed bandage is used with a large firm pad over the decostalised area. This controls any paradoxical movement and must be carefully watched.
2. The maintenance of the posture and arrangement of the pillows are very important, so that the patient will have a correct posture when he gets out of bed.
3. Coughing must be encouraged by the nurse as soon as possible so that all sputum is raised. Holding the painful side of the chest renders it easier. Pethidine and adequate oxygen must be administered.
4. Chemotherapy is continued throughout the operative stage and for six to twelve months afterwards.

## NEW GROWTHS OF THE LUNG

Primary new growths of the lung or, more usually, of the bronchus are increasing in frequency due to inhalation of cigarette smoke. Other factors which have been noted are exhaust gas from motor engines and inhalation of radioactive ores. Chromate workers are more liable to carcinoma of the lung, as are arsenical sheep-dip workers. Simple neoplasms and cysts of the mediastinum also occur, but rarely.

### THE CLINICAL FEATURES OF CARCINOMA OF THE LUNG

If the neoplasm arises in one of the main bronchi the symptoms are those of bronchial irritation. If the growth arises in the periphery of the lung pain is a characteristic symptom. Many cases present the same clinical picture as unresolved pneumonia. The early symptoms are those of bronchial irritation:

1. Irritable cough, productive of very little sputum.
2. Haemoptysis (spitting of blood).

At this stage, and this is an important stage at which the diagnosis must be made if cure is to be effected, careful X-ray and bronchoscopic examinations are of the greatest value. Later, sepsis, degeneration and haemorrhage, together with spread of the growth, produce:

1. Purulent, copious sputum.
2. A bloodstained pleural exudate.
3. Cachexia and loss of appetite.
4. Pain, usually due to pressure on important nerves, and invasion of the chest wall.
5. Difficulty in breathing and swallowing.
6. Signs of venous obstruction from pressure give rise to oedema of the face and engorged veins in the neck.
7. Metastases elsewhere.

*Treatment*

Removal of a lobe or entire lung and mediastinal glands offers the only hope of cure. The operation is a severe one and only early cases are suitable.

The preparation and aftercare are similar to that of lobectomy, which is described below. Deep X-ray therapy may be prescribed in inoperable cases, and while some improvement results, it is seldom curative. Chemotherapy may be helpful to relieve pain and shrink enlarged glands.

*Lobectomy or pneumonectomy*

PREOPERATIVE CARE

Infection is controlled and anaemia is corrected. In the case of bronchiectasis this will require postural drainage (p. 311). In all cases preoperative breathing exercises are important in major abdominal as well as in thoracic surgery and are therefore discussed here in some detail.

PREOPERATIVE BREATHING EXERCISES

Breathing exercises are important in preparation for all operations, and deep breathing exercises prevent many of the common pulmonary complications which are liable to follow an operation.

Postoperative pulmonary complications occur in a proportion of cases, particularly after upper abdominal operations. The commonest is collapse of the base of the lung. This is due to:

1. Shallow breathing, which may be caused by:
    (a) Pain in an abdominal wound which restricts the movement of the lower chest.
    (b) Acute circulatory failure.

2. Excessive bronchial secretion which may be produced during anaesthesia. If this is not coughed up, the air entry to the small bronchi is blocked.

3. Inhalation of the stomach contents.

Breathing exercises are designed to make the fullest possible use of the lower chest in the postoperative period without causing pain or discomfort.

Following operations on the chest, particularly if a lobe or an entire lung has been removed, the patient must know how to utilise the remainder of his pulmonary tissues to the greatest possible advantage. It is for this reason that selective and controlled breathing exercises are taught in the preparatory period.

### GENERAL INSTRUCTIONS

The patient lies back against the pillow with the head and body well supported. The legs are drawn up so that the knees are slightly bent. The hands are placed in the position required for the exercise. The patient should relax and breathe quietly for a short time before beginning the exercise. Air should be breathed through the nose and expired through the mouth with a slight blowing sound.

### SIDE EXPANSION OF LOWER RIBS (Fig. 31.8 A)

1. The patient's hand is placed on one side of the body over the lower ribs with the fingers pointing forwards.

2. He then breathes in, expanding the ribs against the firm pressure of the hand, but releasing this as expansion reaches its limit.

3. The patient then breathes out by relaxing and allowing air to escape from the lungs, gradually increasing again the pressure of the hand, but releasing this pressure as expansion reaches its limit.

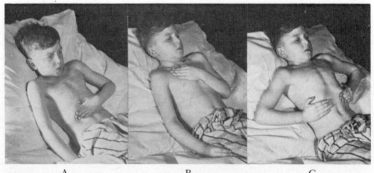

A                              B                              C

FIG. 31.8   A, Side expansion of lower ribs. B, Expansion of upper ribs, one side only. C, Diaphragmatic breathing.

EXPANSION OF UPPER RIBS, ONE SIDE ONLY

1. One hand is placed as shown in Fig. 31.8B.

2. When breathing in, the patient concentrates on expanding that part of the chest under the fingers without moving the shoulders.

3. The patient breathes out by relaxing all effort; at the end the ribs are pressed in farther with the fingers.

DIAPHRAGMATIC BREATHING (Fig. 31.8c)

1. The hands are placed with the palms on the lower ribs and the fingers resting on the abdominal muscles. The fingertips just touch in the midline.

2. The patient breathes in, expanding the ribs against the firm pressure of the hands, but releasing this as expansion reaches the limit.

3. The patient breathes out by relaxing, gradually increasing pressure against the ribs.

Patients should be encouraged to undertake their exercises by themselves as frequently as possible between the regular instructions of the physiotherapist or nurse.

POSTOPERATIVE CARE OF A CASE OF LOBECTOMY OR
PNEUMONECTOMY

ON RETURN TO BED. The patient is nursed in the lateral position because two tubes are usually *in situ* until he has recovered from the effects of anaesthesia and is then propped up with pillows. The greatest care must be taken of the tubes from the chest and of the blood transfusion apparatus. Continuous oxygen which is humified is administered if necessary.

*Fluids* by mouth may be allowed as soon as the patient desires them.

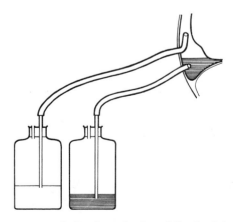

FIG. 31.9   Arrangement of tubes from the chest following lobectomy.

*Pain and exhausting cough* will be relieved by analgesics, but the patient is encouraged to cough.

The respiration, pulse rates, and blood pressure must be carefully observed and charted.

CARE OF THE DRAINAGE TUBE. The wound is closed, but two drainage tubes are brought out through a stab incision below the wound following lobectomy. The lower one is to drain the cavity of blood and the upper tube to remove air so that the remaining portions of the lung can expand to fill the chest completely. Both are connected to separate under-water 'seal' bottles of 2 l capacity containing 500 ml of antiseptic fluid. A blood transfusion is usually kept running after the operation to replace the amount of fluid lost in the bottle. The end of the upper tube to remove air is just below the level of antiseptic fluid so that the patient does not have to displace a large quantity of fluid. The tube must have a clamp on it and if for any reason the closed tube in the bottle is lifted out of the water (for example to change the bottle) the clamp must be closed so as to prevent air entering the chest. The lower tube is removed by the house surgeon usually 48 hours later. If air is still leaking from the upper tube as shown by bubbles on coughing it is retained longer, otherwise it is removed at the same time. The nurse must watch carefully the amount of discharge during the first night, since this is the best guide to haemorrhage, and if excessive (i.e. more than 300 ml in the first six hours) should be reported at once. After the tube has been removed the stab wound must be covered with a sterile airtight dressing *at once*.

FOLLOWING PNEUMONECTOMY. One tube is usually inserted but is kept closed to allow blood to collect in the pleural cavity and keep the mediastinum central. The position of the trachea should be checked by the nurse and if it is deviated blood is released.

The stitches are removed about the tenth day.

RESPIRATORY EXERCISES AND POSTURAL DRAINAGE must be continued after the operation and carried on as required.

The patient gets up on the third day. Attention must be given to the posture and arm movements.

ASPIRATION OF FLUID may be necessary in the first week after the operation.

*Complications.* The complications which may occur are:

1. Haemorrhage.
2. Infection.
3. Bronchial fistula.
4. Non-aeration of the residual lobe (after lobectomy).
5. Congestion of the opposite lung.

*The nursing care of thoracic surgical patients*

After a major thoracic operation the patient is sat up in bed as soon as consciousness is recovered, for in this position the patient can breathe more comfortably. Fluids can be given immediately unless it is an oesophageal operation, and it is important to give adequate fluids, particularly in hot weather, in order to keep the bronchial secretion thin, and prevent areas of lung collapse. The main concentration in the first 24 hours is on coughing, and every hour the wound should be supported and the patient encouraged to cough. Postural drainage may be required in the first 24 hours, and the patient should be moved with great care into the appropriate position and made very comfortable before the foot of the bed is raised.

Any major changes in the hourly pulse, blood pressure and respiration chart should be immediately reported to the medical officer in charge, day or night, as they may indicate a serious complication which may be rapidly fatal.

Most patients require analgesics for the first 48 hours as the pain is considerable. Pethidine is the drug most frequently used as it does not dull the cough reflex.

Thoracic surgical patients require very active nursing. The policy of doing nothing unless something is called for does not pay, as all the time a portion of lung may be quietly collapsing without giving any symptoms. Early mobilisation is the rule and most patients should be up in a chair at least by the third day.

# CHAPTER 32

# Surgery of the Heart

The surgical treatment of various forms of heart disease is now possible and the results are very satisfactory. The heart can be approached and operated upon as simply as any other organ, provided that it is not in a state of cardiac failure.

## CONGENITAL HEART DISEASE

**Patent ductus arteriosus.** The ductus arteriosus connects the pulmonary and systemic circulation in foetal life, so that the blood is short-circuited away from the lungs where it is not required. At birth spontaneous closure usually takes place, but occasionally the ductus remains open and the blood flows in the opposite direction—from the high pressure systemic circulation (120 mmHg) to the low pressure pulmonary circulation (20 mmHg). This results in a constant leak from the systemic circulation, necessitating a continuous high cardiac output to maintain the normal systemic flow. Cardiac failure will occur between 30 and 40 years of age or infective endocarditis may develop. The condition can be cured by undertaking a thoracotomy, exposing the ductus arteriosus and tying it at both ends with silk. The child is then normal.

A large patent ductus may require division because of the danger of recanalisation after a simple ligature.

**Cyanotic heart disease.** A typical form of this condition is the tetralogy of Fallot which is:

1. Pulmonary stenosis.
2. Dextroposition of the aorta.
3. High ventricular septal defect.
4. Right ventricular enlargement.

In this condition, as a result of a ventricular septal defect and stenosis of the pulmonary valve, much of the blood from the right ventricle passes over to the left ventricle and out through the aorta. Only a small portion passes through the pulmonary circulation and only this small portion gets oxygenated. There is no fault in the lungs. The pulmonary circulation can be increased by:

318

(a) Pulmonary valvotomy, in which the stenosed pulmonary valve is cut with a special valvulotome and it then functions normally.
(b) A subclavian artery can be anastomosed to the pulmonary artery to increase the pulmonary blood supply.

Both operations are very successful, permitting greatly incapacitated children to lead a much more normal life. Their colour changes from blue to pink. Later a complete repair of the defect can be made using the heart-lung machine.

**Coarctation of the aorta.** There is a congenital narrowing of the aorta, just distal to the origin of the left subclavian artery, which causes a high blood pressure in the cerebral circulation and the arms. The blood to the lower two-thirds of the body reaches it by a series of anastomotic channels, which run back into the aorta via the intercostal vessels.

Treatment is by excision of the narrowed area and an end-to-end reunion of the aorta. If the ends will not come together, a graft can be inserted. The graft is a tube woven from Terylene or Dacron. Postoperatively the pulses in the arteries of the legs previously not detectable can now be felt.

**Atrial septal defect.** In this condition there is a communication between the two atria resulting in a large flow of blood from the left to the right atrium. This is pumped by the right ventricle through the lungs and returns back again to the right atrium through the defect. As a result there is an excessive amount of blood circulating through the right ventricle and the lungs, resulting ultimately in pulmonary hypertension (rising up to 120 mmHg compared with the normal level of 20 mmHg) and failure of the right ventricle.

Treatment is closure of the defect by suture by an open operation using a heart-lung machine.

**Ventricular septal defect.** There is a communication between the left and right ventricles which results in a large flow of blood passing from the left to the right ventricle (the pressure in the left ventricle is 120 mmHg and the right ventricle 20 mmHg) and then through the lungs. Cardiac failure and pulmonary hypertension supervene.

Treatment is closure of the defect by suture or a patch of plastic material. An open heart operation is necessary and a heart-lung machine is used to by-pass the heart and lungs.

**Pulmonary valve stenosis.** The pulmonary valve is maldeveloped and the opening, instead of being the normal 20 to 25 mm, may be only 4 to 5 mm. Severe strain develops in the right ventricle and sudden death may occur. Often these patients are remarkably free of symptoms.

The pulmonary valve can be exposed by opening the pul-

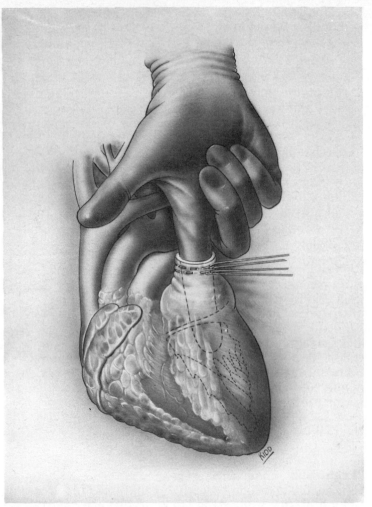

FIG. 32.1  Mitral valvotomy. The surgeon's index finger is in the left auricle.

monary artery and then it is divided with scissors to relieve the stenosis.

## ACQUIRED CARDIAC DISEASE

*Mitral valve disease.* Following rheumatic infection of the heart, the mitral valve may become considerably narrowed, producing the effect of a washer in the circulation. There is a build-up of blood in the lungs, producing pulmonary hypertension and attacks of pulmonary congestion. The valve cusps can be separated and the aperture thus widened. This is performed by inserting a finger into the left atrium via the auricular appendage and passing it through the valve opening, splitting the adherent edges of the cusps on the way. Most cases now have a mechanical splitter inserted through the ventricle or the atrium after the finger split. Many cases of mitral valve disease have associated regurgitation and a satisfactory result can be obtained only by excision of the valve and the insertion of an artificial one.

**Aortic valve disease.** The aortic valve contracts down, similarly to the mitral valve, as the result of rheumatic infection or degenerative changes. This obstructs the outflow from the left ventricle and a very high pressure develops in the left ventricle (up to 300 mmHg compared with the normal 120 mmHg). Left ventricular failure or angina develops.

The pressure in the left ventricle is measured by 'left ventricular puncture' in which a needle is passed directly into the heart in the region of the apex beat, and the pressure read off by an electro-manometer.

Because most patients have regurgitation as well as stenosis valve replacement is usually required. The usual form is the Starr-Edwards valve and is inserted using a heart-lung machine.

**Constrictive pericarditis.** This is the end-result of a tuberculous pericarditis by which the heart becomes encased in a mass of contracting scar tissue in which calcification may occur. The stage of cardiac diastole is interfered with, the heart chambers cannot fill properly, and back pressure occurs on the venous side of the circulation. Distended veins, cyanosis, enlarged liver, ascites, and oedema are the signs. X-ray may show calcification in the pericardium and the heart movements are scarcely visible. Similar symptoms arise in rupture of the heart from injury or disease—cardiac tamponade. The treatment is removal of the thickened pericardium which is done through an anterior thoracotomy. Full recovery is slow, taking many months, but frequently is complete.

**Aneurysms of the thoracic aorta.** These are treated by excision and replacement by grafts.

**Foreign bodies.** Foreign bodies can be removed from the heart by opening the chambers and picking out the object with forceps.

*Preoperative care.*

The preoperative care includes X-ray of the chest, barium swallow, electrocardiogram, and examination of the urine for abnormalities. Fluid balance should be carefully charted. If the urinary output is too low diuretics should be given and if atrial fibrillation is present digoxin will be necessary. The skin preparation includes the area from the neck to the waist back and front, as well as the front and back of the arms to the elbow. The night before operation 120 mg of phenobarbitone may be given. On the morning of the operation the patient may have an early breakfast and if digoxin is being used this is given at 6 a.m.

Most operations on the heart are carried out through a median sternotomy wound in which the sternum is split down the middle and spread widely with a mechanical retractor.

*Postoperative management of the patient following heart surgery*

All patients will require oxygen for at least 12 hours, and many for much longer. The foot of the bed will have to remain raised until the blood pressure is stable over 100 mmHg. Half-hourly recordings of the pulse, the ventricular rate, and blood pressure are required and the blood pressure cuff should be left permanently in place so as not to disturb the patient.

Two pillows only will be necessary for the first 24 hours and after this time a back-rest can be used, but cases of coarctation of the aorta should remain flat (with two pillows) for eight to ten days.

Tachycardia and atrial fibrillation will require the use of digoxin. Most patients with acquired cardiac disease, apart from mitral stenosis, who are got up on the third or fourth day, must remain in bed for at least seven days, but children with congenital heart disease can get up earlier. Drainage tubes are removed in 48 hours. Fluid replacement intravenously must be cautious so as not to overload the circulation. Signs of cardiac failure will require the use of diuretics. Severe restlessness may require the use of morphia. Physiotherapy is important postoperatively.

*Intensive care*

Many patients after an extensive heart or lung operation will require supportive treatment which is best given in a special ward fully staffed day and night.

The use of the mechanical ventilator will enable respiration to be carried on without any effort on the part of the patient and heavy sedation can be administered in the postoperative stage.

The endotracheal tube can be left in place for 24 to 48 hours and then removed. If it is not possible to do so after this time then a tracheostomy can be undertaken and the ventilator connected to this. The patient on a ventilator is completely reliant on this machine, and a continual bedside watch is necessary to ensure that no electrical failure, tube disconnections or kinkings occur. If there is difficulty, then the ventilation must be continued by hand and a doctor called immediately.

Tracheal secretions require constant aspiration by a catheter. This must be done with full aseptic precautions as the introduction of organisms into the bronchial tree may result in a fatal pneumonia.

Tracheostomy is performed by incising the trachea just below the cricoid cartilage and inserting a cuffed plastic or latex rubber tracheostomy tube. If the cuff is blown up, it must be relaxed for two minutes every hour, to prevent damage to the tracheal mucosa. The pressure in the cuff must never be higher than 'just airtight'.

In cardiac cases, and patients with shock, the central venous pressure is monitored by passing a catheter into one of the cavae and recording the pressure on a side tube from the saline drip. The normal is 5 to 10 cm of water and the base-level is that of the right atrium. The arterial pressure is recorded on an oscillograph from a small tube in the radial or femoral artery. A continuous ECG monitor gives an indication of the cardiac action and the heart rate. The urine output is continuously recorded by collection in a measuring bag from an indwelling catheter.

Constant checks of the carbon dioxide, oxygen and pH levels in the blood are taken by puncturing the femoral artery and withdrawing 10 ml of blood for analysis. Other levels can be estimated by taking venous blood.

Recordings of all this data together with $\frac{1}{4}$ or $\frac{1}{2}$ hourly pulse, temperature and respiratory readings are charted so that they are instantly available for examination by the medical officer.

Only by constant control of all these factors can many cardiac patients be satisfactorily brought through their postoperative period.

## HEART-LUNG MACHINES

These are machines designed to bypass the heart and lungs, so that the heart can be opened and intracardiac operations carried out.

Blood is taken from the superior and inferior vena cava, passed through an artificial oxygenator and then returned to the patient via the ascending aorta or the femoral artery.

The use of these machines is technically difficult and requires a large team to control the operation. They are essential, however, to the repair of some forms of intracardiac defect.

### Cardiac catheterisation

In many cases the special investigations of cardiac catheterisation and angiocardiography will be necessary. A catheter, about a metre in length, slightly thicker than a ureteric catheter, is passed via the saphenous or basilic vein into the right atrium, right ventricle, and pulmonary artery. By perforation of the right side of the atrial septum a catheter can be passed into the left atrium and ventricle.

The pressures are taken in the various chambers by recording with a water manometer or electrical pressure recording device connected to the catheter.

The normal systolic pressures are:

| | |
|---|---|
| Superior vena cava | 3 mmHg |
| Right auricle | 5 mmHg |
| Right ventricle | 15–25 mmHg |
| Pulmonary artery | 15–25 mmHg |

Samples of the blood can be taken from each chamber by withdrawal through the catheter and tested in the laboratory for oxygen concentration.

By changes in pressure and variations in the oxygen tension, the diagnosis of congenital disorders of septae and valves and abnormal communications can be made. Heparinised saline is allowed to drip through the catheter during the procedure to prevent intravascular clotting.

### Angiocardiography

Twenty to 40 ml radio-opaque dye are injected via the catheter and the bolus of dye passes through the heart, great vessels, and lungs. During its passage it is X-rayed up to six times a second and study of the plates will demonstrate abnormal pathways of the circulation. Its passage can be watched on an image intensifier—equivalent to closed-circuit television. It is particularly valuable in differentiating the various forms of cyanotic congenital heart disease. As the dye passes through the cerebral vessels a burning sensation in the head will be noticed and the patient should be warned of this beforehand. Anaesthesia is usually unnecessary.

Cine-angiography will give a moving picture of the procedure.

## CORONARY ARTERIAL DISEASE

Degenerative disease of the coronary arteries which carry the main blood supply to the heart may result in gradual occlusion from narrowing or sudden occlusion from thrombosis. It is true, of course, that the disease in the coronary artery is usually part of a general arteriosclerosis, but in many cases the lesion is more advanced in the vital coronary arteries than elsewhere. The provision of a new blood supply to the heart is a subject that has always interested surgeons, and implantation of one or both internal mammary arteries into the myocardium may improve the blood supply to the heart muscle as also may a vein graft between the aorta and the part of the coronary artery distal to the block. Division of the upper dorsal sympathetic chain is of value in the relief of severe anginal pain.

## CARDIAC PACEMAKER

When the conducting mechanism of the heart has been damaged a cardiac pacemaker may be fitted. There are various types. For example, in an axillary pacemaker there is an indifferent lead to the subcutaneous tissues. The cardiac lead is passed into the right ventricle until its tip is in contact with the musculature of the ventricle. Defects which may arise include:

1. Failure of the battery.
2. Breakage of the indifferent lead.
3. Dislodgement of the cardiac lead.
4. Localised fibrosis in contact with the ventricle and failure of transmission of the impulse.
5. Interference from diathermy machines.

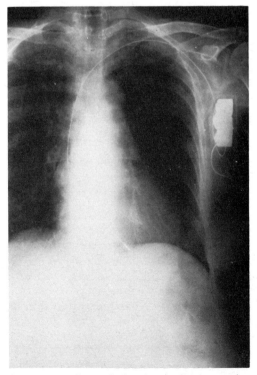

FIG. 32.2   Radiograph showing cardiac pacemaker.

# CHAPTER 33

# Diseases of the Oesophagus

The oesophagus extends from the pharynx to the cardiac orifice of the stomach. It extends through three regions, the neck, the chest, and the abdomen. The principal surgical conditions of the oesophagus are:

1. The lodgement of a foreign body.
2. Perforation (rupture of the oesophagus).
3. Simple strictures, usually due to scarring resulting from the swallowing of corrosive fluids.
4. Cardiospasm, or achalasia of the oesophagus.
5. New growths.
6. Tumours outside pressing on the oesophagus.
7. Hiatus hernia.

## FOREIGN BODIES

Children may swallow coins, marbles, or similar objects which may become impacted and obstruct the oesophagus. In adults, particularly in those without teeth, meat and fish bones may be swallowed. Occasionally, a dental plate is the cause of the obstruction. Should the foreign body perforate the wall of the oesophagus, infection is disseminated in the chest with fatal results, unless immediate operation is undertaken.

*Symptoms and signs*

There is a history that a foreign body has been swallowed. Sudden pain along the course of the oesophagus and dysphagia (difficulty in swallowing) are the usual symptoms.

*Treatment*

The patient suspected of suffering from an impacted foreign body should be given nothing by mouth for fear of stimulating the muscle and causing perforation of the wall.

X-RAY. X-ray examination using gastrograffin will demonstrate the nature and site of the foreign body if it is radio-opaque.

Removal is usually performed through an oesophagoscope. A variety of instruments have been designed for use with the oesophagoscope, one of which is a special coin catcher.

A general anaesthetic is always administered. If the foreign body has sharp edges the oesophagus has to be exposed surgically to remove it.

### POSTOPERATIVE TREATMENT

Penicillin is given because the mouth organisms are always penicillin sensitive.

If the mucosa has been eroded no fluids should be given for 24 hours by mouth, and subsequently if there has been severe damage the patient must swallow no solid food for one week. A fluid diet consisting of milk, soups, and fruit juices should be given during that period.

### PERFORATION OF THE OESOPHAGUS

Perforation of the oesophagus is usually due to a swallowed foreign body or after instrumentation but may occur spontaneously. The perforation occurs in the thinnest portion of the lower third after a severe bout of vomiting. It may be mistaken

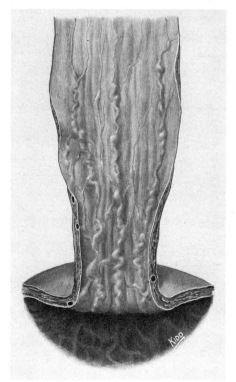

FIG. 33.1   Oesophageal varices. The oesophagus has been opened out and below is a cuff of stomach. The varices are clearly shown extending from the cardio-oesophageal junction.

for a gastric perforation in which pain and not vomiting is the first symptom. Thoracotomy and repair of the perforation are essential.

### SIMPLE STRICTURE

A simple stricture may occur as a remote result of scarring secondary to damage to the wall by a foreign body, as a result of swallowing corrosive fluids or complicating peptic oesophagitis occurring with a hiatus hernia. Increasing dysphagia is the main complaint. The stricture may be examined with an oesophagoscope and may be dilated under direct vision. Otherwise excision may be performed.

The postoperative treatment is similar to that following the removal of a foreign body. The patient is nursed with the head of the bed elevated.

### CARDIOSPASM

This condition is due to failure of the junction of the oesophagus and stomach to open correctly. The bolus of food is held up at the cardio-oesophageal junction, and in an effort to overcome this difficulty the oesophageal wall hypertrophies and dilates above it. There is great discomfort in swallowing, and regurgitation of food occurs in severe cases. The patient loses weight and nutrition generally is impaired. The symptoms develop slowly, and it is usually some years before he seeks relief. X-rays are of great value in distinguishing this condition from a carcinoma.

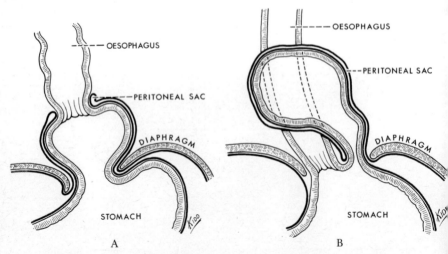

FIG. 33.2   Hiatus hernia. Diagrammatic representation: A, sliding type; B, para-oesophageal type. Peritoneum is indicated by heavy black line.

*Treatment*

HELLER'S OPERATION, which consists of division of the muscle of the sphincter down to the mucous membrane, is performed. It is a procedure similar to Ramstedt's operation, which is performed for congenital pyloric stenosis.

## HIATUS HERNIA

Hiatus hernia is a herniation of the upper end of the stomach through the oesophageal hiatus in the diaphragm. There are two types. First when the stomach passes up by the side of the oesophagus and distension of the intrathoracic pouch causes severe substernal discomfort. In the second type, the oesophagus may become detached from the hiatus and a portion of the stomach passes into the chest giving rise to incompetency of the gastro-oesophageal sphincter with reflux of the acid-pepsin juice of the stomach. This induces oesophagitis, ulceration and eventually stricture formation with substernal pain on lying or bending down. The latter usually occurs in fat women at middle age, and are produced by increased intra-abdominal tension due to pregnancy, cysts or increasing adiposity. The most potent aggravating factor is a corset!

Some relief can be obtained by medical treatment and sleeping on high pillows and elevation of the top of the bed, but the curative treatment is essentially surgical. Restoration of the normal anatomy and repair of the oesophageal hiatus is undertaken. If the condition has advanced to stricture formation then bouginage may be required or resection of the stricture, with less favourable end results. A very light liquidised diet is given.

Operation is usually performed through the chest and the postoperative care is that of a thoractomy (p. 315).

## OESOPHAGEAL VARICES

The veins at the lower end of the oesophagus may be varicose in conditions of obstruction of the portal vein. Rupture of these varices results in severe haemorrhage. The haemorrhage

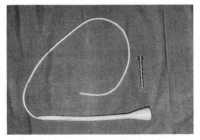

FIG. 33.3  Mousseau-Barbin oesophageal tube for permanent intubation of inoperable carcinoma of the oesophagus.

may be controlled by intravenous injections of pitressin and by passing a Sengstaken tube. This is a rubber tube with an inflatable outer cuff which, when inflated, applies pressure to the bleeding vessels and the patient may be fed through the central lumen. A smaller balloon maintains the correct position of both balloons. Relief of the obstruction may be under taken by anastomosis of the portal vein to the inferior vena cava at a later date.

Contraindications are jaundice or a serum albumin less than 3·0 g per 100 ml.

## CARCINOMA OF THE OESOPHAGUS

The oesophagus is one of the most distressing sites for a new growth, because the patient is unable to swallow sufficient food to keep himself alive and so literally starves to death. In addition his saliva keeps dribbling over into the trachea causing constant 'hawking' and coughing.

### Symptoms and signs

Slight pain or a feeling of 'heaviness' behind the sternum are the earliest symptoms. As time passes, dysphagia increases; first, solid food becomes difficult to swallow and later impossible. Still later, liquids can be swallowed only with the greatest difficulty and in small quantities. The result is rapid loss of weight and dehydration. Radiographic examination after a thick barium meal shows a typical block.

Pneumonia is not uncommon as a terminal complication.

### Treatment

1. REMOVAL OF THE OESOPHAGUS

This is a severe operation. The growth and 6 cm of oesophagus above and a portion of the stomach below, together with the lymphatic glands, must be resected. The stump of the oesophagus is anastomosed to the stomach.

The preoperative preparation consists of correction of the plasma proteins, which are usually low, blood transfusion and breathing exercises. Oesophagoscopy is often necessary preoperatively.

Postoperatively, nasogastric aspiration is performed hourly. As the operation involves opening of the chest the patient is nursed as for a thoractomy including an underwater seal drain (p. 315). Fluid is given parenterally for five to seven days, and the patient is given nothing by mouth, until the bowel sounds are present. Oral hygiene is very important. Water is given hourly for the next 24 hours, followed by milk and water hourly. Fluids are gradually increased until a soft diet is introduced, and the patient is able to take a full diet ten days after the operation. As many of these patients are very old, it is important to get them up and moving about as soon as possible.

## 2. RADIOTHERAPY

Radiotherapy may be used in growths of the upper third of the oesophagus in preference to surgery.

## 3. PALLIATIVE METHODS

Souttar's or a plastic tube is sometimes used to improve swallowing. Should it slip into the stomach it will cause no harm, and is passed per rectum.

A Mousseau-Barbin tube is helpful. A bougie is passed through the stricture into the stomach and the rat-tail end of the tube tied to the end of the bougie. A small incision is made in the stomach and the bougie pulled through drawing the Mousseau-Barbin tube into place in the carcinoma.

A bypass operation, which involves anastomosis of the oesophagus above the growth to the jejunum, is occasionally performed, but it is a very severe undertaking, especially in patients with an inoperable growth who are old, weak and ill.

## 4. GASTROSTOMY

Gastrostomy is the insertion of a tube into the stomach for feeding purposes. It may be performed occasionally as a temporary measure for stricture of the oesophagus.

*The management of gastrostomy*

### PREOPERATIVE TREATMENT

Gastrostomy is not a severe operation in itself, but as the patient is usually dehydrated his condition must be improved by correction of his fluid depletion. It is not frequently performed because in many cases it does not really prolong life and intubation is preferable. The operation can be performed, if necessary, under local anaesthesia.

THE OPERATION. A small opening is made in the stomach, a no. 14 to 16 rubber catheter is inserted, and the wound is closed around the tube. In the theatre a few ounces of citrated milk strained through gauze are run in through a funnel to ensure that the opening is satisfacory. The catheter, or tube, is closed with a wooden spigot.

### POSTOPERATIVE TREATMENT

1. The mouth must be kept clean with sodium bicarbonate solution or liquid paraffin, the teeth cleaned, and the mouth rinsed. Salivation should be encouraged, and for this purpose chewing gum is useful. Barley sugar may also be given.

2. The tube remains in position for about ten days. Four-ounce feeds of strained milk and glucose or, better, Complan

should be run in every three hours. The tube should be cleansed by washing through with water after each feed.

3. As soon as the tube loosens it must be replaced by a similar tube at once, and this should be left in after feeding, otherwise the opening will contract, and then only a tiny tube can be fitted. It is most unusual to leave a patient with a permanent gastrostomy.

# CHAPTER 34

# The Acute Abdomen

The term 'the acute abdomen' covers a large number of important diseases which occur in the abdominal cavity. They have certain characteristics in common, the sudden onset, the presence of abdominal pain and the risk of rapid deterioration in the patient's condition. Abdominal pain which persists for more than six hours is usually due to a condition which is considered here as an acute abdomen. Investigations have only a small but important part to play in the diagnosis and include straight radiography of the chest and abdomen and estimation of the serum amylase (if acute pancreatitis is suspected). An electrocardiograph and estimation of the serum transaminase may be advisable to differentiate an acute abdominal condition from myocardial infarction. Examination of the urine for pus and red blood cells may help to differentiate an acute abdominal condition from a urinary tract infection or stone.

All acute abdominal catastrophes can be resolved into three groups:

1. Peritonitis.
2. Intestinal obstruction.
3. Intra-abdominal haemorrhage. (This forms a very small group of which the symptoms and signs are those of peritonitis in addition to those of internal haemorrhage.)

These conditions almost invariably require emergency operation for their relief. The problem, however, is not as simple as that because many other conditions cause acute abdominal pain. The differentiation of those which require operation from those which do not is of vital importance.

Sometimes a period of observation may be ordered and this time must be used to observe progress. In addition to noting a change of symptoms and the keeping of a half-hourly pulse and temperature chart, nothing must be done to mask symptoms. For this reason sedatives, hypnotics and gastric aspiration are forbidden. The most important of these lesions which do not require operation are:

1. **The colics**
(a) Intestinal—gastroenteritis.

(b) Ureteric (p. 442) }
(c) Biliary (p. 391) } Rarely require urgent operation.

2. **Extra-abdominal causes of abdominal pain**

(a) Pleurisy and pneumonia ⎫
(b) Coronary thrombosis ⎮
(c) Spinal lesions ⎮
(d) Uraemia ⎬ Operation harmful and
(e) Certain blood diseases ⎮    unnecessary.
(f) Arteriosclerosis ⎮
(g) Diabetic hyperglycaemia ⎮
(h) Herpes zoster. ⎭

### ACUTE PERITONITIS

*The peritoneum* is a continuous, thin, shiny, avascular membrane which lines the abdominal cavity. The portion behind the muscles of the anterior abdominal wall and in front of

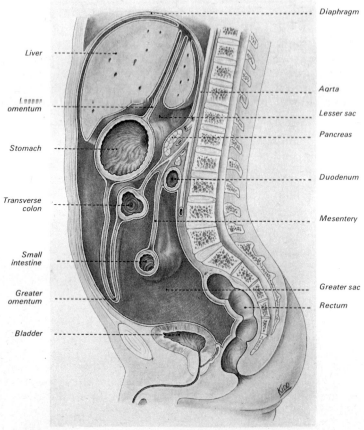

Liver — Diaphragm
Lesser omentum — Aorta
Stomach — Lesser sac
Transverse colon — Pancreas
Small intestine — Duodenum
Greater omentum — Mesentery
Bladder — Greater sac
— Rectum

FIG. 34.1   The peritoneal cavity.

those on the posterior abdominal wall is known as the parietal peritoneum and is richly endowed with nerve endings. Irritation of this portion of the peritoneum gives rise to pain at the site at which it is stimulated.

The visceral peritoneum is the portion which is reflected to envelop most of the abdominal organs. It forms the outer or serous coat of organs like the stomach and the intestines. It has few nerve endings and is almost insensitive.

The peritoneal cavity which is the space between the parietal and visceral layers contains a fine film of sterile fluid. Infection of this cavity is known as peritonitis. The causes are:

1. Blood-borne (rare).
2. Penetrating wounds.
3. Escape of gastrointestinal contents.

The last is much the most frequent cause. If the gastrointestinal tract is healthy its irritant and infected contents make no contact with the peritoneal cavity, from which they are protected by the mucous, muscular and serous coats of the stomach or intestine. If a portion of these organs becomes diseased and their walls infected this infection may spread to the serous covering coat which becomes inflamed. The serous covering coat is part of the visceral peritoneum. If this is inflamed it irritates the adjoining parietal peritoneum and pain is felt at the spot

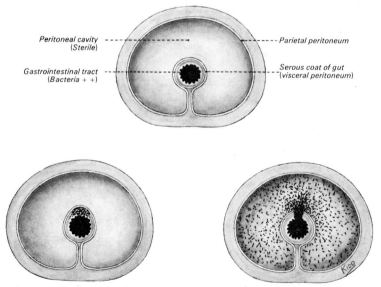

FIG. 34.2   Mechanism of peritonitis. *Lower left figure:* Infected wall of bowel, bacteria spreading in the wall. *Lower right figure:* Perforation of gastrointestinal contents into peritoneal cavity.

where this is inflamed. This is known as a local peritonitis.

If the disease progresses and the organ ruptures the infected contents leak into the peritoneal cavity and a general peritonitis has developed. The peritoneum responds in the ordinary way to inflammation, including an enormous outpouring of fluid. The infection can be overcome provided the supply of toxic material from the gastrointestinal tract is sealed off.

If it is not, the result is:
1. Widespread absorption of toxins.
2. Paralysis of the intestines. Nature tries to limit the outpouring of septic contents by rest.

*Treatment*

The principles of the treatment are:

1. To treat acute circulatory failure. The fluid loss is mainly plasma, water, and electrolytes.
2. To rest the gastrointestinal tract—food and purgatives are forbidden and aspiration of the stomach contents is undertaken.
3. To cleanse or drain the peritoneum of septic contents and pus.
4. To cut off the source of the irritant or infection, e.g. suture of a perforation or removal of a perforated appendix.
5. To counteract infection in the blood stream by antibacterial substances.

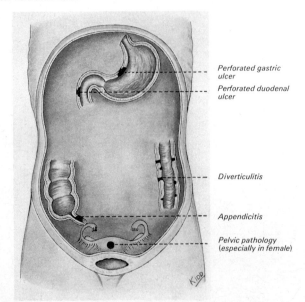

Perforated gastric ulcer

Perforated duodenal ulcer

Diverticulitis

Appendicitis

Pelvic pathology (especially in female)

FIG. 34.3  Common sites of origin of peritonitis.

From all this the lesson which emerges is that lesions which threaten to cause peritonitis should be terminated before peritonitis is established. The commonest causes of general peritonitis are:

1. Perforated acute appendicitis.
2. Perforated gastric or duodenal ulcer.
3. Perforated diverticulitis.
4. Rupture of the intestine, the rectum, or the bladder.
5. Ruptured ovarian cyst. Rupture of the uterus or Fallopian tubes.
6. Perforating abdominal wounds.
7. Haematogenous (blood-borne) infection.

Primary peritonitis, usually pneumococcal in origin, is rare. The sufferers are almost invariably young girls, and the treatment is destruction of the organisms by chemotherapy.

## ACUTE APPENDICITIS

*The cause*

The cause is unknown. Infection commences in the appendix, and in the more severe forms a faecolith may block the lumen of the organ, preventing the drainage of mucus and pus into the caecum. Purgatives increase peristalsis in the organ and cause perforation, i.e., bursting, with leakage of faecal material into the peritoneal cavity. In a smaller percentage of older patients the obstruction may be due to a carcinoma of the caecum. Rarer causes are a carcinoid tumour or matted worms.

*Changes in the appendix as a result of inflammation*

The organ swells as inflammation proceeds. It may be:

1. Red—early appendicitis.
2. Yellow—severe inflammation.
3. Green or black—gangrene.

A faecolith may be found blocking the lumen.

*The course of the disease*

Without treatment the disease may take several courses:

1. Resolution may occur.
2. A localised mass or abscess may form.
3. General peritonitis may develop.

If the attack subsides, recurrence is likely. Early in the attack no one can forecast with certainty how it will progress and, for this reason, the wisest course is to remove the appendix before peritonitis has had time to develop.

*Early symptoms and signs of acute appendicitis*

Sudden colicky pain around the umbilicus is the first symptom. The patient is frequently awakened with pain which comes on in attacks lasting a minute or two. It increases in severity, then passes off completely, only to recur. Vomiting may occur with considerable relief, but as the hours pass by the attacks of pain become more frequent and more severe. Later, the pain settles in the right iliac fossa, where it is no longer intermittent but constant in type. The temperature may be normal or slightly raised (37·2° C; 99° F), and the pulse rate shows a slight increase. The tongue is usually furred but moist, and no flatus is passed per rectum from the commencement of the attack.

Should the appendix be pelvic in position, diarrhoea may be present, and if it is attached to the bladder frequency of micturition may occur.

On examination the abdomen is tender, with muscle guarding in the right iliac fossa, but elsewhere it is soft and painless. Digital examination of the rectum may reveal tenderness on the right side.

*The clinical features of appendicitis with established*
*peritonitis*

The symptoms become more severe and the general condition of the patient deteriorates. The pain is constant and severe, but it may ease suddenly when the appendix perforates, only to return over the whole abdomen. Rigidity and tenderness are widespread, and vomiting is frequent and profuse.

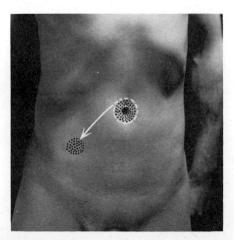

FIG. 34.4  The pain of acute appendicitis is felt first around the umbilicus and later settles over the appendix.

As the patient becomes weaker from lack of sleep, toxaemia and fluid and electrolyte disturbances, the pain and rigidity give way to painless distension of the abdomen, and diarrhoea may be profuse.

The general appearance so typical of late peritonitis sets in. The face is shrivelled and flushed, but the eyes are glistening and bright. The mind is usually clear, but at this stage the patient is frequently too weak to give a coherent account of his illness. The result is that it may be impossible to decide with certainty the cause of his peritonitis. The temperature is always raised (38° to 39° C; 100° to 102° F) and the pulse is rapid, irregular, and of poor volume.

## APPENDIX MASS

An attack of appendicitis may terminate in the formation of a localised mass, which may form a true abscess. The surrounding coils of small intestine and omentum are bound together: they are also bound to the caecum and appendix by a fibrinous exudate. Instead of contaminating the whole of the peritoneal cavity after perforation of the organ, the infection has been limited to the area around the appendix by the great omentum. In this case, and in cases of over 48 hours' duration which appear to be subsiding, it is sometimes decided to observe their course and to operate at once should their condition deteriorate. This method of observation is known as the Ochsner-Sherren regime.

### THE OCHSNER-SHERREN REGIME

This method should be carried out only in the hospital, so that operation can be undertaken at once if it is considered

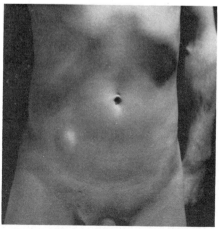

FIG. 34.5   Appendix abscess. A swelling is present in the right iliac fossa.

necessary. It is a technique of observation of an acute attack and not a radical cure. The appendix should always be removed after the attack has subsided:

1. No sedatives or analgesics are given. The size of the swelling in the right iliac fossa should be observed.
2. The patient is nursed in whatever position he is most comfortable.
3. Vomiting or pain are reported at once.
4. Only sips of water are allowed by mouth for 48 hours. Fluid balance is maintained by the parenteral route.
5. The mouth is rinsed out frequently and the teeth kept clean.
6. A fluid balance chart is kept.
7. The pulse is charted hourly and the temperature two-hourly for the first 12 hours. After this time a four-hourly pulse reading is substituted, so as to diminish the disturbance which hourly readings would cause to the patient.
8. The flatus tube is passed every four hours and left in position for at least ten minutes. No aperients are administered.

NURSING PROCEDURE FOR PASSING A FLATUS TUBE. Before this procedure, the patient is offered facilities to pass urine. A tray is prepared containing:

A small, deep bowl (or jug) of water
Kleenex wipes
Lubricant
Inco-pad
Disposable glove
Flatus tube
Paper bag (disposable)

The patient is advised of what is to happen and prepared as for rectal examination.

The Inco-pad is placed beneath the buttocks. The nurse puts on disposable gloves. The flatus tube is lubricated *around* the tip. The other end is placed in and kept below the water level in the bowl. The patient is instructed to take a breath while the nurse gently inserts the tube $2\frac{1}{2}$ inches (approx.) into the rectum. She waits a few moments for air to be displaced from the tube. She then advances it, and then withdraws it slightly. The patient is asked to cough gently. This, and/or extension and flexion of the patient's legs may help to achieve the passage of flatus, seen as the escape of bubbles through the water. These manœuvres may be repeated once or twice, but after seven to 10 minutes, the flatus tube is removed and the anal region gently wiped clean. The patient is repositioned, and made comfortable. The used tube, gloves and tissues are discarded and the tray is cleaned. The nurse washes and dries her hands. A report is made of the result of the procedure.

*Treatment*

The most satisfactory case to treat is one in which the appendix is removed early in the attack. The convalescence is almost invariably smooth, and restoration of the patient to health is rapid.

If general peritonitis is present, however, removal of the appendix and drainage of the peritoneal cavity, usually after the insertion of antibacterial powder, is performed. If a large abscess is present drainage only may be undertaken and the appendix is not removed at the time. The patient is instructed to return for appendicectomy six months later.

## PREPARATION OF THE PATIENT FOR OPERATION IN ACUTE ABDOMINAL CONDITIONS

This is similar to the preparation of a patient for any abdominal operation, but, obviously, it cannot be spread over as long a period as we should like. The orderly preparation of acute abdominal cases for operation is essential, but many are admitted in the small hours of the morning when the ward is relatively understaffed. Frequently the patient has to be ready in the theatre an hour later, and this can be achieved quite easily if the following order of preparation is adopted:

1. The patient is placed in a warm bed, a permission form for operation signed, and, if the patient desires it, a minister of religion summoned at once. Blood is taken for grouping, cross-matching the determination of the haemoglobin level and serum electrolytes. Intravenous infusion of fluid should be instituted if necessary.

2. Morphia (10 mg) and atropine (0·6 mg), or any other preoperative injection which has been prescribed, is given at once, since time is necessary for their optimum effect. Far too often they are given as the patient is leaving the ward for the theatre. If it has been forgotten it is better to tell the anaesthetist who can give an injection intravenously.

3. The bladder is emptied and the urine tested.

4. The suprapubic area and the abdominal wall are shaved. The whole abdomen is washed with 2 per cent hexachlorophane soap and water and dried. Special care must be taken to clean the umbilicus. No antiseptic is applied until the patient has been anaesthetised in the theatre. The whole area from the

nipples to the knees must be prepared, since a lesion of the upper abdomen may resemble appendicitis, and should a second incision be necessary great delay would ensue.

5. A nasogastric tube is inserted and the stomach contents are aspirated if necessary or as prescribed.

6. The head is covered with a disposable paper theatre cap and a theatre gown placed on the patient. The patient's name and unit number are written on a label and attached to the wrist.

7. Dentures are removed and kept in a place of safety.

8. The patient is lifted on to a trolley and protected by warm blankets on his journey to the theatre. On arrival at the theatre the ward blankets are changed for theatre blankets.

9. The patient's case papers and a small bowl are also taken to the theatre.

General washing of the patient is not essential, and may be too exhausting.

After operation, the ward nurse returns to the theatre and accompanies the patient back to bed. She must see that the nature of the operation and any special instructions of the surgeon are recorded and understood before she leaves.

### Postoperative care

If the patient is suffering from established peritonitis intravenous fluid replacement is continued. As soon as he recovers from the anaesthetic he should be allowed to assume whatever position he finds most comfortable. As soon as possible, and usually by the following day, the patient is got out of bed.

ACTIVE MOVEMENTS of the calves of the legs are commenced as soon as possible.

*Pain.* Postoperative analgesics, usually morphia (10 mg) or pethidine (50 mg), if ordered by the doctor are given as soon as the patient complains of pain.

*Immediate postoperative vomiting.* Vomiting is prevented by regular nasogastric suction. If persistent, perphenazine (5 mg) or chlorpromazine (25 mg) intramuscularly is usually effective.

*The bowels.* The passage of a flatus tube every four hours prevents the usual 'distensive' pain of which these patients often complain and helps in the prevention of paralytic ileus (p. 344). About the third day a Dulcolax or Beogex suppository is administered if the bowel has not acted.

*Oral hygiene.* This is important, particularly if the patient is not drinking. The mouth is cleaned four-hourly and before and after each feed.

THE DRAINAGE TUBES (usually a split rubber tube or tubes) are removed when ordered by the surgeon, but all should be rotated and shortened a little each day. Shortening is performed by withdrawing the tube slightly and cutting its external end and always transfixing the remainder with a sterile safety pin. Removal should be recorded.

THE STITCHES are removed when the wound has healed, usually between the eighth and tenth days.

OBSERVATIONS
1. An hourly pulse for 12 hours.
2. A four-hourly temperature reading.
3. Blood-pressure chart.
4. A fluid balance chart.

## COMPLICATIONS

These are many.

*Immediate:*
1. Difficulty with micturition.
2. Chest complications—massive lobar collapse, bronchitis and pneumonia.
3. Persistent hiccough.
4. Paralytic ileus.
5. Haemorrhage. (The signs and symptoms are those of internal haemorrhage. This condition is very rare.)

*Intermediate:*
1. Septic wound.
2. Residual abscesses—pelvic or subphrenic.
3. Faecal fistula.
4. Pulmonary embolism.
5. 'Burst abdomen.'
6. Complications caused by antibiotics.
7. Deep vein thrombosis.

*Remote:*
1. Intestinal obstruction from bands and adhesions.
2. Incisional hernia.

IMMEDIATE COMPLICATIONS

**Difficulty with micturition.** The bladder is palpated to see if it contains urine—not much urine will be secreted if no fluid has been taken. The patient should be encouraged to pass urine half an hour after his second postoperative injection of morphia or other analgesic, and after a flatus tube has been passed. Should all methods of persuasion fail after 12 to 24 hours postoperatively and, only then, a catheter is passed, the bladder emptied and the catheter is left in for 24 to 48 hours.

**Chest complications.** Bronchitis is not uncommon after the inhalation of an anaesthetic, and is frequently the cause of slight pyrexia. Coughing increases pain in the wound and must be treated symptomatically. Massive lobar collapse may occur due to small plugs of mucus blocking the bronchi, and is fairly common. Deep breathing exercises are important in its prevention and in severe cases a bronchoscope may have to be passed to aspirate the mucus which is blocking the bronchi. Pneumonia is a less common although serious complication and must be treated with great care.

**Paralytic ileus.** This is an important and not infrequent complication due to temporary loss of motor tone in the smooth muscle of the gut which is a normal response to surgery. The intestines are paralysed and dilated. Their contents regurgitate into the stomach, which may also be dilated, so that no vomiting occurs, until the stomach is overdistended with fluid. No flatus is passed per rectum. Factors responsible for persistent ileus are:

1. Excessive handling of gut.
2. Unrelieved intestinal distension.
3. Attempts to stimulate intestinal activity by means of drugs when paralysis is still present.
4. Overdosage of drugs producing hypotension.
5. Infection (intraperitoneal).

Paralytic ileus is in large measure preventable. In cases where it is anticipated that it may develop, treatment is commenced from the end of the operation until the bowel has recovered.

*Symptoms and signs*

The abdomen is distended, but usually there is no pain. The distended abdomen makes breathing difficult and embarrasses the action of the heart. The pulse rate is always rapid, and in severe cases the patient is very toxic in appearance.

*Treatment*

Given time and rest the bowels will recover their tone. A flatus tube is passed per rectum four-hourly or, better, left in the rectum continuously. The stomach contents are aspirated continuously or every half-hour through a nasogastric tube and the volume recorded. Some surgeons use instead a Miller-Abbott tube, which is similar to a nasogastric tube and has an inflatable balloon to facilitate its passage into the intestine for a considerable distance. Some cases of paralytic ileus are due to loss of potassium. The serum electrolytes are estimated and any electrolyte deficit corrected.

Morphia (15 mg) is injected intramuscularly every eight hours and intravenous infusions commenced so that the fluid balance is maintained.

*The sign of recovery*

The return of the bowel sounds and the passage of flatus per rectum, normally or by a flatus tube, are the signs that the bowel has recovered its tone. The function of the flatus tube is to overcome the resistance of the anal sphincter.

INTERMEDIATE COMPLICATIONS

**Infection of the wound.** Stitch abscesses and slight degrees of infection are not uncommon after the removal of a septic appendix. This occurs because a septic, and frequently perforated, appendix has to be drawn through a clean wound. The wound, which is clean until the peritoneum is opened, is inevitably contaminated by pus from the peritoneum. Free drainage of any septic pocket is essential and a small strip of rubber drain is secured to the dressing by a large safety-pin.

**Residual abscess.** The commonest situation for a residual abscess is in the pelvis, in the pouch of Douglas in the female or in the rectovesical pouch in the male. More rarely a subphrenic abscess may develop.

**Pelvic abscess.** The early diagnosis of this condition depends on the report from the nurse that she has observed the passage

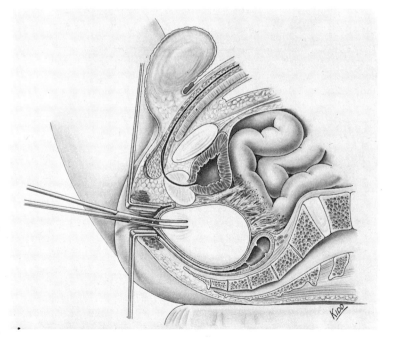

FIG. 34.6 A pelvic abscess showing method of drainage through the rectum.

of a large quantity of mucus in the patient's stools. The temperature and pulse rate are increased, and the patient complains of hypogastric pain, that is, pain in the centre of the lower abdomen.

*Treatment*

The abscess is drained by the insertion of a pair of sinus forceps through the anterior rectal wall in the male or the posterior vaginal wall in the female, when a large quantity of foul-smelling pus drains away. A tube is inserted, but usually stays in position only about twelve hours. The patient's temperature subsides rapidly, and very shortly a marked improvement in the general condition is apparent.

**Subphrenic abscess.** Pus may collect in the spaces under the diaphragm. The presence of pus in this situation is not easy to detect. The patient may complain of a pain under the ribs or in the shoulder, but more commonly the main complaint is of difficulty in breathing. X-ray examination is of value in confirming the diagnosis.

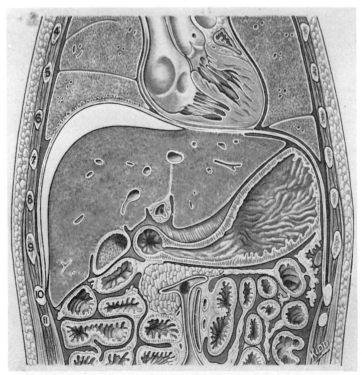

FIG. 34.7   Subphrenic abscess.

*Treatment*

The pus is drained by a small abdominal incision if placed anteriorly, or by the resection of a rib if situated posteriorly. Occasionally it is drained by an incision below the lowest rib. The abscess cavity requires prolonged drainage, and the after-treatment is similar to that of a case of pyothorax (p. 304).

**Faecal fistula.** A gangrenous appendix frequently involves a portion of the caecal wall in the inflammatory process. After operation a small portion of the wall may slough, and faecal contents contaminate the wound and excoriate the skin. The vast majority heal spontaneously in two or three weeks, but the skin must be protected from the discharge by Baltimore paste, silicone vasogen or Orobase (methyl cellulose). The persistence of the fistula with 'sulphur granules' in the effluent suggests that actinomycosis may have been the underlying cause.

**Pulmonary embolism** (p. 131)

**Burst abdomen.** This is an occasional complication of any abdominal operation. It is very rare following a gridiron incision but much commoner with longitudinal incisions. There is a sero-sanguineous discharge from the wound which separates and the intestines prolapse on to the abdominal wall. It is predisposed to by:

(a) Severe coughing.
(b) Infection of the wound.
(c) Deficiency of vitamin C, resulting in failure of the wound to heal.
(d) Removal of stitches before the wound has healed.
(e) Anaemia and malnutrition.
(f) Cortisone therapy preoperatively.

*Treatment*

The prolapsed intestines are wrapped in a sterile towel which has been soaked in warm saline, and the surgeon is informed at once. The patient is taken to the theatre, anaesthetised, and the wound is resutured. It is remarkable that the condition usually causes little or no circulatory failure, and the patient has an uneventful convalescence.

If a wound has not actually burst but there is a danger of this happening, a corset dressing is advisable.

REMOTE COMPLICATIONS

**Intestinal obstruction.** This complication is more likely to occur as a result of adhesions in a patient who has recovered from extensive peritonitis. Occasionally this complication may occur a few days after the operation. The treatment is further operation to relieve the obstruction.

**Incisional hernia.** An incisional hernia may occur after any operation, but if it has been necessary to drain the wound the chances of it arising are greatly increased. Infection and pulmonary complications also predispose to the development of an incisional hernia because of the strain of coughing.

## PERFORATED PEPTIC ULCER

An ulcer developing on a surface exposed to the action of acid-pepsin is known as a peptic ulcer, and includes gastric and duodenal ulcers. Perforation of a gastric ulcer is usually a more severe condition because the acid gastric juice is extremely irritant to the peritoneum and a much larger quantity of fluid leaks from a perforation in the stomach than from a similar ulcer in the duodenum. Apart from this, the clinical features and treatment are the same. Circulatory failure may be profound, and peritonitis becomes established after some hours.

A chronic ulcer may perforate but acute ulceration which is part of a widespread gastritis may also perforate. Aspirin and alcohol are recognised causes of acute ulceration. Steroid therapy is liable to reactivate a latent peptic ulcer. The most dangerous place for a patient to perforate is in hospital where an exacerbation of ulcer pain is anticipated and the patient may be sedated.

*Symptoms and signs*

The sudden onset of violent, constant, generalised abdominal pain is the outstanding symptom. The patient lies perfectly still where he has been smitten with pain. He feels as though he has received a powerful blow in the abdomen. Vomiting may occur. The face is pale and anxious and the skin feels cold and clammy. The temperature is invariably subnormal at first and the pulse rate is elevated. The whole abdomen is tender and extremely rigid or board-like. It does not move with respiration and there is no distension. If unrelieved the pain ceases after about 24 hours as the abdomen distends from general peritonitis. Not all patients give a history suggestive of previous indigestion.

*Treatment*

Every hour is vital. The tempo of deterioration is much faster in this condition than in a case of acute appendicitis. After 24 hours the patient suffering from acute appendicitis is still in a comparatively early stage because peritoneal contamination has not usually occurred. The mortality rate in patients suffering from untreated perforated peptic ulcer of 24 hours' duration is about 90 per cent.

Treatment is usually confined to closure of the perforation. If the symptoms before perforation were such that definitive surgical treatment such as vagotomy or gastrectomy was indicated this may be carried out instead of simple suture.

### PREOPERATIVE TREATMENT

If the patient is collapsed a transfusion of plasma is commenced at once, and the pain is relieved by an injection of morphia. As soon as possible the patient receives the usual preparation for an acute abdominal operation. The stomach preoperatively is aspirated, and every millilitre of gastric contents recovered lessens the damage to the peritoneal cavity.

### POSTOPERATIVE TREATMENT

The general treatment is similar to that for acute appendicitis.

The hygiene of the mouth is even more important in this condition, since fluids by mouth are usually forbidden for the first 24 hours after the operation.

DIET. For the first 24 hours only parenteral fluid is given. After this a fluid diet is prescribed on return of the bowel

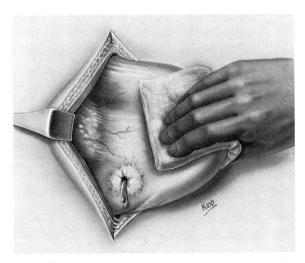

FIG. 34.8    A perforated gastric ulcer. Appearance at operation. The stomach is held out with a warm moist swab by the assistant. Gastric contents are leaking through the perforation.

sounds and is gradually increased to include suitable proportions of carbohydrate, fat and protein. The dietician is an important team member.

The *complications* just after the operation are similar to those following acute appendicitis (p. 343) and those of a case of peptic ulcer (p. 369) more remotely.

*Instructions to the patient on discharge*

It should be explained that the operation was a life-saving measure and that there is a 70 per cent chance that he will have further trouble. He can improve his chances of cure by avoiding undue stress and tobacco.

**Postoperative peritonitis.** Postoperative peritonitis is a very important condition. It is one of the major causes of fatality following abdominal operations. It is peculiarly difficult to diagnose and in not a few cases post-mortem examination reveals that deaths which have been attributed to cardiac failure and respiratory infection are, in fact, cases of true peritonitis from leakage of an anastomosis or rupture of the intestine. The real difficulty is that the severe pain and dramatic suddenness with which most peritoneal symptoms commence are clouded by:

1. Postoperative analgesics and hypnotics.
2. Some pain in the abdominal wound ⎱ which are usual
3. Some degree of pyrexia ⎰ postoperatively.

The important observations are:

1. Any complaint of undue pain should be reported.
2. Tenderness after the second day should be minimal.
3. Abdominal distension should be either responding to the usual measures or, if it is becoming worse, peritonitis should be suspected.

At an advanced stage these patients pass into acute circulatory failure and die very rapidly.

## ACUTE INTESTINAL OBSTRUCTION

There are few conditions in which the real gravity of the patient's condition is more belied by his apparent well-being than in acute intestinal obstruction. The obstruction may affect the large or the small intestine; obstruction of the small intestine is always more severe than obstruction of the large intestine because of the great loss of fluid by vomiting in the former.

There are innumerable causes of intestinal obstruction, which are considered under Diseases of the Small and of the Large Intestine, but to illustrate the two main types a typical case of obstruction in each of·the two portions of the intestines is discussed here.

## Small bowel obstruction

*Symptoms and signs*

*Colicky abdominal pain* commencing around the umbilicus is the first symptom. The pain waxes and wanes, is temporarily relieved by vomiting, but recurs again and again, and never moves from the centre of the abdomen.

*Vomiting* is constant. At first food is returned, later bile-stained gastric juice, and, in the late stages, the foul infected contents of the intestine above the obstruction. This fluid smells of faeces and is described as 'faeculent' vomit.

The loss of fluid, rich in chlorides, is considerable.

*The bowels.* There is usually absolute constipation, i.e. no flatus is passed after the administration of an enema or a Dulcolax suppository.

*On examination* the temperature is normal, but the pulse is rapid. Tenderness is unusual, unless gangrenous gut is present in the abdomen, but there is fullness of the lower abdomen. Only in very late cases is gross distension present.

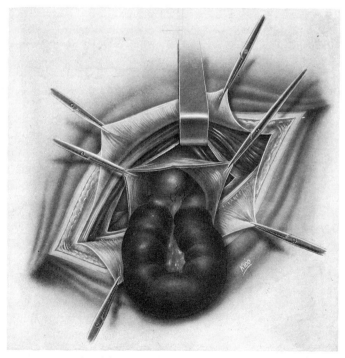

FIG. 34.9 Strangulated hernia. The intestine has just been released and is viable. Note the distended loop above the obstruction.

*Peristalsis* (worm-like movements) of the bowel may be visible through a thin abdominal wall.

If an external strangulated hernia is the cause of the obstruction a tense, tender, painful irreducible swelling which has no impulse on coughing will be felt over one of the hernial sites. On the other hand, if the obstruction is due to some other cause, for example, a peritoneal band, the signs previously described will be present alone.

**Large bowel obstruction.** The commonest cause is a growth narrowing the lumen of the bowel. The acute attack develops when a faecal mass blocks the already narrowed lumen.

*Symptoms and signs*

Obstruction in the large bowel is much better tolerated than obstruction in the small bowel. The main complaint is a feeling of abdominal distension and sometimes breathlessness, for the distension impairs the action of the heart and lungs.

Intestinal colic and vomiting appear only when a fair degree of distension has already occurred and prevents the contents of the large intestine flowing through the ileocaecal valve to the small intestine. A history of increasing constipation is almost invariable before the 'acute stoppage'.

The physical contents of the large intestine can be compared to a coal fire which consists of smoke and embers. If the chimney is blocked the real trouble arises in the room from the smoke. In the large intestine it is the gas which fills the bowel and all the striking symptoms are due to the retention of flatus and not to the presence of faeces.

*The treatment of acute intestinal obstruction*

The mortality rate of this condition is very high indeed, so that every care must be taken if it is to be reduced. If the

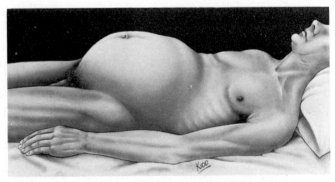

FIG. 34.10   Abdominal distension. Large bowel obstruction.

patient is in a state of acute circulatory failure, resuscitative measures must be instituted forthwith.

A Dulcolax suppository or a disposable phosphate enema is given on admission. This serves the dual purpose of confirming the diagnosis and of clearing the bowel below the obstruction so that there is no unnecessary difficulty in the passage of the intestinal contents after the obstruction has been relieved.

A patient suffering from intestinal obstruction is given nothing by mouth before the operation. Another very dangerous practice is to aspirate the stomach contents from a patient suspected of suffering from intestinal obstruction. This relieves symptoms but delays the diagnosis because vomiting does not occur. A nasogastric tube and morphia are valuable aids in the preparation and after-treatment, but used indiscriminately they may cost the patient his life.

If the obstruction is subacute, and there is no sign of gangrene an obstruction may be treated for a trial period by nasogastric suction and intravenous fluid replacement. Some patients with multiple adhesions may recover if the obstruction is due to kinking of a loop of bowel.

Very occasionally a volvulus of the pelvic colon may be reduced by passing a rectal tube through a sigmoidoscope. An intussusception (p. 406) may also be reduced by retrograde pressure from a barium enema given under X-ray screening control.

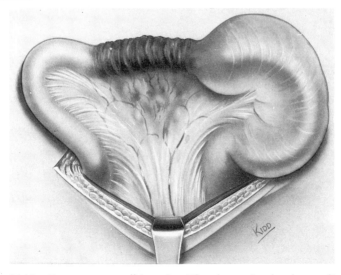

FIG. 34.11  Gangrenous small intestine. The obstruction has been relieved but the gut is gangrenous and must be resected. The bowel above is still distended because it is paralysed.

IMMEDIATE PREOPERATIVE PREPARATION

This is similar to the preparation for any acute abdominal operation, but special stress is laid on fluid and electrolyte replacement. A transfusion commenced in the ward is usually continued on the journey to the theatre, during and after operation.

A nasogastric tube to aspirate the stomach contents is left in the stomach for 24 hours or longer after the operation. This relieves vomiting while the patient is being prepared, and prevents vomiting during the induction of anaesthesia. The aspiration of vomited material into the lungs may be fatal. If the obstruction is so severe that fluid is welling up in the stomach very rapidly, the patient is placed on the operating table in the slightly head-down position and the theatre nurse must aspirate the stomach contents even while the anaesthetist is inducing anaesthesia.

THE OPERATION

This is always confined to the simplest and quickest procedure necessary to relieve the obstruction. Division of a band or reduction of a strangulation is all that is necessary if the bowel wall is not gangrenous. If gangrene is present, however, resection will be necessary, and this is a severe undertaking.

In the large intestine the most frequent method of relief is to form an artificial anus proximal to the obstruction, usually a colostomy—on rare occasions a caecostomy. The care of these fistulae is described on page 417.

POSTOPERATIVE TREATMENT

Parenteral fluid replacement is continued. Continuous aspiration of the stomach for 24 hours is frequently necessary, and the passage of a flatus tube per rectum is also important. These patients are sometimes very breathless from abdominal distension and are more comfortable when nursed sitting upright.

The general care of the patient and his wound is similar to that in any abdominal operation.

**Postoperative complications.** Particularly important in acute obstruction:

1. *Recurrence of the obstruction.* The symptoms are similar to the original lesion.
2. *Paralytic ileus* is very common, since, although the mechanical obstruction has been relieved, the bowel wall may have developed paralysis as a result of the distension.

## INTRAPERITONEAL HAEMORRHAGE

Intraperitoneal haemorrhage is not a very common cause of an acute abdomen. The only common lesion is an ectopic gestation. This is fully described in Chapter 52. Other causes include laceration of the spleen (p. 250) and of the liver.

The principles of treatment are:

1. Replacement of blood.
2. Control of haemorrhage by suture or removal of the affected organ.

## EXTRAPERITONEAL HAEMORRHAGE

The commonest causes of *retroperitoneal* haemorrhage are:

1. A ruptured aneurysm of the abdominal aorta (p. 225).
2. Acute haemorrhagic pancreatitis (p. 397).

## ANTEROPERITONEAL HAEMORRHAGE

The only common cause of a haemorrhage in front of the peritoneal cavity is rupture of the inferior epigastric artery which may cause sudden swelling behind the lower rectus sheath and in front of the peritoneal cavity. It is sometimes associated with severe coughing or handle-bar injuries.

## CHRONIC PERITONITIS

General acute peritonitis has already been described. Chronic disease of the peritoneal cavity is described briefly to complete diseases of the peritoneal cavity.

This is usually tuberculous in origin. It may take three clinical forms:

1. Diffuse tuberculosis of the surface of the intestines and parietal peritoneum with the exudation of free clear fluid.
2. Diffuse adhesive changes which may cause intestinal obstruction.
3. Multiple cold abscesses and fistulae usually pointing at the umbilicus.

Operation is only indicated if intestinal obstruction develops, otherwise the treatment is rest and anti-tuberculous chemotherapy.

## CARCINOMA OF THE PERITONEUM

Carcinoma of the peritoneum is common, and is almost invariably secondary to growths elsewhere in the abdomen. The whole peritoneal surface may be studded with nodules of growth, and ascites is frequently abundant. No treatment of a curative nature is possible, but symptomatic relief may be given by tapping the abdomen and allowing the fluid to drain away. Radioactive gold and cytotoxic drugs are now being used in the relief of the ascites associated with this condition. A suspension of the colloidal form of the metal or drug is introduced through the aspirating needle. In 50 per cent of cases there is relief of the ascites. It does not cure the primary condition.

## ASCITES

A collection of free non-purulent fluid in the peritoneal cavity is known as ascites. The term 'free' means that the fluid can move around the peritoneal cavity instead of being contained in one part of it—when it is described as encysted.

*Causes*
1. Carcinoma peritonei.
2. A failing heart.
3. Certain forms of renal failure.
4. Cirrhosis of the liver.
5. Some forms of tuberculous peritonitis.
6. Splenic anaemia.
7. Portal vein thrombosis.
8. Inferior vena cavae obstruction.
9. Meigs' syndrome.
10. Escape of chyle.

*Treatment*
The treatment is that of the cause where possible. Locally, tapping (paracentesis) may be performed. A small trocar and disposable cannula are inserted into the peritoneal cavity after the injection of a local anaesthetic (1 per cent Lignocaine). The bladder must be emptied in preparation for the operation,

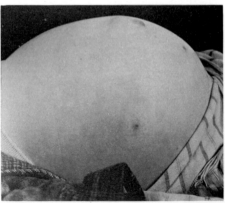

Fig. 34.12    Ascites. The puncture marks indicate the sites for paracentesis.

and the skin of the abdominal wall is prepared in the usual way. Several pints of fluid may be withdrawn and a specimen is sent for pathological examination. A firm binder is applied after the operation to lessen further collection and assist with the drainage of fluid. If the cause is one of disseminated carcinomatosis a cytotoxic drug may be injected through the cannula.

NURSING PROCEDURE FOR PARACENTESIS ABDOMINIS:

A basic dressing trolley is prepared, additional items on the bottom shelf are:

    Local anaesthetic and syringe
    Scalpel
    Trocar and cannula (or other apparatus)
    Extra tubing
    Adjustable clamp
    Receiver
    Drainage bag
    'Green' Savlon
    Iodine
    Green towels
    Gown, mask, gloves
    Binder or many-tailed bandage
    Specimen jars
    Stimulant, e.g. brandy.

The nature of the procedure is explained to the patient, and his co-operation is obtained.

The doctor prepares himself. The trolley is taken to the bed-side. Privacy is ensured. The patient is made comfortable in the semi-recumbent position.

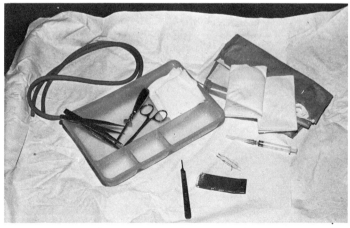

FIG. 34.13    Pack for paracentesis.

The bladder is emptied. Otherwise this is reported to the doctor. Catheterisation may be necessary.

The binder (or many-tailed bandage) is placed in position. The bedclothes are turned down.

The nurse opens the outer wrappings of the basic dressing pack, opens other packets as required, and assists the doctor to assemble the apparatus. The doctor performs the procedure, assisted by the nurse. The nurse observes the patient, giving help and reassurance as appropriate.

The tubing is connected to the cannula and to the drainage bag. The clamp is adjusted to allow the rate of flow ordered by the doctor. The binder is fastened in position, and readjusted as necessary.

The nurse looks after the patient whilst the drainage continues. Special observations are made on the general condition of the patient, the rate and flow of the fluid, the amount and the nature of the fluid.

The apparatus is taken down on instruction from the doctor. The wound is sealed, e.g. with Nobecutane. The trocar and cannula are rinsed in cold water, placed in the appropriate container and returned to C.S.S.D.

## PSEUDOMYXOMA PERITONEI

This is a most unpleasant condition which occurs following rupture of a pseudomucinous cyst of the ovary.

# CHAPTER 35

# Stomach and Duodenum

Ulceration is the main lesion which affects the duodenum. The stomach is liable to a much greater variety of disease and carcinoma, almost unknown in the duodenum, is quite common. The stomach is a J-shaped organ with an upper opening from the oesophagus known as the cardia and a lower, or pyloric, opening to the duodenum. The openings of the stomach may be narrowed by disease occurring at these sites. The mucous membrane of the stomach secretes acid pepsin in response to the nervous stimulation from the vagus nerves and also by the release of a hormone in the pyloric antrum, known as gastrin.

Division of the vagi diminishes the secretion of acid pepsin but because the vagi are also the motor nerves to the stomach, the gastric musculature is paralysed or so weakened that it is unable to overcome the resistance of the pyloric sphincter with the result that dilatation of the stomach occurs. It is for this reason that a procedure which facilitates the emptying of the stomach is undertaken to 'drain' the stomach after vagotomy. This may be a gastroenterostomy or a pyloroplasty. On the other hand when a portion of the distal stomach has been removed, including the pyloric sphincter, and the portion of remaining stomach is joined to the jejunum, emptying is more rapid than usual.

The first part of the duodenum is exposed to the action of acid pepsin and in susceptible subjects an ulcer may form. The lower oesophagus is free from the action of gastric juice unless there is incompetence of the cardio-oesophageal junction and regurgitation of stomach contents may occur. This causes oesophagitis, going on to ulcer formation with all its complications, including narrowing (stricture) and haemorrhage.

## PYLORIC OBSTRUCTION (STENOSIS)

The outlet of the stomach may be obstructed by:
1. Congenital hypertrophy of the muscle (congenital pyloric stenosis).

2. Simple ulceration proximal or distal to the pylorus. An ulcer may cause obstruction by its size, with considerable oedema when it is active, or by scarring when an active ulcer has healed.
3. A carcinoma in the pyloric antrum.

Whatever the cause, obstruction to the pylorus prevents food from leaving the stomach easily—solid food is retained and stagnates. As the condition becomes more severe fluid is slow to leave the stomach.

Because the stomach is nearly always full the patient has no appetite, feels distended in the epigastrium, vomits large quantities of foul material, loses weight and is constipated. Vomiting results in fluid and electrolyte depletion. On examination the patient's skin is dry and wrinkled, there is evidence of gross loss of weight and peristalsis may be visible. A hypertrophied pyloric sphincter may be palpated in the ten-day-old infant and an epigastric mass from carcinoma may be detectable in the adult suffering from carcinoma of the stomach. A barium meal will reveal delay in the emptying time of the stomach.

*Management*
Whatever the cause:

1. The stomach is emptied of its contents by a nasogastric tube and kept empty by frequent aspiration. If the contents are very foul a stomach washout, using a solution of sodium bicarbonate, is performed.
2. Fluid and electrolytes are replaced by intravenous infusion.

Finally, definitive treatment depends on the cause. This may be division of the pyloric sphincter (Ramstedt's operation) in the infant, gastrojejunostomy in a simple pyloric stenosis, or a partial gastrectomy for carcinoma of the stomach.

GASTRIC WASHOUTS
*Equipment required.* This includes that for passing an intra-gastric tube (p. 366), with the following in addition:

Tubing 24 inches in length
Connection
Funnel
Small jug—1 litre
Large jug containing 4 litres fluid (e.g. tap water)
    at 100° F (37·8° C)
Bucket
2 Large polythene sheets.

The procedure is carried out very much as detailed for passing an intragastric tube (p. 366).

When the patient is unconscious, the position of the patient may be semiprone, prone or recumbent, with the head lower than the trunk. Usually, in such patients, the doctor intubates the patient and carries out the stomach lavage.

The polythene sheets are spread to protect the patient, bedding and floor. The bucket is placed on the floor. The stomach tube is passed into the stomach.

The small jug is filled with fluid. The funnel, tubing and connection are assembled. Some fluid is run through to expel air, and then stopped. The connection is attached to the stomach tube. The funnel is raised above the level of the head (or stomach if the head is low); 300 ml (half pint) of fluid is run into the stomach. Before the funnel is empty it is inverted over the bucket, and the fluid siphoned back. A specimen of the first washing is sometimes saved for analysis of gastric contents particularly drugs.

The process is repeated until the fluid returns clear, or the 4 litres of prepared fluid have been used.

Afterwards, the tube is compressed and withdrawn quickly. The patient's face is wiped, he is given a mouthwash and left comfortable in bed. An unconscious patient is kept under observation, and any alteration in the level of unconsciousness noted and reported.

Used equipment is discarded. The siphoned contents are measured and recorded, and saved for inspection.

The nurse washes and dries her hands and makes a report to the nurse in charge.

## CONGENITAL PYLORIC STENOSIS

Excessive thickening of the pyloric sphincter with narrowing of the pyloric canal may occur as a malformation in a newborn infant, which is almost invariably a male.

*Symptoms and signs*

At birth the infant is apparently quite fit, but after two or three weeks projectile vomiting and deterioration of his general condition occur. The vomit is large in quantity and consists of more than one feed. Weight is lost rapidly, and the face becomes wizened in appearance due to dehydration. Tetany may develop if vomiting is severe. The thickened pyloric sphincter can usually be felt as a mass in the epigastrium, and visible peristalsis may be present. The child is constipated.

The differentiation from pure duodenal atresia is easily made. In this condition vomiting occurs almost immediately after birth, while in congenital pyloric stenosis vomiting does not occur until the child is two to three weeks old.

*Treatment*

MEDICAL TREATMENT consists of gastric lavage with normal saline to wash out stagnant stomach contents. This may be necessary once or twice daily. Eumydrin (atropine methonitrate), an antispasmodic drug, is administered. The dosage is 1 ml of a $\frac{1}{10000}$ solution 20 minutes before each feed. This can be increased to 3 ml if necessary.

SURGICAL TREATMENT in most centres is now the treatment of choice as medical treatment is tedious and never certain. The operation, which consists of division of the pyloric sphincter (Ramstedt's operation), is never an emergency and in a dehydrated baby adequate preparation must be carried out.

PREOPERATIVE CARE

1. The electrolytes and blood urea are estimated as well as other chemistry of the blood.

2. A scalp drip is set up, usually $\frac{N}{5}$ saline and 5 per cent dextrose is transfused. Sometimes Darrow's solution and plasma may be ordered depending on the biochemical findings.

The subcutaneous administration of fluid, the absorption of which is greatly increased by the use of hyaluronidase, has been largely abandoned in favour of an intravenous scalp drip.

3. Gastric lavage is carried out with normal saline before the operation. The stomach is emptied and the nasogastric tube is left in position.

4. The operation is undertaken. An incision is made through the muscle of the pylorus but not through the mucosa.

POSTOPERATIVE CARE

Feeding can be started four hours after operation unless the mucosa has been inadvertently opened by the surgeon when he will order feeds to be withheld for 24 hours. The feeding regime is as follows:

| *Hours postoperatively* | *Amount* | |
| --- | --- | --- |
| 4 | 4 ml | Glucose water |
| 6 | 4 ml | Feed |
| 8 | 8 ml | Glucose water |
| 10 | 8 ml | Feed |
| 12 | 16 ml | Glucose water |
| 14 | 16 ml | Feed |
| 16 | 32 ml | Glucose water |
| 18 | 32 ml | Feed |
| 20 | 48 ml | Glucose water |

Feeds are continued two-hourly for about the next six hours and gradually increased to 90 ml every three hours depending on the age and weight of the baby. Should any feed be vomited it is repeated in two hours rather than proceeding to the next stage.

Following successful operation the child grows up normally and it is unusual to see a patient in adult life, who has had an operation for congenital stenosis, suffering from serious surgical stomach disorders.

### PEPTIC ULCER

A peptic ulcer is an ulcer which occurs on a surface exposed to the action of acid pepsin. The common sites are:

1. The first part of the duodenum—duodenal ulcer.
2. The lesser curvature of the stomach—gastric ulcer.

Less common are:

1. The jejunum after anastomosis of the stomach to the jejunum—stomal ulcer.
2. Lower oesophagus usually associated with hiatus hernia causing a reflux oesophagitis and going on to an oesophageal ulcer.
3. An ulcer in a Meckel's diverticulum (p. 403), which will contain ectopic fragments of gastric mucous membrane.

All peptic ulcers are similar in pathology, basic clinical features and complications with the exception that a gastric ulcer may become, or may be mistaken for, a malignant (carcinomatous) ulcer of the stomach.

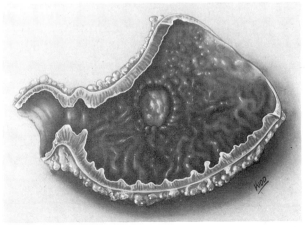

FIG. 35.1    Gastric ulcer. Specimen from subtotal gastrectomy.

The cause of a peptic ulcer is unknown, but certain conditions are said to aggravate an existing ulcer or predispose to its formation in susceptible patients:

1. The presence of sepsis elsewhere in the body, e.g. septic teeth, chronic appendicitis.
2. Smoking, particularly on an 'empty' stomach.
3. A diet which contains excessive meat or meat extract.
4. Emotional factors undoubtedly play an important part.
5. Duodenal ulcer has a higher incidence amongst patients of blood group O than in the population in general.
6. Zollinger-Ellison syndrome (a pancreatic gastrin-secreting tumour which causes hyperchlorhydria).

### Signs and symptoms of an uncomplicated peptic ulcer

1. Burning epigastric pain appearing half an hour to two hours after food. Food may relieve the pain of a duodenal ulcer.

2. The appetite is usually good, but the patient is often afraid to satisfy it for fear that the pain may recur.

3. Vomiting is much more common in the case of a gastric ulcer, but it is not a prominent symptom in uncomplicated cases. Nausea and heartburn are not unusual. Many patients feel distended after a meal.

4. Weight alteration is variable. Many patients are well nourished, since food relieves the pain; others have lost weight.

5. Remissions (freedom) of all symptoms for several months are usually due to healing occurring spontaneously or as a result of medical treatment.

*Investigations*

The investigations which are performed are:

#### 1. RADIOGRAPHIC EXAMINATION

Radiographic examination of the stomach and duodenum after a barium meal is of the greatest value in proving the presence of an ulcer. In addition, considerable information about the function of the stomach is obtained, for example, the rate of emptying of the organ.

*Preparation of the patient for a barium meal.* An aperient should be given two evenings before the barium meal examination. No food or drink is taken from midnight before the examination so that the stomach is empty of food at the time of radiological examination (say 10.00 hours).

After the barium meal is given no further solids or fluids

must be given to the patient until instructions are received from the radiologist, a period covering about six hours.

## 2. TESTS OF GASTRIC SECRETORY FUNCTIONS

In all these tests a gastric tube is passed, preferably orally, into a fasting stomach.

The patient should be as relaxed as possible. He should have been fasting for 12 hours. After spraying the throat with a local anaesthetic the tube is passed via the mouth into the stomach. An X-ray is then taken to ensure that the tube is in the pylorus.

The patient is now positioned in bed on his left side. A suction pump is used to withdraw the stomach contents at regular intervals, air being pumped in through a bleeder tube if the tube appears blocked.

Resting juice is aspirated and put into the first container—three quarter-hour basal specimens are then collected under continuous suction.

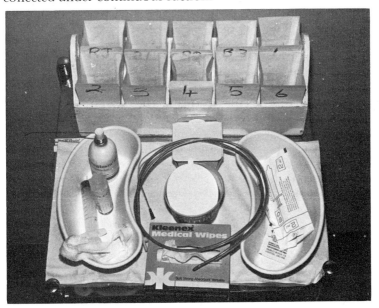

FIG. 35.2    Requisites for gastric secretion test:

Labelled specimen box
Rayx Porges gastric tube
Ribbon gauze
Gingicain spray
   (oral anaesthetic)
Liquid paraffin or glycerine
Denture box
Saliva box

Medical wipes
Syringe, needle, injection
   S.W.P.
Robert's pump
2 Flasks
1 Bung with attached
   tubing
1 Hand pump

Drug used—pentagastrin, according to body weight.

(a) *Pentagastrin*. A subcutaneous injection of pentagastrin is then given (6 μg per kg body weight). Six further specimens are then collected at quarter-hour intervals. Pentagastrin has virtually no side effects.

(b) *Insulin*. This procedure is similar to the pentagastrin test. Three quarter-hour basal specimens are collected, a blood sample being taken with the third. Intravenous injection of soluble insulin 0·25 units per kg body weight is given. Six quarter-hour specimens are again collected and blood samples are taken half an hour and three-quarters of an hour after the insulin injection. The patient may become hypoglycaemic and sweat profusely after insulin injection. Oral or intravenous dextrose should be available but is rarely necessary.

(c) *Night secretion volume*. After suitable sedation such as phenobarbitone, the total amount of juice secreted over a period of the 12 hours of the night is aspirated hourly or by continuous suction and the acidity is estimated. A volume in excess of 400 ml is suggestive of a duodenal ulcer while a volume of a litre suggests a gastrin-secreting pancreatic tumour.

Gastric secretion tests are particularly indicated for:

(i) X-ray negative dyspepsia.
(ii) Recurrent dyspepsia after vagotomy and drainage.
(iii) If the diagnosis of the Zollinger Ellison syndrome is considered. In this condition the level of serum gastrin is greatly raised.

Four terms are used to describe the nature of gastric juice:

Hyperacidity—excess of total acid
Hyperchlorhydria—excess of hydrochloric acid
Achlorhydria—no hydrochloric acid
Achylia—no pepsin.

*Nursing procedure for passing an intragastric tube.* Equipment required:

Tube—Ryles, oesophageal (Lenin) stomach or other
   Paper towel (Kleenex roll)
Cleansing material for nose—sinus forceps
Cleansing material for nose—cotton wool swabs
Cleansing material for nose—sodium bicarbonate
   solution
Lubricant—KY jelly, liquid paraffin
Spatula and torchlight
Litmus paper
Vomit bowl, mouthwash
Medical wipes

Strapping
20 ml Syringe
Receiver
Spigot
Other apparatus, e.g. meal, suction according to reason for
   procedure.

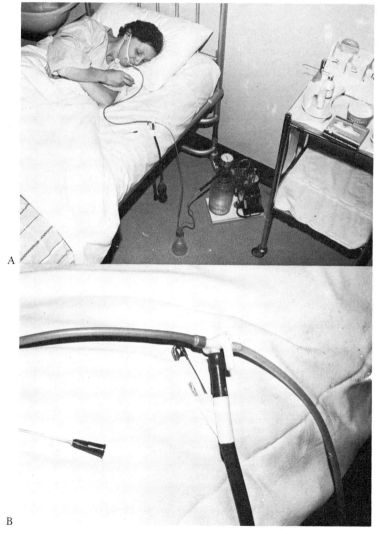

A

B

FIG. 35.3   Test of gastric secretory functions. A, Position of patient and
assembly of equipment pump to register at a pressure not exceeding
40 mmHg. B, Close up view of 3-way tap system.

The procedure is explained to a conscious patient, and his co-operation obtained. Privacy is ensured. Dentures are removed, if necessary.

When possible, the patient sits straight up, supported by pillows, and his head tilted forward. An unconscious patient lies in the semiprone position. A paper towel is placed under the chin. If he can do so, the patient is asked to blow his nose, otherwise the nurse carefully cleanses the nostrils.

The tip of the tube is lubricated. When the nasal route is used, it is gently inserted along the floor of the nose into the pharynx. When the oral route is being used, the tongue is depressed and the tube is passed over the side of the mouth and tongue into the pharynx, care being taken not to touch the uvula. When the tube is in the pharynx, the patient is asked to swallow, and the tube is gently pushed each time he does so. Sips of water may be given to assist in swallowing. In between swallows he is encouraged to take a deep breath. The nurse observes the patient for any coughing, apnoea, cyanosis or vomiting. If the tube is entering the larynx or trachea, it is removed, and the nurse passes it again when the patient has recovered from the coughing etc.

To ensure that the tube is in the stomach, the mouth is opened, the tongue depressed and the torch used to see the position of the tube in the pharynx. Using the syringe, some of the contents of the stomach are aspirated and tested with litmus paper. An acid reaction would most probably indicate that the tube is in the stomach.

A spigot is inserted into the end of the tube, and the tube is attached to the face with a piece of strapping.

When a patient has an indwelling nasogastric tube, it is necessary to attend to the cleanliness and condition of the nares and the mouth at regular intervals.

### 3. TEST FOR OCCULT BLOOD IN THE FAECES
Red meat and green vegetables must be excluded from the diet for three days previous to the collection of the specimen. It is not necessary to submit the patient's entire stool for testing. A disposable plastic container should be used, with a tin spoon attached to the under surface of the lid.

### 4. GASTROSCOPY
Gastroscopy is the examination of the stomach under direct vision by the use of an instrument known as a gastroscope. The modern fibreoptic endoscope enables the duodenum and the stomach to be viewed as well as taking specimens for biopsy. In preparation for gastroscopy the patient should have no food during the morning. It may be necessary to empty the

stomach. The examination is carried out between 08.00 and 09.00 hours. Before the examination the patient is given morphia (15 mg); under a local anaesthetic the gastroscope or flexible fibroscope is passed. No food or drink is allowed for half an hour afterwards, because the pharynx is anaesthetised and a little may run into the larynx.

5. GASTRIC CAMERA

6. CYTOLOGICAL EXAMINATION
After filtration of aspirated contents.

*Treatment*
The principles of treatment of a peptic ulcer are the same whether medical or surgical measures are employed. Basically they aim at the dilution, neutralisation or diminution of acid pepsin.

1. Dilution by frequent meals, milk drip or short circuit operation, for example, gastrojejunostomy.
2. Neutralisation:
   (a) Alkalis.
   (b) Buffers, such as milk.
3. Diminution:
   (a) Drugs inhibiting vagal action, including sedatives which diminish anxiety. Rest in bed has a similar effect.
   (b) Drugs inhibiting acid secretion locally, e.g. Nactan.
   (c) Vagotomy.
   (d) Gastrectomy.
   (e) Avoidance of smoking.
4. Increasing mucosal resistance—agents such as carbenoxolone sodium stimulate protective mucorrhoea in gastric ulcer.

The main indications for surgical treatment are:

(a) The occurrence of complications.
(b) The failure to respond to careful medical treatment. This requires fine judgement and the treatment of an uncomplicated ulcer requires a multidisciplinary approach including close co-operation between the physician and surgeon.

### THE COMPLICATIONS OF A PEPTIC ULCER
The principal ones are:

Perforation (p. 348).

Haemorrhage
Pyloric stenosis and hour-glass contracture
Penetration of adjacent organs
Carcinomatous change in a simple gastric ulcer is rare.

**Haemorrhage.** When blood accumulates in the stomach the colour changes rapidly from red to black due to the action of gastric acid. It may be vomited (haematemesis) as black coffee-ground material or, if the haemorrhage is so severe that no mixing with gastric acid occurs, fresh red blood may be vomited. Alternatively the blood may pass into the duodenum and because it is irritant in the stomach and intestine it is passed very rapidly from the rectum as a tarry stool (melaena). The main causes of gastrointestinal bleeding are illustrated in Fig. 35.4.

The onset of haematemesis or melaena may be the first symptom or may be the sign of a revealed haemorrhage after

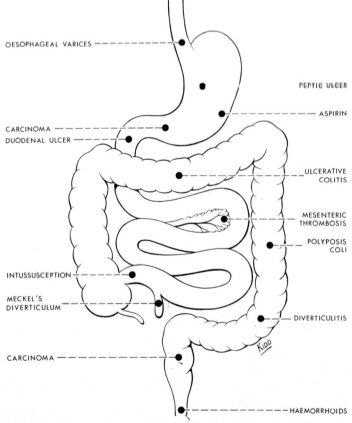

OESOPHAGEAL VARICES

PEPTIC ULCER

ASPIRIN

CARCINOMA
DUODENAL ULCER

ULCERATIVE
COLITIS

MESENTERIC
THROMBOSIS

POLYPOSIS
COLI

INTUSSUSCEPTION

MECKEL'S
DIVERTICULUM

DIVERTICULITIS

CARCINOMA

HAEMORRHOIDS

FIG. 35.4   Common causes of haemorrhage into gastrointestinal tract.

the patient has had a mild or severe collapse following the loss of blood into the stomach and duodenum. All patients with gastric bleeding are best admitted to hospital, however mild the symptoms and signs, because no one can forecast the outcome. It may be a trivial incident or it may be the beginning of a haemorrhage that will never cease until it is controlled by extensive surgical measures. The patient's history is taken with special reference to any symptoms of indigestion and anything to suggest a systemic bleeding condition such as purpura.

Corticosteroids may have activated a latent ulcer and some drugs taken as tablets by mouth are particularly liable to erode the gastric mucous membrane. Aspirin and certain rheumatic and arthritic remedies are particularly suspect.

*Management*
1. The patient is reassured and unnecessary noise is eliminated. The haemoglobin is estimated and the patient is grouped and several units of blood are cross-matched. In more severe cases more blood is cross-matched.

2. PULSE AND BLOOD PRESSURE. Half-hourly pulse chart is kept and a careful note should be made of its volume and any irregularity. A rising pulse rate and a falling blood pressure indicate continued bleeding. In more severe cases the central venous pressure is monitored.

3. THE BED. Only one pillow is allowed but if the patient is very collapsed, the foot of the bed will have to be elevated.

4. BLOOD TRANSFUSION is usually necessary and the rate and amount is decided by consideration of the blood pressure, the central venous pressure, blood haemoglobin, pulse rate and urinary output. Ten ml of 10 per cent calcium chloride has to be given after every 4th unit of blood and many of these patients require large volumes of blood. If rapid transfusion is necessary a blood warmer should be used.

5. NASOGASTRIC SUCTION. Nasogastric suction should be commenced at once to prevent the accumulation of clots in the stomach, which increases bleeding. Observation includes measurement of the volume and recording of the nature of the aspirated fluid.

6. MORPHIA is given to secure rest.

7. ANTIBIOTICS. Because the haemorrhage is of the secondary type, antibiotics may be prescribed.

In the older patient or in the patient where the haemorrhage is not controlled by these measures, surgical treatment may have to be undertaken to prevent the patient bleeding to death. A barium meal may be advised. But an oesophago-gastro-duodenoscopy enables a precise visual diagnosis to be made in 80 to 90 per cent of all patients, when the final diagnosis lies within the stomach or the first two parts of the duodenum. It should be performed within 24 hours of admission.

**Pyloric stenosis and hour-glass contracture.** The ulcer may cause constriction of the area of the stomach in which it is situated, and since the vast majority are in the neighbourhood of the pylorus, and this is the narrowest portion of the stomach, pyloric stenosis is not uncommon. At other sites the stomach is much larger and ulceration much more rare. Occasionally, however, contracture does occur, and is known as an hour-glass contracture.

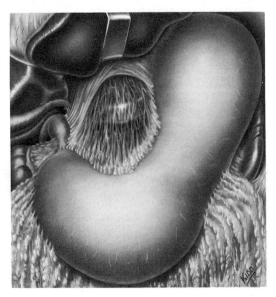

FIG. 35.5  Pyloric stenosis. The appearance of the stomach at operation.

*Symptoms and signs*

Vomiting is frequent, profuse, and projectile in type. Food consumed on the previous day may be recognised in the vomit, since it cannot pass through the pylorus. This stagnation of food results in still greater infection in the stomach, and since the pylorus is blocked no bile enters the stomach. In a severe case the tongue is dry and furred and the skin wrinkled and dry. Pain is usually constant. Loss of weight is considerable and is directly attributable to undernourishment and dehydration.

*Treatment*

The treatment is always surgical, after careful preparation (p. 374).

**Penetration of adjacent organs.** A chronic ulcer may invade locally the pancreas, the liver, or the intestine. The ulcer pain is usually more constant and more severe than usual, and is referred to the back.

Penetrating ulcers usually require surgical treatment. Ulceration into the colon is a serious condition, and usually results in what is known as a gastrocolic fistula.

## NEW GROWTHS OF THE STOMACH

Simple growths are rare, the commonest being a leiomyoma—a benign tumour of smooth muscle. Malignant growths are common and are relatively painless until far advanced. Their incidence in patients of blood group A is commoner than in the general population.

While surgery offers the only hope, the survival rates, even in early cases, are extremely low. It is one of the most unfavourabe sites in the whole body in which to develop a neoplasm.

*Symptoms and signs*

The early symptoms are few and very general in type. A feeling of malaise, increasing fatigue, and slight loss of appetite are the most common. Later pain, vomiting, and anaemia may develop. Loss of weight is usually rapid, and occasionally there may be a small haematemesis. An acute onset, such as a large haematemesis or a perforation, may occur exceptionally.

On examination of the abdomen there are no physical signs in early cases, but later the malignant growth can be palpated as a hard mass in the epigastrium. The liver may be enlarged and irregular from the presence of secondary deposits.

*Investigations*

1. Radiographic examination after a barium meal shows the typical appearance of a filling defect.

2. Gastric secretion tests usually reveal the absence of hydrochloric acid (achlorhydria), but when the growth causes pyloric obstruction total acidity from fermentation may be increased. In all cases the amount of free hydrochloric acid is reduced. Examination of the gastric aspirate may reveal malignant cells.

3. Occult blood is usually present in the faeces.

4. Gastroscopy and the gastric camera are valuable aids to diagnosis in doubtful cases.

*Treatment*

Removal of the stomach (gastrectomy) is the only operation which offers any hope of cure. If the growth is inoperable but pyloric stenosis is present or impending, considerable relief may be achieved by the performance of a gastroenterostomy. Should the growth be inoperable, careful nursing can do much to render the remaining days of misery more tolerable. Analgesic and hypnotic drugs will relieve pain, and vitamins by injection will delay deterioration. Antiemetics such as perphenazine (5 mg) may be prescribed. The diet should be light and nutritious, and in particular it must be what the patient fancies from day to day.

## ACUTE DILATATION OF THE STOMACH

In this condition the stomach loses its tone and may fill almost the whole abdomen. Several pints of fluid are exuded into the cavity of the organ from its own walls and from the duodenum. The condition is similar to paralytic ileus with which it is in fact often associated.

*Causes*
1. After operations on the stomach.
2. Occasionally it follows severe injury especially·fractures of the dorsolumbar spine treated in a plaster jacket.
3. Sometimes the condition arises without any obvious cause.

*Symptoms and signs*
Symptoms and signs are identical with those of paralytic ileus.

*Treatment*
The stomach must be emptied and rested, but the fluid balance must be maintained. These objects can be achieved by:

1. Nasogastric suction for at least 24 hours or longer if necessary and intravenous fluids.
2. Elevation of the foot of the bed and turning the patient on his left side facilitate drainage of the stomach contents.

## OPERATIONS OF THE STOMACH

1. GASTROSTOMY. This is performed very rarely for a growth of the oesophagus. It may be used to feed an unconscious patient on whom a tracheostomy has been performed.

2. GASTROJEJUNOSTOMY. In this operation the stomach is joined to the upper portion of the small intestine.

3. PARTIAL GASTRECTOMY. This operation is performed for gastric or duodenal ulcer. Two-thirds to three-quarters of the stomach and the first inch of the duodenum are removed. The stump of the stomach is usually sutured to the jejunum (Bill-

roth II type). It may be sutured to the duodenum (Billroth I type). The great disadvantage of the extensive removal of the stomach is an obvious one, that the patient is left with little or no reservoir for food and the portion which remains is unguarded by a sphincter.

4. TOTAL GASTRECTOMY. This is the most severe operation which can be performed on the stomach, and is done for carcinoma. It may be approached through an incision in the abdomen extending on to the chest wall and known as abdominothoracic total gastrectomy.

5. VAGOTOMY. The vagus nerves are divided in the chest or in the abdomen to diminish the acid secretion. Because the stomach muscle is paralysed defective emptying of the organ occurs in a proportion of patients. For this reason gastroenterostomy or some form of drainage operation such as pyloroplasty is normally combined with this procedure. This is known as truncal or total vagotomy. If only the fibres of the vagus nerve to the stomach are divided it is known as 'selective'

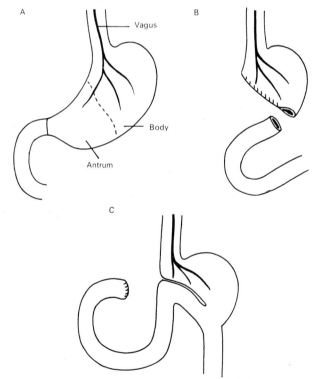

FIG. 35.6  Examples of radical surgical operations on the stomach. A, Normal stomach. B, Partial gastrectomy with gastroduodenal anastomosis (Billroth I). C, Partial gastrectomy with gastrojejunal anastomosis (Polya).

vagotomy. If only the fibres to the acid-secreting parietal cell mass are divided it is called 'a highly selective' vagotomy.

6. PYLOROPLASTY consists of division of the pyloric sphincter longitudinally and sewing the wound up in the opposite direction (transversely) so that an enlarged opening is produced.

### Preoperative care

Many patients benefit from a preliminary course of medical treatment. As a result the ulcer becomes smaller and less septic, and the operation is safer and easier.

The preoperative correction of anaemia and vitamin deficiency is important.

*Smoking* must not be allowed—it aggravates the ulcer and predisposes to pulmonary postoperative complications.

*Breathing exercises* are also important.

*Dental sepsis* should be cured before operation is undertaken.

*Fluids and electrolytes* must be replaced if the patient is deficient in them, and preliminary blood transfusions undertaken if necessary. A blood count is performed before the operation and the patient's blood is grouped and cross-matched.

*The stomach* must be empty at the time of operation. Normally this occurs in three hours, and if emptying is not delayed it is unnecessary to pass a stomach tube. If pyloric stenosis is present, the stomach is emptied and washed out the evening before operation so that the patient is disturbed as little as possible the next morning. In severe pyloric stenosis gastric aspiration over several days is advisable.

*A nasogastric tube* is passed through the nose and left in position before going to the theatre. Some surgeons prefer to have the nasogastric tube passed by the anaesthetist if its use is not necessary until after the operation. The end is plugged with a tiny disposable spigot. Although the tube is usually passed through the nose some nurses and doctors who have had a gastrectomy performed have felt that intubation was rendered less intolerable by having it placed through the angle of the mouth. A further point to be borne in mind about passing the tube nasally is that staphylococci are often harboured in the nose and, if a nasogastric tube is to be indwelling for some days, it is advisable preoperatively to take a nasal swab to make sure that staphylococci are not present.

The preparation of the skin, etc., is similar to that for any other abdominal operation.

### Postoperative treatment

Swabbing with glycerine and borax and the rinsing of the mouth are very important.

During the operation a transfusion is sometimes commenced and this is continued until the blood volume has been restored. After this the patient usually requires no fluid by mouth or parenterally until the following morning. This ensures a good night's rest. On the day following operation a litre of fluid plus a volume equal to the amount of urine secreted and fluid aspirated from the stomach should be given intravenously. This will usually be of the order of 2 litres in all. Half a litre may be given as normal saline and the rest as 5 per cent dextrose. If this can be given over eight hours during the day the patient should again have a more restful night and, in most cases, no further intravenous fluid will be necessary. The exact type and amount of fluid administered intravenously will be prescribed on assessment of all results of electrolyte estimations.

The relief of pain, the care of the bladder, the promotion of sleep, care of the pressure areas, and careful charting of the pulse receive the same attention as in any severe operation. Most patients prefer to be propped up in bed.

CARE OF THE NASOGASTRIC TUBE

This tube, which was passed before or during the operation, is left in place afterwards and the stomach contents are aspirated hourly and the amount recovered is measured and recorded. The early aspirations consist of bright red blood which, in a few hours, changes to dark blood and which, in 24 hours, should be bile-stained. The amount aspirated diminishes until only a few millilitres of fluid are recovered, and the bowel sounds have returned. This indicates that the gastrointestinal tract has recovered its normal activity and that it is now safe to give fluid by mouth.

Thirty ml of sterile water are given. The stomach is aspirated an hour later and, if it is emptying satisfactorily, the total amount of fluid may be increased slowly to 90 ml each hour. On the day after operation the patient is allowed up and the nasogastric tube is removed as soon as normal emptying of the stomach occurs over several days. The diet is gradually built up with citrated milk, eggs and strained soup. By the sixth day the patient is eating most foods, but he should also drink large quantities of milk.

Excessive aspirate may occur because:

1. The tube is too low and protruding through the stoma. It should be withdrawn so that it is just below the cardio-oesophageal junction. This position is attained by withdrawing the tube until no aspirate is recovered and then pushing it down again very cautiously 1 cm at a time until the stomach contents are again recovered.

2. Over-infusion of fluids in the two or three days following operation.

GASTRIC ASPIRATION

A nasogastric tube is passed as in procedure on page 366.

1. *Intermittent aspiration.* A tray is prepared containing:

Receiver
20 ml syringe

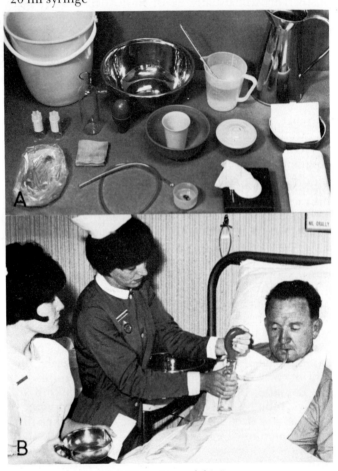

FIG. 35.7    Stomach lavage.

A, Equipment

| | |
|---|---|
| Disposable stomach tube | Bucket |
| Disposable Medi-wipes | 2 Jugs plus lotion thermometer |
| Disposable impermeable sheet | Specimen containers |
| Disposable towel | Disposable polythene bag |
| Sendran's evacuator | Denture bowl |
| Bowl | Gallipot and lubricant |

B, Sister demonstrating the procedure to a student nurse.

Measure jug
Medical wipes/tissues
Disposal bag.

It is kept on the patient's locker, covered by a paper/green towel.

The patient is advised of what is to happen. The nurse holds a tissue around the junction, she removes the spigot and places it in the receiver. She ensures that there is no air in the syringe, attaches the tip to the tube and applies gentle suction. She holds the end of the tube and detaches the syringe. The aspirate is measured while still in the syringe, and then emptied into the jug. The aspiration is repeated until no fluid is aspirated. The spigot is reinserted. The total amount of aspirate is charted. The nurse leaves the tray clear, placing used tissues in the disposal bag. She reports to the nurse in charge.

2. *Continuous drainage.* The tube is connected to a drainage bag. The amount of drainage is measured and charted as instructed, e.g. hourly or when the bag is emptied or changed.

*Removal of nasogastric tube.* The patient is advised of what is to happen. The adhesive tape holding the tube is gently detached. The nurse tells the patient to take a deep breath, smoothly withdraws the tube, and places it in a disposable bag. The patient's face is cleaned and his oral hygiene attended to. Used equipment is discarded.

ALTERNATIVES AND MODIFICATIONS OF
NASOGASTRIC INTUBATION

Some believe that a nasogastric tube is unnecessary and can be dispensed with. There is no doubt that, in the majority of cases, this is correct. In a significant minority, however, dilatation of the stomach occurs quietly and sometimes disastrously and this is preventable by an indwelling tube.

Morris Lee's two-way intubation tube is a double-barrelled tube, one barrel of which is much longer than the other. The larger one is manipulated into the jejunum (or duodenum) at the end of the operation and the nasal end is connected to a reservoir of fluid. This obviates the need for intravenous fluid. The shorter barrel is in the stomach and can be aspirated in the ordinary way. The underlying principle of its use is that the jejunum is often active and functioning while the stomach is still paralysed.

Kay uses a special tube from the cavity of the stomach to the abdominal wall to obviate the need for a nasogastric tube. It is a modified gastrostomy procedure.

THE DRAINAGE TUBE. If a corrugated tube has been inserted it should be removed on the fifth day, but if there has been a discharge of bile or intestinal contents this should be reported at once and the tube should not be removed.

The bowels may be opened by a Dulcolax or Beogex suppository on the third day. An enema is not usually necessary, but a flatus tube relieves abdominal distension in the 48 hours following operation. Superficial sutures are removed as soon as the wound has healed, usually about the eighth to tenth day, and if deep tension sutures have been inserted, on the fifteenth day.

Postoperatively vitamin C is frequently administered intravenously.

## COMPLICATIONS

1. **Haemorrhage.** Small quantities of blood are usually aspirated in the first 12 hours. Larger quantities of loss, however, require treatment. Morphia is administered and the foot of the bed is elevated. A nasogastric tube is usually in position and the stomach contents aspirated.

Treatment for haematemesis (p. 371) is instituted. If the bleeding persists the wound may have to be reopened and the bleeding point ligated.

2. **Vomiting.** Some vomiting may occur after return from the theatre, and usually diminishes very quickly. All material vomited should be measured and specimens kept for inspection.

Occasionally severe persistent vomiting occurs, due to the obstruction of the intestine which has been joined to the stomach. It may be necessary to reopen the wound when this complication is present. Acute dilatation of the stomach may follow gastric operations and the nasogastric tube must not be removed until the stomach has recovered its tone.

3. **Staphylococcal diarrhoea,** due to a pure growth of *Staphylococcus pyogenes*, may occur as a complication of any operation, but more than 50 per cent of cases are subsequent to gastrectomy. It should be stressed that:

(a) It may be epidemic.
(b) The patient is usually receiving broad-spectrum antibiotics.
(c) A nasogastric tube has been used.

Clinically the condition may simulate internal haemorrhage, coronary thrombosis or pulmonary embolism until the diarrhoea appears. There is a gross loss of fluid. In suspected cases a specimen of faeces is sent for immediate microscopic examination for Gram-positive cocci, to confirm the diagnosis. The culture is also performed for antibiotic sensitivity.

*Treatment*

The antibiotics in current use are discontinued. Erythromycin (0·5 g) four times daily is given intramuscularly but in severe cases 250 mg doses should be given by slow intravenous injection. Fucidin (500 mg) six-hourly is also of value. Fluid loss is replaced by intravenous fluid. The patient is nursed in isolation.

4. **Pulmonary complications.** These are common. Bronchopneumonia and massive lobar collapse are the most common. All may be prevented in a considerable measure by deep breathing exercises and free movement in bed. Antibiotics are administered in established disease.

5. **Peritonitis** may occur from leakage at the anastomosis or from rupture of the duodenal stump. Rupture results in a duodenal fistula, which can also occur from damage to the duodenum in the operations of right hemicolectomy or nephrectomy on the right side. A small abdominal drainage tube will always discharge bile-stained fluid if the duodenum has ruptured. The commonest day for a rupture is the fourth or fifth postoperative day. It is impossible to resuture the ruptured duodenum because the ferments are already eating away its very substance. Therefore treatment consists of:

   (a) Gastric aspiration.
   (b) Suction drainage through the stab wound.
   (c) The parenteral administration of fluid to maintain the fluid balance.
   (d) The administration of antibiotics.

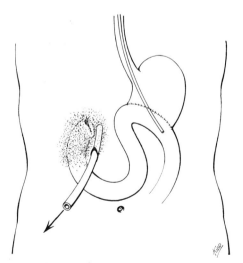

FIG. 35.8 Rupture of the duodenal stump following gastrectomy is the commonest fatal complication. The escaping enzymes destroy so much of the wall that suture is impossible and the only hope lies in removing the enzymes by nasogastric tube and suction through the fistula.

6. **Stomal ulcer.** A more remote complication, its onset is heralded by recurrence of the original symptoms of indigestion.

A stomal ulcer is an ulcer at the line of junction (the stoma) with the small intestine. Strict medical treatment is usually prescribed, but if this is not successful a more extensive removal of the stomach or vagotomy (p. 375) is performed.

A stomal ulcer may cause a gastrojejuno-colic fistula by perforation into the colon.

### THE POST-GASTRECTOMY SYNDROME

A proportion of patients develop symptoms of varying severity after the main meal. They include:

Dizziness
Sweating
Palpitation
Epigastric discomfort
Extreme weakness, and, on occasion, loss of consciousness.

These symptoms may appear one-half to three hours after food, and may be relieved by lying down.

The patient is advised to avoid a large meal if any of the above symptoms appear. His diet must be revised to ensure adequate nutrition by means of smaller but more frequent meals.

Other post-gastrectomy syndromes which may appear are:

1. Bilious vomiting.
2. Malnutrition.
   (a) Anaemia.
   (b) Vitamin deficiency, particularly vitamin B.
   (c) Gross loss of weight.
   (d) Osteoporosis.

*Treatment.* Vitamin deficiency and anaemia can be treated medically by giving the appropriate vitamin preparation or iron. A gluten-free diet is sometimes of help.

### Advice on leaving hospital

It should be explained to the patient that at his operation the ulcer and a large portion of his stomach have been removed, or some other operation performed, but his tendency to form another ulcer remains.

The fundamental principles of aftertreatment must be rest, relaxation, a calm attitude to life and its incidents, plenty of soft non-irritating food, taken at frequent intervals, and not lacking in any of the essentials of a good normal diet. More important than the exact diet is the mental attitude of the patient who eats it.

The precise constitution of the diet should be varied to suit the patient's needs and tastes. The regularity and frequency of the feeds are as important as their composition. If irritants such as mustard, spices, vinegar, and alcohol are avoided, and if other food is free from gross roughage, all the common foods may be safely taken from the beginning of treatment. An elaborately graded diet is unnecessary. Meals should be served as attractively as possible and efficient mastication is essential.

# CHAPTER 36

# Diseases of the Liver, the Gall-bladder, and the Pancreas

The liver and the pancreas are mixed glands which pass their internal secretion into the blood and their external secretions into the duodenum by means of ducts. The two ducts join at the ampulla of Vater in the duodenum. The surgical diseases of these organs are caused mainly by lesions obstructing or invading the ducts. Jaundice is a frequent symptom of disease in this region, and some of the surgical aspects of jaundice must be considered.

## JAUNDICE

Jaundice is not a disease but a sign of disease. It may be classified by the site at which it is effectively caused, viz.:

**Prehepatic.** Haemolytic jaundice, which is a condition produced by the too rapid breaking up of the red blood corpuscles. It may be treated medically with cortisone or cured in some cases by removal of the spleen (p. 250).

**Hepatic** (diseases of the liver)

1. Viral jaundice is considered in more detail on p. 385.
2. Cirrhosis.
3. Multiple secondary deposits.
4. Acute yellow atrophy.

**Posthepatic** (cholestatic jaundice). Due to obstruction of bile ducts:

1. Canalicular obstruction—largactil.
2. Bile ducts—stones; carcinoma of the head of pancreas.

Jaundice is due to the retention of bile pigments in the tissues and in the blood. It is caused by a variety of diseases fully dealt with in medical textbooks. The important surgical form is due to obstruction of the common bile duct. This may result from:

(a) A stone impacted in the duct; or
(b) A carcinoma of the head of the pancreas obstructing the duct or a tumour growing in the common duct.
(c) Chronic pancreatitis (rarely).

Operative interference on a patient who is jaundiced is dangerous, because the blood has a lessened coagulability, due to the lack of vitamin K and consequently haemorrhage may be extremely difficult to control. Vitamin K is fat-soluble and therefore is not absorbed from the intestine in the absence of bile salts. For this reason vitamin K should be administered by intramuscular injection some days before and after operation. In addition, large quantities of glucose are necessary to prevent further liver damage.

After operation a jaundiced patient requires special care, since not only is internal haemorrhage more likely to occur, but it may be more easily overlooked because *pallor cannot be observed*. The pulse volume and rate should be carefully watched. As the condition improves, the colour of the stools is carefully noted each day, for they are a guide to the amount of bile reaching the intestine. When the patient is severely jaundiced the stools are almost white, and, as recovery occurs, tend to become more and more their normal colour. The urine is very dark in colour due to the presence of bile pigments.

There is an increased risk of renal failure and Mannitol is used to prevent it (p. 396). Wound healing is delayed and the susceptibility to infection is greater. Intolerable itching from retention of bile salts can be very distressing in persistent jaundice. Cholestyramine, which binds bile salts, is effective in relieving this symptom.

Jaundice in any form is very depressing mentally, and the nurse must make every allowance for irritability on the part of the patient. It is part of his disease. The bleeding and coagulation times are increased. The degree of jaundice may be measured by an examination of the serum bilirubin (normal 0·5 to 1 mg per cent).

## THE LIVER

Injury to the liver usually takes the form of laceration, and is due to a crush injury of the abdomen in the majority of cases. Pain in the right hypochondrium, tenderness, and the signs of internal haemorrhage will be present. It is frequently combined with multiple abdominal injuries.

TREATMENT. The treatment is laparotomy and suture of the lacerated liver.

### VIRAL HEPATITIS

Viral hepatitis comprises two microbiologically separate diseases, serologically distinguishable from each other.

1. **Infective hepatitis.** Epidemic and believed to be transmitted by the faecal oral route.

2. **Serum viral hepatitis.** This is transmitted by physical procedures and arises from:

  (i)  A pool of infected plasma or serum;
  (ii)  Diabetic or venereal clinics;
  (iii)  A renal dialysis unit.

Serum hepatitis is associated with the serological entity Australian antigen (AuAg), much more commonly indicated as HB Ag, ie hepatitis B. It is acquired primarily within the walls of a hospital.

*Sources*
  1. Blood donors. All donors are tested for HB Ag.
  2. Symptomless carrier. When methods of testing on a large scale are available all patients admitted to hospital may be tested.
  3. Patients who should be specially tested are those (a) with liver disease; (b) who have had previous transfusions; (c) who receive frequent treatment; (d) drug addicts and the sexually promiscuous.
  All blood and serum products are potentially infected.

*Prevention*
  Preventive measures which should be taken include:
  1. Screening of all patients and blood in dialysis units.
  2. Spilt blood should be disinfected with a hypochlorite solution such as Chloros or Domestos. Metal, which these solutions corrode, should be soaked in a 10 per cent formalin solution.
  3. Specimens of blood from suspected patients should carry a distinguishing mark on the tube such as a yellow label.
  4. The sterilisation of syringes must be adequate (p. 85).
  5. After surgical operation on these patients the linen should be destroyed.
  6. Similar precautions should be borne in mind if the patient dies and a post-mortem examination is performed.

### LIVER ABSCESS

An abscess of the liver may take two forms:
  1. *A solitary abscess*, which is usually a complication of amoebic dysentery. Surgical drainage of the abscess may be performed, but in most cases treatment consists of chloroquine or metronidazole (Flaygl) with tetracycline for the secondary infection.
  2. *Multiple abscesses* of the liver may occur as a complication of peritonitis or pyaemia. The condition is frequently fatal. It is associated with mild jaundice, a high temperature, and rigors. Chemotherapy offers the best prospect of cure.

## PORTAL HYPERTENSION

Cirrhosis of the liver may be caused by alcoholism or as a late result of infective jaundice. In addition to malnutrition the scarring which results in this condition strangles the veins in the liver. The result is that dilatation or varicosity develop in the veins of the portal system. The most marked effect is in the veins at the cardio-oesophageal junction called oesophageal varices where haemorrhage may occur. Shunting of the blood from the portal system into the systemic system by anastomosis of the portal vein to the inferior vena cava may be undertaken.

## HYDATID CYST OF THE LIVER

Hydatid disease is due to an infection caused by a parasite known as the *Taenia echinococcus*. The liver is one of the commonest sites for the infection. Surgical treatment consists of excision of the lining of the cyst and drainage of the cavity.

## CARCINOMA OF THE LIVER

Carcinoma of the liver is almost invariably secondary to an intra-abdominal primary growth and is fatal.

*Investigations*
LIVER PUNCTURE BIOPSY

This enables liver tissue to be obtained for histological examination without open operation. It is helpful in the study of patients with liver disease when clinical signs and laboratory tests do not give a definite diagnosis. It is seldom indicated in jaundiced patients and is performed when sarcoidosis, Hodgkin's disease, or brucellosis are suspected.

Before the puncture is made the bleeding, clotting and prothrombin times are estimated and must be normal, liver function tests are performed, 2 units of blood are crossmatched and premedication with 15 mg morphia or 60 mg phenobarbitone instead of morphia is given if there is gross liver damage. The patient lies on her back with a pillow under her left buttock, the right hand behind the head. The skin is cleansed, a local anaesthetic infiltrated and the liver biopsy needle is plunged into the liver. The biopsy specimen is placed in normal saline, labelled and sent to the pathologist. Postoperatively a watch should be kept for signs of internal haemorrhage.

LIVER FUNCTION TESTS

Liver function tests are carried out to determine the extent of disease of the liver and to help to differentiate between obstructive jaundice which requires surgery and liver disease in which surgery is unnecessary. The tests are non-specific and difficult to interpret. Even after performing a series of tests, diagnosis may still be impossible and a laparotomy may have to be undertaken.

The numerous chemical reactions which occur in the liver form the basis of some of the tests. Others depend on whether or not the various bile ducts are blocked. Over three-quarters of the liver may be destroyed before many of the tests show abnormality.

*Bromsulphophthalein test* is the most sensitive test of liver function. A reading of more than 30 per cent of the dye in the serum one hour after injection indicates liver damage. In the presence of jaundice the value of the test is diminished.

*Galactose or laevulose tolerance test.* If the sugars galactose or laevulose are given orally or intravenously they are quickly converted into glycogen by the healthy liver and their level in the blood does not rise very much. If, however, the liver cells are diseased, the sugars cannot be converted into glycogen, so they pass unchanged through the liver and their level in the blood rises considerably. Glucose, the natural sugar of the blood, is not used in this test, for the blood sugar (glucose) level depends on many other factors than the state of the liver.

METHOD. The patient fasts overnight and in the morning a sample of blood is taken. Galactose (40 g), dissolved in a cupful of warm water, is then given by mouth and further blood samples taken every half-hour for two hours. Some laboratories prefer the galactose to be given intravenously as a sterile 50 per cent solution, the dose being 0·5 g per kg body weight. If laevulose is given the dosage is 50 g orally dissolved in warm water.

*Plasma proteins.* Albumin and fibrinogen are synthesised in the liver. In severe liver disease therefore their level in the blood falls. The albumin may fall as low as 25 g per litre (normal 36–50 g per litre). The globulin level, however, remains unchanged, so the normal ratio of albumin to globulin (2 : 1) may be reversed. Globulin is not a single substance but a series of similar proteins called a(alpha), β(beta) and γ(gamma) globulins. When the liver is diseased the ratio of these globulins to one another in the plasma is altered. The thymol and zinc flocculation and turbidity tests are positive when these ratios are abnormal. Prothrombin is synthesised in the liver. Vitamin K is necessary for the liver to make prothrombin. If there is no bile in the intestine vitamin K cannot be absorbed and therefore in obstructive jaundice the prothrombin level is low (prothrombin time prolonged). If an injection of vitamin K is then given the prothrombin level becomes normal in 12 hours. In severe liver disease, however, the prothrombin level is low because the diseased liver cannot synthesise it and an injection of vitamin K will have no effect. The plasma proteins are normal in obstructive jaundice unless the obstruction is so longstanding that severe secondary liver damage has occurred.

*Serum alkaline phosphatase* is removed from the blood by the liver and excreted in the bile. Normal values are about 2 to 10 King Armstrong units per 100 ml of serum. When the liver cells are diseased it may rise to 30 units but if the bile ducts are blocked very high levels of 100 units or more will occur. It should be noted that very high values of serum alkaline phosphatase also occur in bone diseases when osteoblastic cells are over-active, e.g. rickets, Paget's disease, hyperparathyroidism, bone tumours.

*Bile metabolism.* Jaundice (yellowness) is due to an increased amount of bilirubin in the blood which may be due to liver disease, blockage of the bile ducts or increased red cell haemolysis. Bilirubin is formed from haemoglobin in the cells of the reticulo-endothelial system (spleen, bone marrow, liver) where old red cells are broken down. The bilirubin becomes attached to albumin in the plasma and is carried by the circulating blood through the liver. The bilirubin becomes conjugated (joined) to a substance called glucuronic acid in the liver and is passed down the bile ducts into the intestine where bacteria act on it and convert it into stercobilinogen most of which is excreted in the faeces where, on exposure to air, it darkens to brown and is called stercobilin. Some of the stercobilinogen, however, is reabsorbed from the intestine into the bloodstream and excreted in the urine which, on exposure to the air, darkens to urobilin (the same substance as stercobilin).

*The serum bilirubin* is normally less than 15·4 $\mu$mol per litre (1 mg 100 ml). The level rises much more in obstructive jaundice than liver disease or haemolytic jaundice. Several estimations are more valuable than single tests. In infective hepatitis the serum bilirubin rises to a peak and then steadily returns to normal. Where the obstructive jaundice is due to gall-stones the level of serum bilirubin fluctuates as the obstruction is usually intermittent. The intensity of the jaundice varies. If the obstruction is due to carcinoma of the pancreas, blockage of the common bile duct is complete. The serum bilirubin rises to a high level and remains high and the jaundice deepens.

TESTS FOR BILE PIGMENTS IN THE URINE. Bilirubin is found in the urine in obstructive jaundice and in jaundice due to hepatitis.

*Urobilin in the urine.* In complete obstructive jaundice there is no bilirubin in the intestines for the bacteria to convert to urobilinogen. Therefore there is no urobilin to reabsorb into the bloodstream and none to pass into the urine. Tests for urobilin therefore are negative though the urine is dark due to a high content of bilirubin glucuronide.

*Urobilin (stercobilin) in the faeces.* The dark colour of the faeces depends on the amount of bilirubin entering the intestine. The stools are pale in obstructive jaundice.

*Bile salts* also appear in the urine in obstructive jaundice as they are drained back into the blood and excreted by the kidneys. Bile salts are detected by sprinkling flowers of sulphur on the surface of the urine in a test glass. If bile salts are present the sulphur sinks due to the lowering of surface tension.

## THE GALL-BLADDER

The most common disease of the gall-bladder is caused by gall-stones formed by the precipitation of the constituents of bile. A gall-stone gives rise to symptoms when it moves. Movement may result in its obstructing the cystic duct with resultant acute cholecystitis, or the stone may migrate into the common

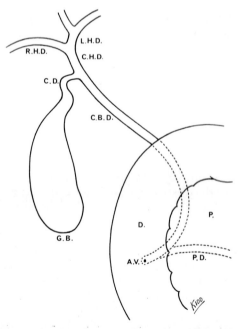

FIG. 36.1   Diagram showing the normal anatomy of the biliary tree. G.B., gall-bladder; C.D., cystic duct; H.D., hepatic ducts; C.B.D., common bile duct; A.V., ampulla of Vater; D., duodenum; P., pancreas; P.D., pancreatic duct.

bile duct causing obstruction to the main outflow of bile from the liver. There is a strong hereditary tendency in gall-stone formation.

### SYMPTOMS AND SIGNS OF GALL-STONES

It has long been said that the most typical patient is a fat parous woman about the age of 40. This, however, is far from true. Gall-stones are equally common in the thin. They are certainly more common in the female than the male but they are by no means rare in men and are occasionally seen even in children.

*Severe pain in the epigastrium* radiating to the tip of the right shoulder-blade is the most usual symptom. When severe pain between the shoulders is frequently complained of by the patient, he has a stone in the common bile duct. This is sometimes followed by rigors due to infection and obstruction of the smaller ducts in the liver. After the severe colic has passed, the pain continues as a dull ache, associated with a distaste for food. The patient may complain of shortness of breath and feels distended.

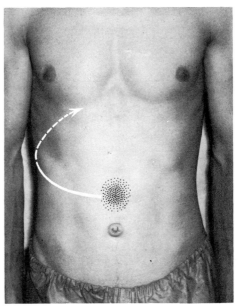

FIG. 36.2   Gall-bladder pain commences in the epigastrium and radiates to the back and shoulder.

*Vomiting* is common during the acute attacks, and in less severe cases takes the form of nausea associated with eructation of air.

*Jaundice* is a comparatively rare symptom, and occurs only when a stone is obstructing the common bile duct. In this case it varies from day to day and usually disappears completely only to recur at a later date.

### SIGNS AND SYMPTOMS OF SPECIAL LESIONS

**Acute cholecystitis.** The pain is usually constant in type, increasing in severity from time to time. The temperature is high, 37·8° to 38·3° C (101° to 102° F), but the pulse rate is usually in the region of 100. The abdomen is tender and rigid in the right hypochondrium. Slight jaundice may occur, and, in some cases, rigors. Most cases subside satisfactorily with rest and analgesics. Occasionally the patient develops an empyema of the gall-bladder, and drainage may be necessary.

**Chronic cholecystitis.** Indigestion with pain of the gall-bladder type is usual. Fatty foods aggravate the pain. The patient may be tender in the right hypochondrium. The symptoms are very much milder than those of acute cholecystitis. The gall-bladder is occasionally the site of typhoid organisms and the patient who may be symptom free is a carrier.

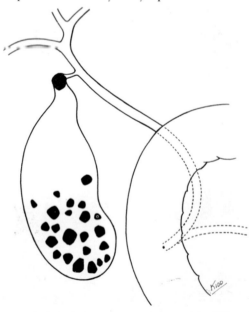

FIG. 36.3   Acute cholecystitis. A stone is impacted in the cystic duct. The gall-bladder, which contains numerous stones, is tense and distended.

*Investigation of gall-bladder disease*

1. DIRECT RADIOGRAPHIC EXAMINATION of the abdomen reveals gall-stones only in 5 per cent of cases in which they are

present, because the majority of gall-stones are not radio-opaque. Therefore, only a positive X-ray will be of value.

2. CHOLECYSTOGRAM. The cholecystographic examination varies according to the opaque medium used and the technique employed.

The material, usually orablix, telepaque, or biloptin, is given by mouth the evening before. A radiograph is taken at 9 a.m. and if the gall-bladder functions a fatty meal is then given and a further radiograph taken half an hour later. The patient will already have been prepared with the colon free from gas and faecal shadows. The material should be administered according to the makers' instructions, which should be closely followed. It is very important to be certain that the patient has not vomited the drug, as this renders the examination valueless.

The test is of little value in the presence of jaundice. The medium is excreted in solution by the liver and concentrated by the gall-bladder. A diseased gall-bladder fails to concentrate.

3. CHOLANGIOGRAM (outlining of the common duct). This may be done:

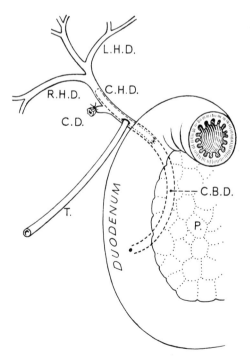

FIG. 36.4   The gall-bladder has been removed and the cystic duct (C.D.) ligatured. A tube (T.) is sutured into the common bile duct (C.B.D.).

   (a) When the abdomen is open at operation or before a tube is removed from the common duct.

   (b) By the intravenous injection of biligrafin. Frequent radiographs are taken as the liver excretes the biligrafin.

   4. PERCUTANEOUS TRANSHEPATIC CHOLANGIOGRAPHY is a useful procedure in obstructive lesions. It is usually done as an immediate preoperative investigation in the theatre.

### COMPLICATIONS OF GALL-STONES

   1. Acute cholecystitis, which may be further complicated by an empyema or mucocele of the gall-bladder.

   2. Biliary colic.

   3. Jaundice.

   4. The development of carcinoma of the gall-bladder due to long-standing gall-stones.

   5. Intestinal obstruction by a gall-stone.

   6. Pancreatitis.

   7. Adhesions.

   8. The formation of multiple fistulae.

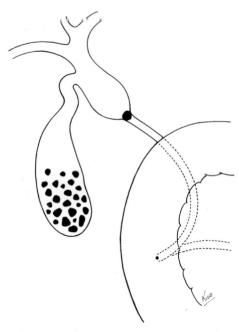

FIG. 36.5   Obstruction of the common bile duct by a stone. Note the duct above the stone and also dilatation of the hepatic ducts. This patient would be jaundiced.

*Treatment*

ACUTE CHOLECYSTITIS AND BILIARY COLIC

Most surgeons do not advise operation in the acute stage, and the treatment usually prescribed is:

1. Rest in bed.
2. Pethidine (100 mg) by injection. Morphia is not recommended since it is said to produce spasm of the sphincter of Odii which guards the common bile duct and pancreatic duct at the ampulla of Vater.
3. Fluids only by mouth.
4. Antibiotics.

*Complications.* The only urgent complication is perforation of the gall-bladder and, although it is uncommon, it must be constantly borne in mind. When the tenderness has passed—about six weeks later—removal of the gall-bladder can be undertaken at a quiescent stage of the disease.

RADICAL CURE OF GALL-STONES

Gall-stones can be dissolved by the administration of Chenodeoxycholic acid but its use is far too dangerous for clinical practice.

The gall-bladder is usually removed (cholecystectomy) after ensuring that the common bile duct is patent.

Removal of the gall-bladder removes the stones, the site of their formation, and a potential site for a new growth. If excision of the organ is impossible, operation is confined to the removal of the stones and drainage of the gall-bladder (cholecystostomy).

CARE OF THE PATIENT FOR GALL-BLADDER OPERATIONS

The usual preparation for any major abdominal operation is necessary. The main specific points concern the care of the drainage tube, and the nurse attending the patient in the theatre should take special care to note the exact position of each tube.

In all patients for cholecystectomy a nasogastric tube should be passed before operation. Patients after cholecystectomy tend to vomit a good deal of bile, and aspiration through a nasogastric tube for 24 hours eliminates this complication with its accompanying distress.

1. DRAINAGE TUBE IN THE SUBHEPATIC POUCH. The tube is usually inserted after operation to drain the oozing of blood from the liver bed. It is also useful to reveal internal reactionary haemorrhage, and is usually removed after 48 hours.

2. TUBE IN THE COMMON DUCT. Bile flows along this tube, which is connected to a plastic bag as illustrated in Fig. 36.6.

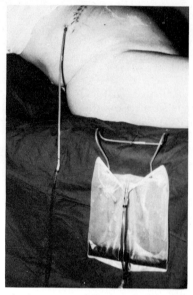

FIG. 36.6   Tube in common bile duct draining into plastic bag.

It is sewn in position with catgut sutures and must not be removed until at least the seventh day, by which time the catgut
has loosened and allows easy withdrawal. An analgesic is advisable one hour before this is undertaken. A cholangiogram
may be performed to outline and test the patency of the duct.
For a day or two before withdrawal the tube may be clamped
off and any complaint of pain is noted. After removal of the
tube the bile then drains through the resulting sinus and diminishes each day until the discharge ceases and the wound
heals. Fluids by mouth are allowed as soon as desired postoperatively.

A specimen of bile may be sent for bacteriological examination. Where there has been severe cholangitis an antibiotic
may be prescribed.

If the patient has been jaundiced or is jaundiced due to a
stone in the common bile duct, vitamin K (10 mg) must be administered by injection preoperatively for three days and continued for several days after the operation. The jaundiced
patient is liable to develop hepatorenal failure. This is now
largely preventable by the administration of 500 ml of 10 per
cent mannitol one hour before operation and this should be
continued postoperatively. As mannitol produces a heavy
diuresis, the fluid balance and electrolytes should be watched
with great care.

3. TUBE IN THE GALL-BLADDER is inserted only if a cholecystostomy has been performed. It is removed about the 10th day.

## Complications

1. *Pulmonary complications* are very liable to occur, particularly in the base of the right lung. They are diminished by breathing exercises and free movement of the patient in bed.

The patient is usually nursed propped up during the 24 hours after the operation, and should sit out of bed next day.

2. *Pulmonary embolism* may occur, since many of these patients are unwilling to move about in bed because of pain.

3. *Haemorrhage* may be very severe if a ligature slips, and in the first 48 hours the pulse rate should be carefully observed.

4. *Backache* may be due to using a bridge on the operating table and this should be avoided particularly in elderly patients with osteoarthritis.

5. *Liver failure.*

6. *Delayed postoperative pain.* In the convalescent stage some patients develop severe pain, probably due to mucus or grit in the common bile duct, but this usually passes.

DIET. Immediately after the operation only fluids should be given for 24 hours, but after this period the diet should be as normal as possible. The restriction of fats results in the stagnation of bile, and is probably an important factor in the causation of pain which sometimes occurs when the patient gets up.

7. *Recurrent stone in·the common bile duct.* This will require further exploration.

### CARCINOMA OF THE GALL-BLADDER
The new growth usually occurs in a gall-bladder which contains gall-stones. The rapid invasion of the liver by the growth renders most cases hopeless.

## THE PANCREAS

The principal pancreatic diseases of surgical importance are acute and chronic pancreatitis and carcinoma. Rarely cysts, calculi, insulin and gastrin secreting tumours occur.

### ACUTE AND RELAPSING PANCREATITIS
The great danger of this condition lies in the fact that the pancreatic juices, so potent in the digestion of fat and protein, digest the tissues with which they come in contact.

*Causes*
1. Reflux of infected bile.

2. Viral infection—mumps.
3. Pancreatitis resulting from the hypercalcaemia of hyperparathyroidism—rare.
4. Excessive alcoholic consumption.
5. Aminoaciduria—rare—caused by an inborn error of metabolism.

*Symptoms and signs*

There is a sudden onset of epigastric pain and collapse, frequently after a meal. The face may be slightly cyanosed and the patient does not lie absolutely still as in the case of a perforated peptic ulcer, but tends to roll about. The temperature is subnormal in the first hours of the attack and the pulse rate is elevated. The abdomen is tender, but not always rigid.

*Investigation*

1. THE ESTIMATION OF THE SERUM AMYLASE by the laboratory is of the greatest value. The normal is 40 to 200 Somogyi units, and in acute pancreatitis a reading of over 1000 units is usual. It should be performed within the first 24 hours.

2. A WHITE BLOOD COUNT is usual.

3. THE SERUM CALCIUM. An estimate of the amount of calcium fixed in the formation of calcium soaps is some guide to progress.

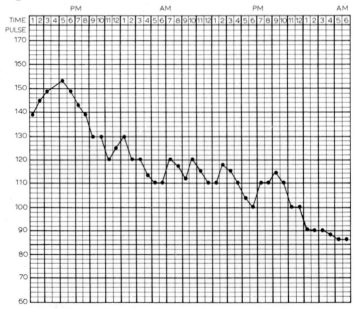

FIG. 36.7 Postoperative hourly pulse chart—always important. Vital in jaundice, as pallor from haemorrhage is unobservable.

4. CHOLECYSTOGRAPHY is performed when the attack has subsided.

**Complications**

1. *Pancreatic abscess* which may require drainage.
2. *Pseudocyst formation* which is drained by joining it to the stomach.
3. *Recurrence or relapse.*

*Treatment*

1. Maintenance of fluid and electrolyte balance—loss of fluid into the retroperitoneal space may be very great. Massive transfusions of whole blood and plasma may be vital.
2. Alleviation of pain—this may be very severe and intractable. Codeinephosphate by injection is the best analgesic as it relaxes the sphincter of Oddi, but pethidine may also be required.
3. Antibiotics—one of the tetracyclines or ampicillin as they are excreted in bile is the antibiotic of choice.
4. Suppression of pancreatic secretion by the use of continuous gastric suction to suppress the secretion mechanism is essential. Anticholinergic agents such as Pro-Banthine to suppress the vagal stimuli on secretion.
5. Calcium gluconate 10 ml 10 per cent solution i.v. daily.
6. Aprotinin (Trasylol)—a protease inhibitor—has been shown to reduce considerably the mortality in acute pancreatitis.
7. Surgical interference is rarely undertaken.

### CHRONIC PANCREATITIS

This is a condition in which the pancreas is slowly destroyed. It does not follow acute pancreatitis but is a separate condition. It may present with:

Pain in the upper abdomen
Symptoms and signs of malabsorption
Jaundice
Diabetes

*Investigations*

Investigations include cholecystography, sophisticated tests to determine the secretory capacity of the pancreas and chemical examination of the stools to measure malabsorption. Duodenoscopy and cannulation of the papilla of Vater and retrograde choledochpancreatography may be performed.

*Treatment*

Treatment is very unsatisfactory. Pancreatic enzymes and a high calorie, high protein diet may help.

SURGICAL PROCEDURES undertaken for pain or persistent jaundice include division of the sphincter of Oddi.

## CARCINOMA OF THE PANCREAS

Carcinoma of the pancreas may develop:

(i) *In the head;*
(ii) *In the body and tail*—persistent pain is the prominent symptom. The diagnosis may be made only by isotope scanning or at laparotomy.

*Treatment*

If jaundiced the patient will require vitamin K and mannitol preoperatively (p. 396). Anastomosis of the gall-bladder to the duodenum relieves the jaundice (cholecystoduodenostomy). Should the growth be operable, it may be excised three weeks later. This is a long, difficult operation and carries a high mortality rate.

## ISLET CELL TUMOUR

A tumour of the islet cell results in an excessive secretion of

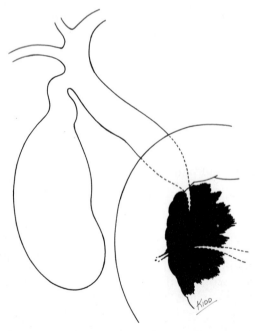

FIG. 36.8   A carcinoma of the head of the pancreas showing obstruction of the common bile duct and pancreatic duct. The gall-bladder is distended due to back pressure.

insulin. The patient suffers from recurrent hypoglycaemic attacks. Cure is effected by excision of the tumour.

## GASTRIN-SECRETING TUMOUR

This tumour causes intractable duodenal and jejunal ulceration. The treatment is removal of the tumour if it can be
located or total gastrectomy to cut off the acid response to
gastrin.

# CHAPTER 37

# Diseases of the Small Intestine

The small intestine commences at the pylorus and terminates at the ileocaecal valve. The proximal intestine or jejunum is wider than the ileum or distal intestine.

New growths of the small intestine are very rare indeed. The inflammatory conditions are common, but respond to medical measures, although their complications occasionally require surgical aid.

Obstruction of the intestine has already been considered but its causes and the special features of particular conditions are reviewed here.

**Abdominal injuries.** Intraabdominal injury may occur as a result of a penetrating wound or a closed injury. The liver, spleen or the mesentery may be lacerated causing haemorrhage or the intestinal tract may be penetrated. In severe cases the patient is shocked and signs of peritoneal irritation such as pain, tenderness or rigidity may be present.

Investigation includes radiograph of the abdomen for the presence of free gas or fluid. The pulse rate is raised, hypotension may be present, a falling haemoglobin may indicate haemorrhage, and aspiration with a needle of the four quadrants of the abdomen may be undertaken. Laparotomy is necessary if there is severe bleeding or perforation. Rupture particularly delayed clinically up to four days after injury may occur from seat belts.

## INJURY TO THE SMALL INTESTINE

The small bowel may be injured as the result of a blow on the abdominal wall or from a penetrating wound. The loop of bowel may be torn across completely or partially, or the blood vessels supplying the part may be damaged. One or several loops may be damaged.

*Symptoms and signs*

The patient complains of sudden abdominal pain, and this continues after the injury. Vomiting usually occurs. If the blood vessels are torn the symptoms and signs of concealed internal haemorrhage will be present.

The abdomen is rigid and tender from leakage into the peritoneal cavity of the intestinal contents and the exudation of blood. (See the signs of peritonitis on p. 338.)

*Treatment*

After careful preoperative treatment of acute circulatory failure the skin is prepared and the patient taken to the operating theatre. Fluid by mouth is forbidden, because it would leak into the peritoneal cavity.

*Operation*

Lacerations of the intestine are trimmed and sutured. If the blood supply is destroyed, resection of the affected loop and anastomosis must be performed after the haemorrhage has been controlled.

The postoperative treatment is similar to that of acute intestinal obstruction (p. 354).

# INFLAMMATORY CONDITIONS OF THE SMALL INTESTINE

## PERFORATION OF SPECIFIC INFECTIVE ULCERS

Occasionally typhoid and tuberculous ulcers perforate. The symptoms and signs are similar to those of a perforated peptic ulcer. Immediate operation is necessary. Special care must be taken to see that gloves, gowns, and instruments are packed and marked afterwards so that they can be separately sterilised.

## MECKEL'S DIVERTICULUM

In the last 60 cm of the ileum a diverticulum of the bowel, not unlike the appendix, may be present. It varies in length from 5 cm to 50 cm and, like the appendix, it may become inflamed. The symptoms, signs, and treatment are similar to those of appendicitis. On other occasions it may be the cause of intestinal obstruction by ensnaring a loop of the intestine, and the clinical features are those of intestinal obstruction. An important feature of the histology of Meckel's diverticulum is the frequent presence of ectopic epithelium such as gastric and pancreatic tissue. Ectopic gastric epithelium is very apt to cause the adjacent epithelium to bleed and a bleeding Meckel's diverticulum is one of the commonest causes of rectal bleeding in children.

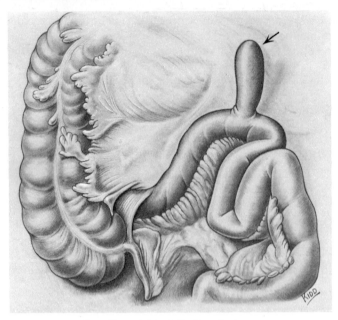

FIG. 37.1   A Meckel's diverticulum.

### CROHN'S DISEASE OR REGIONAL ENTERITIS

This is an inflammatory condition of the wall of the lower portion of the small intestine, and may involve the caecum and colon. It may give rise to symptoms similar to appendicitis due to inflammation, or it may give rise to obstructive symptoms. Ninety per cent of all cases come to surgery eventually. Corticosteroids and immuno-suppressive drugs such as azathioprine may be prescribed but are of doubtful value. Obstruction, perforation or fistula formation are complications which occur.

### INTESTINAL OBSTRUCTION

The main clinical features and treatment of acute intestinal obstruction we have already considered on page 350. Chronic intestinal obstruction is a condition in which the obstruction is incomplete, and usually terminates in acute obstruction.

*Causes*

The bowel may be obstructed because:

1. Its lumen is blocked by a foreign body or a gall-stone.
2. Its wall is altered by disease such as Crohn's disease, a stricture due to an old tuberculous ulcer, or drugs such as potassium chloride in certain preparations, or to an intussusception.

3. The wall is constricted by something outside it; by a loop twisting around itself—adhesions or connective tissue bands. The neck of a hernial sac is the commonest cause of all.

1. **Blockage by a foreign body.** The most frequent cause is a gall-stone. The fundus of the gall-bladder becomes adherent to the duodenum, and slowly a fistula between the two organs is formed. A large gall-stone may pass through the fistula and become impacted in the narrowest portion of the small intestine, the ileum. If the stone is small it may pass without difficulty. An impacted stone is removed after incision of the bowel and then the wall is re-sutured.

Another interesting cause of blockage of the lumen of the bowel is unchewed dried fruit.The patient has failed to follow the instructions and has not soaked the fruit. When swallowed whole, instead of disintegrating, the fruit enlarges in size and blocks the intestine. In some conditions of intestinal hurry, digestion has not time to occur and inadequately chewed food may block the lower ileum. This may result after gastrectomy or gastrojejunostomy. Swallowed foreign bodies such as marbles are occasionally the cause of blockage in the case of children.

2. **The wall is altered by disease.** Crohn's disease, which we have discussed on page 404, is one cause. An important cause, particularly in infants under 2 months, is intussusception.

*Intussusception.* This is due to a small portion of the bowel becoming invaginated into the portion distal to it. As a result of peristalsis, the process is carried further until, as it were, the bowel, instead of being a single tube, now has three layers. The bowel is, in fact, telescoped into itself.

SYMPTOMS AND SIGNS. The child is usually a healthy male infant about 9 months old. His good health is probably the cause of excessive peristalsis driving one loop of bowel into the one below. The change of diet at the time may be a causal factor, and in the infant the Peyer's patches are enlarged so that they form a small tumour-like mass, disturbing the normal peristaltic wave. An alternative theory is that it is due to enlargement of Peyer's patches from an adenovirus which could account for its seasonal occurrence. The child screams with pain, which is typical of intestinal colic. The face becomes very pale when the colic is at its height and brightens in the intervals between the spasms. Vomiting is invariably present, and the passage of a small amount of bright red jelly-like blood clot per rectum is almost diagnostic. Careful examination of the abdomen reveals a sausage-like mass. Treatment consists of reduction of the bowel usually by operation, but retrograde pressure by barium enema may effect reduction. It should be given only under X-ray screening control. The nurse must watch especially for recurrence of symptoms on the first night after operation.

In the adult, intussusception occasionally occurs due to an adenoma, a Meckel's diverticulum, or a growth.

3. **Lesions outside the bowel.**

*Causes*

   Strangulated hernias (p. 352)
   Bands
   Adhesions.

Bands and adhesions may form as a result of previous operations, particularly for peritonitis. Tuberculous peritonitis also causes extensive adhesions which may cause intestinal obstruction.

As in all acute obstructions, urgent operation is essential.

### MESENTERIC THROMBOSIS

This condition presents with acute abdominal pain, circulatory collapse, the passage of blood from the rectum and abdominal tenderness. It is increasingly common as a manifestation of atherosclerosis. The main vessel or branch of it

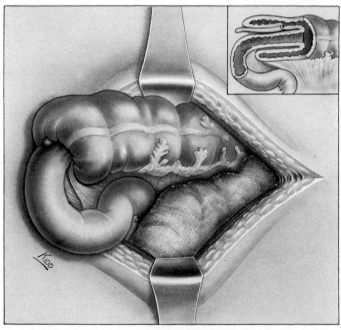

FIG. 37.2   An intussusception.

may be involved with gangrene of the segment of intestine supplied. The outlook is very poor however it is treated. Treatment includes resection, removal of the thrombus and anticoagulant therapy.

## OPERATIONS ON THE SMALL INTESTINE

*Enterostomy*

1. FOR FEEDING PURPOSES. This is performed:

   (a) Sometimes for inoperable cancer of the stomach.
   (b) Very occasionally for intractable gastric ulcer where the condition of the patient is too poor for radical operation, yet relief from medical treatment is very slight.

2. FOR ULCERATIVE PROCTOCOLITIS. The ileum is brought to the surface (p. 409)—an ileostomy.

*Enterectomy*

A loop of bowel is removed. The continuity of the intestine is then restored by suture.

This is usually performed for a gangrenous small intestine or for injury. Postoperatively the important points are the relief of flatus by the passage of a flatus tube and aspiration of the stomach to relieve any distension above the anastomosis as well as parenteral fluid replacement.

*Enteroanastomosis*

This is the short-circuiting of one portion of the bowel into another beyond a pathological lesion without removing the cause.

This is frequently performed for an obstruction which is not causing gangrene of the intestine, such as tuberculosis of the small intestine, severe adhesions, or Crohn's disease.

# CHAPTER 38

# Diseases of the Caecum and the Colon

The large intestine extends from the ileo-caecal valve to the anus. The colon is that portion of large bowel distal to the ileocaecal valve, and terminating at the beginning of the rectum. The caecum is the portion of large intestine immediately below the level of the ileocaecal valve.

The main diseases which attack all portions of the large intestine in varying degrees are the inflammatory conditions and the new growths.

New growths of the colon are very important indeed. They are sometimes elusive to diagnose both on clinical and radiographic examination, yet they remain one of the most favourable sites for treatment.

### INFLAMMATORY CONDITIONS OF THE COLON

**Ulcerative proctocolitis.** Non-specific ulceration of the colonic and rectal mucous membrane is a condition which is usually treated medically. The aid of the surgeon is sought when it is considered that the bowel is so diseased that excision is advisable. The usual operation consists of making an

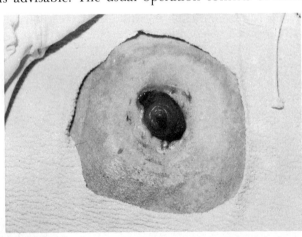

FIG. 38.1    Ileostomy showing coaptation of mucosa to skin.

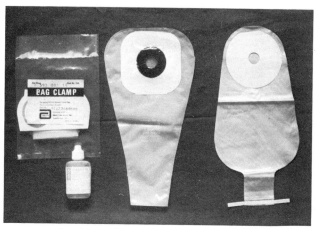

FIG. 38.2 Ileostomy bag and equipment.

artificial opening in the terminal ileum known as an ileostomy (Fig. 38.1) after total colectomy. An alternative procedure is anastomosis of the ileum to the rectum. The problems arising in the care of these patients are two in number:

1. THE MAINTENANCE OF NUTRITION. The patients are usually very wasted, dehydrated and anaemic. They require blood transfusion as well as a diet rich in protein, glucose and vitamins and low in residue. In the immediate postoperative period only fluids are given until the second or third day. A light

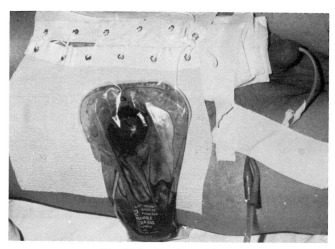

FIG. 38.3 Bag in position.

diet is then commenced. By the tenth day the patient is given a full diet with limited roughage. Up to this time the bowel movements are extremely frequent, but they should now have diminished to three or four changes of the bag each day. Isogel and Celevac granules are of value to thicken the effluent. At this time the patient should be making rapid progress. The ileostomy contents should be thickening and weight should be increasing. Additionally they require all the care associated with abdomino-perineal resection of the rectum (p. 435).

2. THE CARE OF THE ILEOSTOMY. The skin round the ileostomy is sometimes very sore, but can be protected by Karaya gum, Tinct. Benzoin Co. or Siccolam cream which is a silicone vasogen. The ileostomy discharges thin fluid and it cannot be controlled. Over the ileostomy stump is fitted a bag such as the Koenig-Rutzen bag (Fig. 38.2). The flange of the bag is made to adhere to the skin by means of a cement containing a latex rubber mixture. The patient should be instructed in changing the bag and the flange. In particular he should be warned that : (i) ether meth. which is used to loosen the

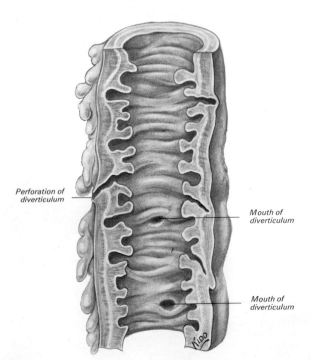

Perforation of
diverticulum

Mouth of
diverticulum

Mouth of
diverticulum

FIG. 38.4  Segment of the colon showing diverticula, inflammation, and perforation.

adhesive is inflammable, but special solvents are now available, (ii) the skin must be perfectly dry before the flange is stuck back to the skin, (iii) soreness of the skin is liable to occur if the flange becomes loose. An application of Baltimore paste, stoma adhesive or Orabase to the skin will be of help.

A very striking feature of these patients as a group is their fortitude and courage. They have formed ileostomy societies at which they meet and discuss methods of overcoming their difficulties and it is advisable for the patient to be visited by one of their members before and after the operation.

### DIVERTICULAR DISEASE OF THE COLON

This is a condition of disorder of muscle function of the bowel. There is an increase in the tone of the longitudinal muscle and contraction of the circular muscle. The result is muscular hypertrophy. Diverticulum formation is a complication of this muscle abnormality and infection is a complication which may occur in a diverticulum. The corrugations of the bowel are very striking in a dissected specimen (Fig. 38.4). A diverticulum may perforate causing peritonitis or several diverticula may form a conglomerate inflamed mass, sometimes with abscess formation. The inflammatory mass may form a stricture and obstruct the bowel, which can be easily mistaken for a new growth. The inflammatory process may involve the bladder, and a fistula between the colon and the bladder is most commonly due to this condition.

*Clinical features*

The patient is usually past middle life, and, according to the course of the disease, the clinical features vary.

1. *Peritoneal symptoms* may be most prominent:

(a) Pain, particularly in the left iliac fossa.
(b) Constipation and some urgency of micturition.
(c) Vomiting is usually present.
(d) The temperature and pulse rate are elevated.

On examination a localised mass may be felt in the left iliac fossa.

2. *Obstructive symptoms.* A fibrous stricture may form, and the symptoms are those of large bowel obstruction (p. 352).

*Treatment*

The majority of cases subside with rest. The Ochsner-Sherren regime (p. 339) is instituted. If general peritonitis is present the peritoneal cavity must be drained, omentum sewn over the area of leakage, and a colostomy performed proximal to the inflamed area of bowel.

A low or non-residue diet is desirable during the acute stage and convalescence. As a long-term regime it is now considered inadvisable because it causes constipation and obesity and therefore a normal or high residue diet is given.

Myotomy, that is division of the hypertrophied muscle as far as the mucous membrane, has occasionally been undertaken instead of resection. Resection is undertaken after perforation, fistula formation for severe haemorrhage, stricture or for intractable disease.

### NEW GROWTHS OF THE COLON AND CAECUM

Carcinoma of the large bowel causes 14,000 deaths each year in the United Kingdom. It is commoner in north-west Europe and North America. The areas of large incidence of disease, with the exception of Japan, have a high standard of living. Several studies indicate a possible relationship of large bowel cancer to diet, either excess of fat or protein. The theory is that intestinal bacteria produce carcinogens from dietary fat and from bile steroids.

Familial polyposis of the colon is a condition in which carcinomatous change is inevitable and only a total proctocolectomy will save the patient. It should be undertaken before ma-

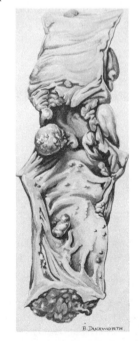

FIG. 38.5  Polyposis coli. The condition is hereditary, invariably becomes malignant and can be cured only by total protocolectomy.

lignant changes occur and all members of the family must be examined regularly.

Malignant growths, usually carcinomas, are extremely common. They may occur in any portion of the large bowel, but the most common sites in order are the rectum, the pelvic colon, and the caecum. Although some growths, particularly in the caecum, are soft and proliferative, the vast majority grow around the bowel and eventually cause obstruction by forming a ring stricture (see Fig. 38.6).

*Symptoms and signs*

*Increasing constipation* is the most important symptom. At first, aperients give relief. Later the dose has to be increased, with a diminished effect, and finally the bowel action ceases. Many patients present themselves suffering from acute obstruction.

*Pain* is not prominent, and is usually described by the patient as being due to 'wind'. This is quite an accurate description, since his difficulty arises in his inability to pass flatus. The passage of small quantities of blood is an occasional complaint, but severe haemorrhage is uncommon.

*Anaemia* particularly hypochromic in type may be the presenting and only symptom of carcinoma of the caecum.

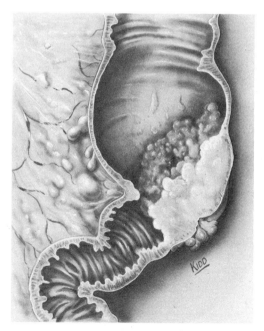

FIG. 38.6   Carcinoma of the colon. Note the distended bowel above the growth and the secondary deposits in the lymphatic glands.

*A lump* in the right ilial fossa felt by the patient is unfortunately not an uncommon symptom in carcinoma of the right colon and caecum.

*Other symptoms.* The increasing size of the abdomen is a frequent complaint, and is due to distension of the bowel. In later cases the distension is further increased by secondary deposits which cause ascites (free fluid in the peritoneal cavity).

Diarrhoea with mucus, particularly alternating with constipation, is not uncommon and is due to ulceration of the bowel above the growth by retained faeces. Loss of weight appears slowly, and vomiting is a late symptom usually indicative of acute intestinal obstruction. The patient is sometimes pale and 'muddy' in appearance and runs a slight temperature. The temperature is not due to the growth but to the infection in the bowel above and around the growth.

Examination of the abdomen may reveal a palpable mass or a distended large bowel. In early cases nothing abnormal can be made out on abdominal or rectal examination.

### Investigations

RADIOGRAPHIC EXAMINATION of the colon after the administration of a barium enema or barium meal may be performed. Exfoliative cytology (p. 215) may be undertaken.

SIGMOIDOSCOPY is of value for growths in the lower bowel, and the test for occult blood in the faeces is also performed.

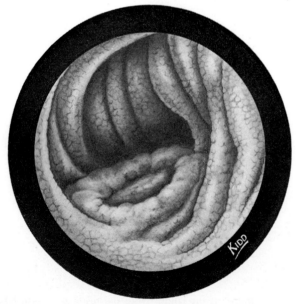

FIG. 38.7   A growth visualised through the sigmoidoscope.

FIBREOPTIC COLONOSCOPY enables a large area of the colon to be visualised. The patient is prepared with a careful bowel washout in addition to any laxative deemed to be advisable.

PREPARATION OF THE PATIENT FOR A BARIUM ENEMA. Preparation may be for 48 hours, or shorter preparation (an enema given the previous night, and a colonic washout next morning at least two hours before examination) may be satisfactory. Occasionally in the ambulant patients preparation by Dulcolax suppositories is satisfactory.

### Treatment

The ideal treatment is to excise the loop of bowel and mesentery containing the growth and lymph glands and to join up the divided bowel. If obstruction is present a colostomy is performed and later, when the growth is excised, the bowel is restored in continuity and the colostomy is closed then or later.

## THE CARE OF THE PATIENT FOR COLONIC OPERATIONS

The main operations for colonic conditions are:

1. The formation of an artificial anus, viz. colostomy or caecostomy.
2. Excision of a portion of the colon. If one half of the colon is removed the operation is known as a hemicolectomy.

### GENERAL PREPARATION

It is important that the patient be in the best possible condition, and, particularly for an excision of the colon, anaemia should be corrected by blood transfusion preoperatively.

### PREPARATION FOR COLECTOMY

In addition to the general measures for any major operation mentioned in Chapter 4, the following special points are of great importance:

1. *The relief of mild obstructive symptoms.* If these can be overcome a one-stage operation may be performed with great benefit to the patient.
   (a) The diet should be light and of low residue but high protein content—meat soups, fruit juice, custards, and milk puddings.
   (b) Liquid paraffin, 15 ml t.d.s., ensures a soft stool.
   (c) Gentle enemas or colonic lavage may be administered.
2. *The diminution of infection in the intestine.* It is impossible by any method to sterilise the lumen of the large intestine.

The single most effective procedure in reducing infectivity is to ensure the colon is empty of faecal material.

Infection can be further diminished by the administration by mouth of:

(a) Phthalysulphathiazole or Sulfasuxidine, 2 g four-hourly, for five days preoperatively. In addition, phthalylsulphacetamide retention enemas (180 ml) may be given each evening, followed by a soap enema next morning.

(b) Neomycin, 1 g each hour for four hours, then 1 g 4 hourly until theatre time.

(c) Neomycin 1 g
Bacitracin 100,000 units ⎫ is said to be the most effective
Nystatin 500,000 units ⎭ given 6 hourly for 48 hours.

### POSTOPERATIVE CARE

Enemas should *not* be given.

Similarly, since the suture line in the intestine is so near to the rectum, *rectal infusions should not be given*, and it is preferable that the patient should drink as soon as possible.

Liquid paraffin, 15 ml thrice daily, should be given on the second day, and at all stages it is important to relieve the distension of the bowel, and therefore of the suture line, by the regular passage of a flatus tube four-hourly while the patient is awake. Some surgeons perform a three-finger anal dilatation at the end of the operation.

The general postoperative care described in Chapter 4 is necessary.

### COLOSTOMY AND CAECOSTOMY

The formation of an artificial anus consists of bringing a portion of the bowel to the surface so that the patient excretes faeces on to the abdominal wall.

This may take the form of either a colostomy or a caecostomy. Of the two, the colostomy is undoubtedly preferable because the faeces become more solid as they approach the rectum.

The faecal discharge from a caecostomy opening is thin and extremely irritant, so that, as a permanent arrangement, it is unsatisfactory. It is occasionally performed as an emergency measure in a patient who is so ill from obstruction of the distal bowel that exploration of the abdomen is impossible.

A colostomy is performed either as a temporary or permanent measure for growths of the pelvic colon or rectum. It is almost invariably performed in cases of wounds of the rectum, so that the faecal flow is deviated from the wound. Congenital

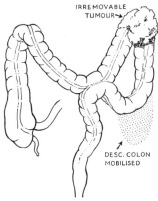

FIG. 38.8   Colocolic anastomosis, short-circuiting an irremovable tumour of splenic flexure.

absence of the rectum or paraplegia in young adults is occasionally an indication.

**Caecostomy.** A caecostomy is performed by the insertion of a tube into the caecum. The opening is usually valvular in type and frequently closes spontaneously after the tube has been removed.

The tube is connected to a Bardic bag by the bedside so that the discharge does not irritate the skin. After ten days, however, the tube drops out, and every effort must be made to prevent the skin from becoming inflamed and excoriated. Moist and petroleum jelly dressings tend to make the skin soggy. The following preparation, known as 'Baltimore paste', is useful to prevent the skin irritation caused by a caecostomy or ileostomy:

> Powdered aluminium, mixed with sufficient liquid paraffin to produce a stiff paste, 1 part
> Ung. zinc oxide, 4 parts.

A permanent caecostomy, except on the lines of an ileostomy, is almost unmanageable from the patient's point of view and if at all possible it is avoided by anastomosis of the ileum to the transverse colon. It is occasionally used as a 'safety valve' in some cases of anastomosis in the lower pelvic colon or upper rectum.

**Colostomy.** There are many varieties of colostomy.

1. *Loop colostomy.* A loop of colon is brought to the surface of the abdominal wall and held in position by a glass rod passed through the mesocolon. The wound is then sutured. The colostomy is opened immediately if the patient is suffering from acute intestinal obstruction or

perforation in the bowel beyond, otherwise the colostomy is opened several days later when the wound has healed.

2. *Defunctioning colostomy*. The loop is exteriorised and then divided so that there is no communication between the two orifices. This provides complete rest to the distal colon.

3. *End or terminal colostomy*. The colonic mucous membrane is sutured to the skin. Since this is usually performed only when all the distal bowel has been removed there is only one orifice. It is performed in conditions such as abdomino-perineal resection of the rectum and there is no possibility of subsequent closure. The patient should not be given any false hope that the colostomy can be removed.

The bowel is covered with petroleum jelly gauze, and if the case is not one of acute obstruction the dressings may be left undisturbed for five days so that healing in the surrounding wound will advance rapidly. In all types of colostomy it is usual to fix a disposable bag on the skin at the end of the operation.

A colostomy may be performed in the transverse colon or in the pelvic colon.

OPENING OF A COLOSTOMY. The colostomy is opened with a diathermy knife or by a thermocautery. No anaesthetic is needed because the bowel is insensitive to all stimuli except distension.

The surrounding skin is carefully covered with sterile gauze. The patient is greatly relieved by the opening of the colostomy, which expels a large quantity of flatus.

For some time the bowel motions are irregular and uncontrolled. The diet should be light, and liquid paraffin (15 ml t.d.s.) should be given until a regular action of the bowel is attained.

THE ROD. The rod is removed on the tenth day.

REGULATION OF THE BOWEL. Normally the bowel will act without any special measures. Liquid paraffin by mouth may be necessary. If the bowel is obstinate a Dulcolax suppository may be inserted into the opening of the colostomy and this usually produces a good result. Exceptionally, a washout through the colostomy may be given in the same way as rectal washouts are performed.

Once the bowel has been regulated, washouts and enemas are unnecessary, and excessive lavage may result in colitis.

When a loop colostomy has been opened there are two orifices:

1. The '*active*' orifice through which faecal material is discharged and which leads proximally from the growth.

2. *The 'non-active' orifice*, which leads distally towards the growth. Usually only mucus is discharged from this opening.

The nurse should be able to recognise the 'active' orifice, because it is through this opening that washouts, salines, etc. are normally given. The 'active' orifice in an iliac colostomy is usually the upper opening, the 'non-active' one the lower. In a transverse colostomy the opening towards the right side of the abdomen is the active orifice and towards the left the non-active. A terminal colostomy has only an active orifice as the bowel below it (usually the rectum) has been removed. If the nurse is in any doubt, or the colostomy performed is not one with which she is familiar, she should have no hesitation in asking the surgeon which is the active orifice.

A washout should also be given through the non-active orifice:

1. Before a second stage operation for excision of the rectum or colon. (In this case the active orifice must, of course, also be washed out.)
2. If the patient with a colostomy is troubled by excessive mucus or pus from a fungating growth.

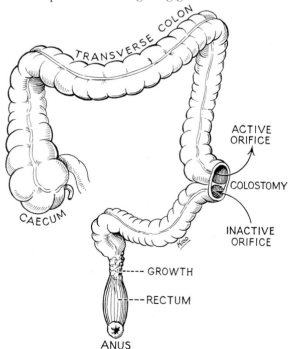

FIG. 38.9   Diagram of colostomy orifice (loop colostomy).

Many surgeons open the colostomy as the last step in the operation and cover it with a disposable bag.

THE STITCHES. The stitches are removed on the tenth day. The patient can be allowed out of bed as soon as possible preferably on the first postoperative day.

INSTRUCTIONS TO THE PATIENT

There are 100,000 patients with colostomy in Great Britain. Certain basic amenities are essential for the management of colostomy, and these include an indoor lavatory, a bath and hot water. A patient with a colostomy should have top priority for housing. They also require more home help and modern cleaning and laundry methods. Some form of incineration is necessary for dressings. The laundry service for the incontinent should be used but, in most areas, it does not function at the week-end. The community services can be a tremendous help to the patient with a colostomy.

The patient should be taught how to attend to the colostomy. A colostomy is compatible with a useful and happy life but the initial training is most important. Routine washouts are unnecessary and harmful. There is a danger of colitis or perforation. With training the colostomy will function once or twice a day. Fruit and pips usually irritate the colostomy but what the patient can eat is largely a matter of intelligent investigation by himself. An agent which retains water and renders the stool soft but formed may be advisable. Agar or methyl cellulose in granules taken with water in the morning may be helpful.

DRESSING. Provided full control has been obtained gauze or lint smeared with petroleum jelly is all that is necessary. A colostomy belt or, probably better, a roll-on is used to keep it in position. Alternatively, disposable plastic bags may be worn attached with adhesive or on a supporting belt. The skin around the stump should be washed with warm soapy water.

*Diarrhoea*, which may be troublesome, may be checked by the administration of kaolin opiates, codeine or amphetamine sulphate. If it is persistent, however, it should be investigated. If this shows no obvious cause and severe 'looseness' persists, spironolactone may be given.

## Complications of a colostomy

1. *Sepsis in the wound.*

2. *Prolapse of the bowel.* In this condition a loop of bowel above the colostomy is blown out through the wound. It is usually due to a technical error in selecting the wrong portion of the bowel at operation. The doctor will usually be able to reduce it in the ward.

3. *Retraction.* The loop may slip back into the abdomen,

particularly if the mesentery is very short. Another cause for this complication is too early removal of the rod.

4. *Intestinal obstruction.* A loop of small bowel may become ensnared at the side of the colostomy. The symptoms are those of small bowel obstruction, and urgent laparotomy is indicated.

5. *Contracture of the colostomy orifice.* This is usually prevented by excision of an area of skin when performing the colostomy opening. Occasionally it may be necessary to dilate the opening by inserting a gloved finger.

*The closure of a colostomy*

When it is anticipated that a colostomy will ultimately be closed it is advisable to train the patient to perform sphincter exercises each day, so that there is no atrophy of the anal sphincter when it comes into action again.

The closure of a colostomy may be a dangerous operation unless the bowel is carefully prepared. It is essential to be certain that the bowel between the colostomy opening and the anus is not obstructed. A barium enema is administered through the anus and the barium is allowed to run out of the

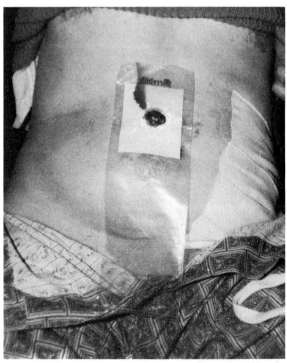

FIG. 38.10   Colostomy with disposable bag attached.

colostomy opening. Radiographs will confirm the patency or otherwise of the segment of bowel.

PREOPERATIVE PREPARATION. The colostomy wound must be firmly and completely healed before the operation can be attempted. The lower bowel must be completely free of hard faecal material. Rectal washouts are given after the instillation of olive oil to soften the material. In an attempt to reduce infectivity of the intestinal contents sulfasuxidine therapy (p. 416) is instituted.   A further X-ray is taken to ensure no barium remains in the colon or rectum.

POSTOPERATIVE TREATMENT. A flatus tube should be passed every four hours, but enemas must *not* be given for fear of perforating the sutured bowel.

A careful watch must be kept for the symptoms of peritonitis.

## CHAPTER 39

# Diseases of the Rectum and the Anus

Diseases of the rectum and anal canal are common. These are favourite sites for a new growth. The intestinal contents have reached the highest degree of infectivity in this region of the alimentary tract, and a crack or injury to the mucous membrane or skin is very likely to result in infection. Hae-morrhoids are another extremely common complaint amongst civilised peoples.

RECTAL EXAMINATION

This procedure is usually carried out by a doctor. A small tray is prepared, containing:

Disposable glove (e.g. Dispos-A-Glove)
Lubricating jelly (e.g. KY)
Kleenex wipes
Paper bag (disposal)
Proctoscope–with light, leads and battery, if available
Torch or portable light.

The patient is informed, privacy is ensured and the patient assisted to lie, if possible, in the left lateral position, with the

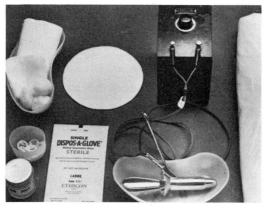

FIG. 39.1   Equipment for rectal examination.
Swabs                    Disposable gloves
Wool balls               Finger cots
Filter papers            Proctoscope and battery
Underpad                 Lubricant.

knees well flexed and the buttocks near to the edge of the bed. The bedclothes are turned back to expose the buttocks and anal region and personal clothing is rearranged.

The person carrying out the examination puts on a Dispos-A-Glove, lubricates the tip of the index finger and anus and gently carries out the examination. If protoscopy is to follow, the nurse assists in this procedure.

On completion of the examination, the anus is wiped with tissues and these, together with the used glove, are discarded into the paper bag. The patient is repositioned and made comfortable.

Used equipment is removed, the tray is cleaned. If the proctoscope is of the electrical variety, the leads are disconnected. The proctoscope is washed and soaked in Savlon 1 per cent (in) for at least 30 minutes.

### PERIANAL ABSCESS

Infection in the rectal or anal wall from an inflamed haemorrhoid or abscess may spread into the ischio-rectal fossa or the infection may be blood borne.

*Symptoms and signs*

Pain may be severe because the pus is under considerable tension. Pain on defaecation is usually present. The affected area is swollen, red, and indurated.

*Treatment*

Very free drainage is necessary, and, as in all wounds around the anus, healing must occur from the depth of the abscess cavity. This is achieved by frequent baths keeping the wound well open with a corner of a square of gauze soaked in Eusol. If this is not carried out meticulously the skin heals over and one or more septic tracks are left in the depth, with resultant fistula formation. The diet should be light, fluid in nature, and of a non-residue type.

### FISTULA-IN-ANO

A fistula is a track lined with septic granulation tissue connecting two epithelial lined surfaces. The surfaces which the track connects in this region are the skin of the buttock and mucous membrane of the anal canal. The commonest cause is an ill-treated or neglected ischiorectal abscess. Rarely multiple fistulae are present when the condition is tuberculous. Fistula-in-ano may be a complication of Crohn's disease, ulcerative colitis or diverticular disease of the colon.

A radiograph of the chest may be taken in all cases of fistula to exclude pulmonary tuberculosis.

*Symptoms and signs*

A mucous or purulent discharge occurs around the anus. There is usually no pain until the opening becomes blocked and an abscess forms in the track behind.

*Treatment*

The two openings are found with a fine probe, and the track is excised. A wide raw area is left to granulate, and the same care is essential as in the case of an abscess to see that healing takes place slowly from the floor of the cavity. The specimen which has been excised is usually sent for pathological examination to exclude tuberculosis and new growth formation. The detailed preparation and aftercare are discussed on page 431.

### FISSURE-IN-ANO

This is the most painful of all rectal conditions. As a result of pressure from hard dry faecal material, a small crack (or fissure) appears in the posterior portion of the anal wall. There is severe pain on defaecation, and this persists for several hours afterwards. The patient dreads another bowel action; the faeces as a result become still harder and drier. When the bowel has to act the pain is more severe than ever. A small pile, known as a 'sentinel pile', is usually present.

*Treatment*

In acute cases three-finger dilatation of the anus under an anaesthetic is sufficient to effect a cure. This requires admission for only half a day. If the fissure is thickened, excision of the crack and partial division of the internal sphincter is necessary.

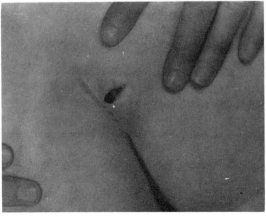

FIG. 39.2   Pilonidal sinus complicated by an abscess. The tiny 'pore-like' openings in the centre are characteristic.

## PILONIDAL SINUS

This is a very common cause of recurrent abscess formation in the area between the tip of the coccyx and the anal margin. Fine tracks lead from the skin into the tissues down to the coccyx.

*Treatment*

1. ACUTE STAGE. An abscess may form, and incision is necessary. Any area seen to contain hair is laid open.

2. RADICAL TREATMENT consists of wide excision of the area. A few millilitres of methylene blue are injected into the track by means of a syringe and cannula—*not a needle*. The wound is closed by uniting the skin and the cavity obliterated by means of several deep nylon sutures tied over a roll of gauze. The wound is left undisturbed for 14 days. After this time it has healed. The patient is nursed lying on the side or the prone position.

More usually, however, surgical treatment is limited to opening up and laying open all visible tracks. The hairy skin of the buttock is shaved and kept shaved postoperatively. Special care is taken to remove any visible hair which may be seen in the granulating wound.

## PRURITUS ANI

Severe irritation and itching (pruritus) around the anus may occur from many causes. The commonest cause is threadworms. Other causes are vaginal discharge, gross uncleanliness, haemorrhoids and diabetes. But it may occur without any obvious cause to account for it. This is known as idiopathic pruritus ani.

*Symptoms and signs*

Severe irritation causes great distress, particularly at night in bed. The buttock area is covered with multiple scratch marks and the loss of sleep results in extreme weariness.

*Treatment*

The urine is tested for sugar because the condition may be caused by mild infection of the skin in diabetic subjects. Any obvious focus of irritation is treated. Warm baths of sodium bicarbonate and painting with 1 per cent gentian violet solution give considerable relief. An antipruritic cream such as Teevex is of value. The injection of local anaesthetic into the affected area is usually advised. Proctocaine is a solution of local anaesthetic in oil. A wide-bore needle is necessary to drain it into the syringe from the ampoule.

## HAEMORRHOIDS

Haemorrhoids are dilated veins covered with a fold of mucous membrane, and in the case of internal haemorrhoids an artery is contained in the pedicle. Great confusion has arisen from a lack of understanding of the terms 'internal' and 'external' haemorrhoids.

*External haemorrhoids* are small dilated veins covered by redundant folds of skin, and are situated on the anal margin. The only complication is a small haemorrhage into the skin folds. This causes severe pain which can be relieved by simple incision through which the haematoma is evacuated.

*Internal haemorrhoids.* Internal, or true, haemorrhoids always originate inside the bowel. There are three stages (degrees) of increasing severity:

1. Early in their development they are soft and bleed readily.
2. Later they become thickened and descend outside the sphincter on defaecation, but return spontaneously afterwards.
3. Still later they remain outside (prolapsed haemorrhoids).

*Symptoms and signs*

Bleeding is the earliest symptom, and severe anaemia may result if it is profuse. The blood is bright red and occurs on defaecation. As they progress, irritation and distress during

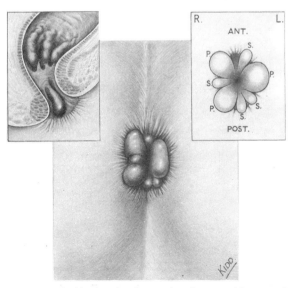

FIG. 39.3   Haemorrhoids showing internal and external haemorrhoids and the position of the three primary and four secondary haemorrhoids.

prolapse are prominent complaints. Prolapse may occur suddenly or gradually. Sudden prolapse is extremely painful, and if the piles cannot be returned the patient is unable to walk. The anus and lower rectum may be examined visually by means of a proctoscope.

### TREATMENT OF PROLAPSED HAEMORRHOIDS

Treatment is directed to the relief of pain and the reduction of the inflammation locally. Rest in bed, preferably with the lower end of the bed raised and the patient lying on his side, is essential. Compresses of lead and opium or cold sodium sulphate are soothing. Morphia (15 mg) eight-hourly should be prescribed, and the diet should be confined to fluids. Anal dilatation may be advised and in many is effective even in painful prolapsed haemorrhoids.

### TREATMENT BY INJECTIONS

Injections can be given only when the haemorrhoids are inside the anal canal. This is most effective for early bleeding haemorrhoids. Five per cent phenol in almond oil is injected by means of a haemorrhoid syringe.

### ANAL DILATATION

Lord believes that the primary defect is narrowing of the outlet of the anal canal. The anal sphincter is unable to dilate to whatever size is necessary to allow the stool to pass and fae-

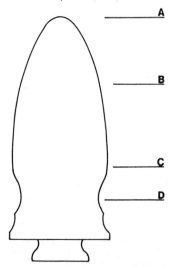

FIG. 39.4 Dilator. A, Blunt nose. B–C, Working part. D, Groove into which sphincter can slip so that patient knows that he has passed the dilator all the way.

cal material has to be expressed. The rise in intraluminal pressure obstructs the venous return from the haemorrhoidal area. The haemorrhoidal plexus dilated with blood further obstructs the outlet. The aim of dilatation is to break this vicious circle.

1. PROCEDURE. Dilatation of the anal sphincter up to eight fingers is undertaken under a general anaesthetic in an operating theatre. When dilatation has ironed out the constriction a sponge is placed in the anal canal to reduce the risk of haematoma formation. It is removed one hour later and the patient can go home.

2. POSTOPERATIVE DILATATION BY THE PATIENT AT HOME. The patient is instructed to pass a specially designed dilator (Fig. 39.4) $1\frac{1}{2}$ inches long each day for two weeks after a hot bath before retiring, and on alternate days for the following month. It should be left in position for one minute. After this time the patient should pass the dilator only if there is any tightness.

*Complications:*
1. Haematoma.
2. Splitting. There is a danger of infection so the patient must be kept in hospital and antibiotics prescribed.
3. Prolapse occurs occasionally and should be reduced.
4. Incontinence. If it occurs it usually clears up in two weeks.

OPERATIVE TREATMENT.
This is a very satisfactory operation and consists of ligation of the three primary haemorrhoids. The preparation and after-treatment are considered on p. 431.

CRYOSURGERY
The need for operation for haemorrhoids has diminished considerably since the introduction of Lord's dilatation. An alternative to surgical ligation is cryosurgery which necessitates hospitalisation for only two days.

## PROLAPSE OF THE RECTUM
Conditions which predispose to rectal prolapse are chronic cough, constipation, phimosis, whooping cough, torn perineum from childbirth, and occasionally threadworms. The essential aim of treatment in these conditions is to treat the cause.

Rectal prolapse may be:

1. *Incomplete.* In this form only the mucous membrane prolapses. This condition is usually seen in infants. In the adult it

may be associated with haemorrhoids and is cured at the same operation. In infants, regulation of the bowels is usually all that is necessary. If the condition persists the buttocks are strapped together after the prolapse has been reduced, and the child is kept in bed.

2. *Complete prolapse* is a distressing condition associated with ageing, weight loss and decreasing muscle tone.

*Treatment*

If possible, the prolapse is replaced and the patient confined to bed. The foot of the bed should be elevated. If the patient's condition is satisfactory cure by operation may be undertaken. This consists of anchoring the rectum by an abdominal approach. In more feeble patients a suture of silver wire or nylon may be inserted around the anus to leave an aperture the size of the base of the operator's index finger. This is sufficient to allow a motion to pass but small enough to prevent the mucosa prolapsing.

### SIMPLE STRICTURE OF THE RECTUM

Simple stricture of the rectum may occur as a result of a gonococcal proctitis, ulcerative proctocolitis or as a complication of an operation for haemorrhoids or radiotherapy. Administration of an enema which is too hot may give rise to rectal stricture and it cannot be stressed too often that the temperature of all fluids used must be taken with a thermometer. Dilatation with special rectal bougies may be advised.

### PROCTITIS

Inflammation of the rectum or anal canal unassociated with haemorrhoids or a new growth may be:

1. *Non-specific.* This is part of the condition known as ulcerative proctocolitis (p. 408) in which the rectum is involved in about 70 per cent of cases.

2. *Specific.* Causes include bacillary and amoebic dysentery,

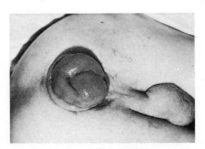

FIG. 39.5   Rectal prolapse.

gonnococcal and tuberculous infection. The treatment is that of the cause.

## RECTAL BIOPSY

Biopsy of a rectal lesion is of great value in the diagnosis of rectal tumours, whether simple or malignant in nature, in the differentiation of Crohn's disease from ulcerative proctocolitis. It is also of value in the confirmation of the presence of amyloid disease (p. 559).

## PREPARATIONS AND AFTERTREATMENT OF OPERATIONS ON THE RECTUM AND ANUS
(Excluding removal of the rectum)

The rectum, the anus, and the surrounding skin are teeming with vast numbers of pathogenic organisms. By any method of preparation it is impossible to have a sterile operating field. It is none the less important to render the area as free of organisms as possible, and operation in this area must be carried out under strict conditions of asepsis so that fresh forms of infection are not introduced. Because absolute asepsis is impossible, all wounds in this area require free drainage, and healing always occurs by secondary intention.

*General preoperative treatment*

1. THE BOWEL

The bowel should be emptied before the operation. A mild aperient should be given two nights before the operation, followed by an enema in the evening and a washout on the morning of the operation day. A rectal washout is given not later than six hours before the patient goes to the theatre.

RECTAL WASHOUT. An enema saponis is given to ensure that the bowel is empty of faeces.

Equipment required (on a trolley):

> Rectal tube or catheter
> Connection tubing 24 inches in length
> Funnel
> Small jug—1 litre
> Large jug containing 4 l fluid (tap water) at 100°F (37·8°C)
> Bucket
> Incopad
> Large polythene sheet
> Disposable gloves
> Lubricating jelly
> Medical wipes/tissues.

The procedure is explained to the patient, and he is told that it may take 15 to 20 minutes. He is allowed to pass urine. He is placed in the left lateral position, with an Incopad under the buttocks. The polythene sheet is spread on the floor, and the bucket placed on it.

The small jug is filled with fluid. The funnel, tubing, connection and catheter are assembled. The tip of the catheter is lubricated. Some fluid is run through to expel air, and then stopped. The patient is asked to take a deep breath, and the catheter is inserted about $2\frac{1}{2}$ inches into the rectum. The funnel is raised above the level of the buttocks; 300 ml (half pint) of fluid is run into the rectum. Before the funnel is empty it is inserted over the bucket and the fluid siphoned back. The process is repeated until the fluid returns clear, or the 4 litres of prepared fluid have been used.

Afterwards, the tube is withdrawn. The anal region is cleansed. If the patient desires, he is allowed to use a bedpan or commode. He is left comfortable in bed.

Used equipment is discarded. The fluid siphoned back and also that passed into the bedpan are measured and added together—the total amount thus returned is usually equal to the amount given.

After washing and drying her hands, the nurse reports on the amount of fluid given and returned, whether the final washout was returned clear, and any untoward effects.

## 2. THE PERIANAL REGION

The skin around the anus, groin, and suprapubic area should be shaved. It is washed with Derl soap.

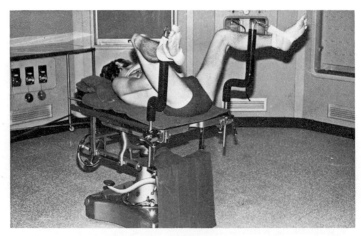

FIG. 39.6   Lithotomy position.

3. THE DIET

During the two days before the operation the diet should be light, nutritious, and of the non-residue type.

4. GENERAL ATTENTION

Warmth, dentures, and other details must be given the attention as for any other operation. In the theatre general or spinal anaesthesia may be used. The usual position of the patient is the lithotomy (Fig. 39.6).

*Postoperative treatment*

A normal diet is allowed as soon as the patient desires food.

*Pain.* This is usually severe, and repeated morphia injections are necessary. Hot baths are valuable for the relief of pain following an operation for haemorrhoids, and many patients like to spend several hours a day lying in a hot bath.

*Haemorrhage* may occur, and will be severe if the ligature of a haemorrhoid base has slipped. It must be reported at once.

A TUBE covered with petroleum jelly is frequently left in the anal canal at the end of the operation for haemorrhoids, partly for the passage of flatus and partly lest haemorrhage should occur and not be revealed owing to the sphincter ani being in spasm. Severe haemorrhage is treated by pressure from the inflated balloon of a Foley catheter in the anal canal and a pack is applied to the anus. The bleeding point has to be secured in the theatre if haemorrhage persists.

THE PACKS. The original packs in cases of fistula are usually removed at the end of 24 hours and replaced, after irrigation of the wound, by a light pack. In most cases flat packs are used, but one corner can be tucked into the wound to ensure that the skin edges are not allowed to fall inwards. Firm, deep packing with ribbon gauze is avoided.

APERIENTS. Liquid paraffin (15 ml t.d.s.) is given on the evening of the operation. The bowel does not usually act until the third day, but the paraffin keeps the faecal material fairly soft. A gentle olive oil enema may be given on the third morning. A bath after a bowel action is very important.

DIGITAL DILATATION OF THE ANUS. This is a particularly important after-treatment following a haemorrhoid operation. It is commenced on the sixth day and performed daily for two days. Its purpose is to separate the 'sticky' surfaces so that stricture formation does not occur.

*Acute retention of urine.* This is particularly liable to occur after a haemorrhoid operation, and, if the simpler methods mentioned on page 467 fail, catheterisation must be undertaken.

## NEW GROWTHS

Simple new growths include polyps and adenomas. The main symptoms are similar to those of haemorrhoids, and the treatment is excision.

### CARCINOMA OF THE RECTUM

Malignant new growths are very common.

*Symptoms and signs*

1. *Constipation.* Increasing constipation alternating with diarrhoea is not uncommon.

2. *Bleeding.* The blood is bright red in colour and is so important a symptom that it must not be attributed to haemorrhoids until carcinoma has been excluded. Pain in the rectum is a late symptom in most cases, but appears earlier in growths situated in the anal canal.

3. *Tenesmus.* With a polypoid growth of the rectum, the patient has a constant sensation of fullness associated with the desire to defaecate, which is not relieved by bowel action.

4. *Sciatic pain.* Sciatic pain is sometimes the presenting symptom, and is due to infiltration of the sacral plexus by the growth.

5. *Intestinal obstruction.* Intestinal obstruction may develop acutely if the lumen of the bowel has been narrowed by the growth.

6. *Mucus and pus.* Discharge of mucus and pus may occur in a large fungating growth filling the rectum.

7. *Digital examination.* Digital examination of the rectum will reveal a palpable growth.

8. *Sigmoidoscopic examination.* The higher reaches of the rectum and the lower colon may be examined by means of a sigmoidoscope (Fig. 39.7) and a portion of the growth taken for biopsy. The bowel should be emptied by a gentle aperient, followed by a Dulcolax suppository, six hours before examination. Some surgeons prefer no preparation at the first attempt.

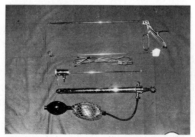

FIG. 39.7   Sigmoidoscope with biopsy forceps at top.

*Treatment*

Removal of the rectum offers the only hope of cure. The patient is usually left with a permanent colostomy. If the growth is inoperable, colostomy is avoided if at all possible.

## THE TREATMENT OF A CASE OF RESECTION OF THE RECTUM
### (Abdominoperineal resection)

The operation consists of removal of the rectum and lower portion of the pelvic colon. Two separate surgical teams combine in these cases, one operating in the abdomen and the other in the perineum at the same time. Resection of the rectum is always a severe operation.

Blood transfusion before operation is usual, and another transfusion is set up before the operation is commenced. The bowel should be emptied by aperients and enemas and sterilised by sulfathalidine or neomycin. After the patient has been anaesthetised a Gibbon or small Foley catheter is inserted into the bladder. This is left in place for four to ten days as temporary disturbance of bladder function results from removal of the rectum.

*Postoperative care*

The abdominal wound is closed and covered with Elastoplast. To the colostomy is attached a disposable bag.

### IMMEDIATE POSTOPERATIVE TREATMENT

The patient is laid on his side and the head is kept low (on one pillow) until he recovers consciousness. Blood transfusion is continued until the general condition is satisfactory.

Systemic antibiotic therapy is commenced after the operation. Sulfasuxidine is not of particular advantage because there is no anastomosis to leak.

Strain by coughing or attempting to pass urine must be limited to the minimum.

There is a great loss of blood serum into the large wound of the perineum, and the patient must have a very high protein diet to compensate for this. Eggs, meat, milk, and cheese are necessary. A transfusion of blood plasma for this specific purpose may be necessary about the seventh or eighth day.

THE BLADDER. A catheter is left in the bladder and connected to a closed drainage. About the fourth to fifth day the catheter can be removed. A good sign that the bladder will function is to see the patient passing urine around the catheter before it is removed.

FLUIDS should be taken as soon as possible by mouth and the diet increased as soon as the bowel sounds are heard. The colostomy frequently does not work for a day or two after operation and, if necessary, a gentle washout through the colostomy opening affords considerable relief. The patient should be given massage to his legs during his convalescence and encouraged to move his joints so that when he gets up he is as fit as possible. He must be instructed in the care of his colostomy (p. 420) and provided with a colostomy belt. If it is difficult to get the colostomy to work a Dulcolax suppository into the mouth of the colostomy is often satisfactory.

THE PERINEAL WOUND may be closed and suction drainage attached. The wound can heal by primary intention in two to three weeks. Alternatively the wound may be packed for 48 hours and will require irrigation each day until it heals.

## CONSERVATIVE RESECTION

Occasionally a sphincter preserving operation is possible for growth of the upper third of the rectum. The postoperative care is similar to a colectomy but special care must be taken to see that the flatus tube is passed no further than 2 cm beyond the anal sphincter.

# CHAPTER 40

# Hernia

A hernia is a pouch of lining membrane protruding itself through a weak point in the covering structures. The most common site of a hernia is the abdominal wall. The term, however, includes a weakness at any point, for example, a defect of the skull results in what is known as a hernia cerebri.

The weak points in the musculature of the abdomen are scars and the canals through which certain structures normally run. The hernias which occur at these sites are named accordingly:

1. Inguinal.
2. Femoral.

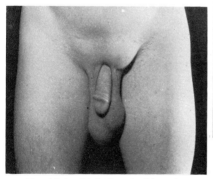

FIG. 40.1    Right inguinal hernia.

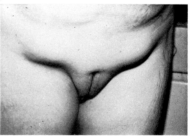

FIG. 40.2    Bilateral femoral hernias.

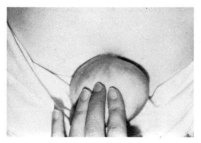

FIG. 40.3    Paraumbilical hernia.

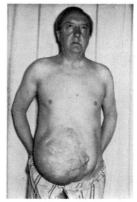

FIG. 40.4    Incisional hernia.

437

3. Umbilical, in the adult usually paraumbilical.
4. Epigastric.
5. Incisional, known as ventral, if arising on the anterior abdominal wall.
6. Obturator.
7. A rarer type of hernia is the diaphragmatic. The abdominal contents herniate into the chest.

The constituents of an abdominal hernia are:

(a) The sac. This is the protruding pouch of peritoneum.
(b) The contents. The most frequent are loops of the small intestine and the great omentum. They slip in and out, provided the hernia is not strangulated or obstructed. Long-standing friction results in adhesion of the contents to the sac. Almost any abdominal organ except the pancreas may be found in a hernial sac.
(c) The coverings include all the tissues superficial to the hernia and consist of the stretched muscles and aponeurosis, the fascia, and the skin.

*The cause of hernia*

A hernia may be congenital or acquired.

The commonest hernia in an infant is an umbilical hernia, from the failure of the umbilicus to seal off satisfactorily. The majority of small congenital umbilical hernias in infants cure themselves and reassurance of the parents is the only treatment necessary. In the larger ones a simple operation is necessary if they do not close spontaneously. In gross cases the whole of the intestines are outside the abdomen, a condition known as exomphalos. This condition requires urgent operation. Combined with an undescended testicle, congenital inguinal hernia is not uncommon in male children.

Hernias are frequently acquired as a result of tearing of the muscles due to strenuous work or play.

### SYMPTOMS AND SIGNS OF UNCOMPLICATED HERNIA

Small hernias are noticed by the patient only after coughing or standing up. A swelling, with a slight dragging ache, is the commonest complaint. The skin over a large hernia may be in folds which tend to become eczematous as a result of friction.

On examination there is an expansile impulse on coughing.

### Complications of a hernia.

1. *Irreducibility* occurs in long-standing hernias.
2. *Strangulation*. The blood supply is cut off, and, in addi-

tion to the local pain, the symptoms and signs of intestinal obstruction are present (p. 351). There is no impulse on coughing, and the hernia is irreducible and tender. Unrelieved, the strangulated loop of bowel becomes gangrenous.

3. *Progression.* Increase in size is usual.

4. *Intertrigo of the skin*, i.e. abrasion due to two folds of skin rubbing together.

*Treatment*

Operative repair is the treatment of choice and many uncomplicated hernias are suitable for 'day' surgery and patients can get up next day at home. The sac is excised after the contents have been reduced into the abdomen and the weakness repaired by suture of the muscles or by the introduction of special suture material if the muscles are weak. The patient is kept in bed for only one day, but in large recurrent hernias three to four days in bed are advisable. He is advised against very heavy lifting for three months. There are special cases, however, where this ideal course of treatment is not possible, nor can it be carried out at once if certain aggravating factors are present, for example, an enlarged prostate or a chronic cough. If these conditions are not treated first, recurrence of the hernia is inevitable.

1. SPECIAL AGGRAVATING FACTORS:

(a) Enlargement of the prostate.
(b) A urethral stricture.
(c) Constipation.
(d) A persistent cough.

2. THE PATIENT IS TEMPORARILY UNFIT FOR OPERATION

(a) In an infant the operation for hernia is undertaken at three months or even earlier.
(b) During pregnancy, provided the hernia is reducible, operation is best deferred until after parturition.
(c) After a severe illness such as pneumonia.
(d) Chronic bronchitis with an acute exacerbation.

3. THE PATIENT IS UNFIT FOR OPERATION

(a) Extensive pulmonary tuberculosis.
(b) Extreme age.

In all these conditions a truss may be advised, provided the hernia can be reduced and is not a femoral hernia. No truss so far designed will control a femoral hernia.

In babies an umbilical hernia is reduced by supporting with strapping. This is the only type of hernia support which may 'cure' the hernia, because obliteration of the umbilicus is a physiological process and adequate support may enable it to proceed to completion.

SPECIAL ADVICE TO A PATIENT WEARING A TRUSS

Careful washing and powdering of the skin are necessary. The pad must be maintained in good repair, and if a spring is used in the truss it must be renewed before it becomes too weak.

The patient must be instructed to apply his truss while he is lying down in bed after the hernia has been reduced.

THE CARE OF THE PATIENT FOR A HERNIA OPERATION

Careful shaving of the suprapubic area and cleansing of the skin are essential. Slight cuts from shaving are very likely to give rise to infection, which will ruin the operation.

Abdominal exercises are commenced on the day following the operation. Retention of the urine may occur and must be relieved. Abdominal distension must be prevented by passing a flatus tube.

If the patient is very fat and the hernia is large it is usually wise to prescribe measures to reduce his weight before the operation.

Some patients have two very large hernias, and it is frequently decided to operate on them one at a time as the sudden reduction of the contents of two large hernias into the abdomen may give rise to cardiorespiratory embarrassment.

Certain terms connected with hernia operations give rise to some difficulty:

1. HERNIOTOMY means opening of the sac.
2. HERNIORRHAPHY refers to the repair of the defect in the musculature.
3. HERNIOPLASTY is a herniorrhaphy in which extra material, e.g. fascia lata, is introduced.

# CHAPTER 41

# Diseases of the Kidney and Ureter

The urinary system is composed of the kidneys, the ureters, the bladder, and the urethra. The diagnosis and treatment of diseases or injury in the urinary system demand a knowledge of:

1. The exact anatomy of the organs in the patient. For example, a patient may have been born with only one kidney.

2. The efficiency of the renal function. This is determined by a consideration of the patient's history, symptoms, and clinical examination together with an investigation of his urinary tract by special methods. The retention of $K^+$ and non-protein nitrogenous products occurs with renal failure and these are estimated by examination of the blood.

## SYMPTOMS AND SIGNS OF URINARY DISEASE

### PAIN

1. **Renal pain.** This may be of two varieties:

(a) A fixed dull aching in the loin. Lesions which distend the kidney frequently give rise to pain of this type. If the outer surface of the kidney is inflamed, as is commonly the case in

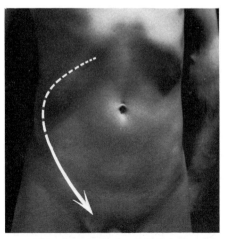

FIG. 41.1    Ureteric colic radiates from the loin towards the groin.

441

pyonephrosis, adherence of the organ to the muscles in the loin may give rise to very severe pain.

(b) Renal colic or, more strictly, ureteric colic. The pain commences in the loin and radiates to the testicle in the male or the vulva in the female. It is severe and violent. The expression of a small stone or clot frequently results in this type of pain. Atypically, the pain may shoot to the leg, to the opposite kidney, or to the chest.

2. **Bladder pain.** Bladder pain may be felt as a suprapubic discomfort, but more commonly is felt as a burning pain in the urethra at the end of micturition.

## HAEMATURIA

The passage of blood in the urine is known as haematuria. Haemorrhage arising in the bladder usually results in the passage of bright red blood, more marked at the end of micturition. Bleeding originating in the kidney is more intimately mixed with the urine, and the urine passed is usually described as 'smokey'. In addition to gross bleeding, the presence of small quantities of blood may be discovered only by microscopic examination of the urine.

*Causes*
RENAL
1. Injury to the kidney.
2. Haemorrhage into a cyst of a congenital cystic kidney.
3. Acute nephritis.
4. A stone.
5. Tuberculosis.
6. A neoplasm, e.g. innocent—angioma; malignant— hypernephroma, or nephroblastoma.

EXTRARENAL
1. Hypertension.
2. Anticoagulants in excess.
3. The sulphonamide drugs.
4. Certain blood diseases.

BLADDER
1. Foreign body.
2. Severe cystitis.
3. A stone.
4. Neoplasms.
5. An enlarged prostate.

URETHRA
1. Trauma.

2. A stone.
3. Urethritis.

Following operation on any portion of the urinary tract haematuria is common and aggravated if clot formation occurs.

### INCREASED FREQUENCY OF MICTURITION

Under nervous strain increased frequency of micturition is
not an uncommon symptom. Irritation of the mucous membrane of the trigone of the bladder by infection, a stone or a
growth are the usual urological causes. In tuberculosis of the
urinary tract the mucous membrane is not only damaged but
contraction of the bladder may result in unbearable frequency. Increased frequency is a prominent symptom of
overflow retention (p. 444).

### DIFFICULTY IN MICTURITION (Dysuria)

Difficulty with micturition is usually due to an enlarged prostate or to urethral stricture in the male. In the female it may
be due to a painful urethral caruncle, a retroverted gravid
uterus, or an impacted pelvic tumour.

### STRANGURY

Strangury is the desire to pass urine when only a few drops
are present in the bladder and is unrelieved by micturition.
This symptom is fairly commonly associated with renal colic.

### SCALDING

Scalding, or pain on micturition, is usually due to infection.

### RETENTION

Retention is the inability to pass urine.

### OLIGURIA

Oliguria means that the urinary output is diminished—usually less than 300 ml in 24 hours.

### INCONTINENCE

Incontinence is the patient's inability to control the emptying
of the bladder. It may be:
1. **True incontinence.** The sphincter is damaged, or the nervous control is eliminated so that co-ordinated micturition is
impossible. The patient is always wet and damage to the skin
occurs very rapidly. Pelvic floor exercises may help but the
skin must be kept dry by a dribble bag or an incontinence
clamp in the male, or, in either sex, by a fine Gibbon catheter
inserted into the bladder and connected to a bag. Any ob-

vious surgical defect is remedied. In some cases a muscle sling operation may be advised. The care of the paraplegic bladder is best undertaken in a special centre.

2. **False or paradoxical incontinence.** The patient suffering from prostatic obstruction may develop acute retention, with the result that a litre or more of urine may accumulate in the bladder. After a certain point 60 or 90 ml may overflow. The condition is really one of retention, and the incontinence is only a complication of this condition. Retention with overflow is a common description of this condition. This condition may also occur in women with an incarcerated gravid uterus.

3. **Stress incontinence.** Stress incontinence is a condition, usually seen in women, in which coughing, sneezing, laughing, or any condition which increases intra-abdominal pressure results in some escape of urine from the bladder. It occurs because the supports of the sphincter have been damaged, usually due to injuries sustained during childbirth, and some element of cystocele is present.

### ANURIA

This is a condition in which no urine is formed by the kidneys or if glomerular filtrate is formed it is totally reabsorbed so the patient passes no urine, and on catheterisation none is recovered from the bladder. It is frequently due to a stone or other lesion blocking the ureter of the only kidney which the patient possesses.

Other causes are:

*Acute tubular necrosis.*

*Acute circulatory failure.* The urinary output is diminished, but as the patient responds to treatment kidney function is resumed.

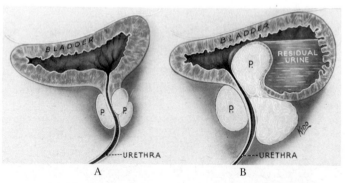

FIG. 41.2    A, Normal bladder after micturition. B, Bladder obstructed by an enlarged prostate after micturition.

*Nephrotoxic drugs* such as gentamicin.

*The sulphonamide drugs.* The crystallisation of the sulphonamide drugs in the renal tubules is liable to occur if the patient does not drink sufficient fluid when taking the drugs.

## RENAL INVESTIGATIONS

### 1. COLLECTION OF SPECIMENS

Collection of specimens of urine must be undertaken with great care.

Urine for routine examination is collected in a clean urinal or bedpan. Observations of colour, smell, deposits, specific gravity and pH are made. Tests for abnormalities (glucose, ketones, albumin, bile and blood) are carried out in the ward.

If bacteriological examination is required, a midstream specimen of urine is collected from a male patient. Prior to this the genital area is cleansed with soap and water. The patient is instructed to pass a little urine into the urinal, to interrupt the stream and pass a little urine into a sterile container, and then to complete micturition into the urinal. Female patients are asked to pass urine directly into the sterile container or a sterile receiver. The container is then sealed, labelled and sent to the laboratory.

If the patient has an indwelling catheter a fresh specimen is obtained by spigotting the catheter for 20–30 minutes and

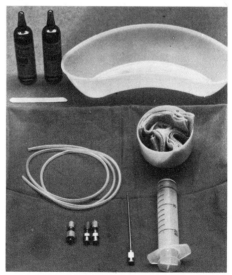

FIG. 41.3   Tray for intravenous or retrograde pyelogram.

| | |
|---|---|
| Sterile polythene tubing and connections | Swabs |
| Syringe, 20 ml | Ampoules |
| Filling needle | Urografin. |

then releasing the spigot and collecting the urine in the sterile container. The specimens may be collected in two portions for routine examination and specimens kept for inspection in two separate glasses.

## 2. RESIDUAL URINE

The presence of residual urine is a most valuable sign of prostatic enlargement. The correct method of estimating residual urine is as follows:

(a) The patient is requested to empty his bladder completely by his own efforts. The normal bladder is empty at the end of micturition, and if a catheter is passed no urine will be obtained.

(b) If, after the patient has emptied his bladder to the best of his ability, a catheter is passed and urine is obtained, this is known as 'residual urine'. The volume should be measured and charted.

If for any reason it is undesirable to pass a catheter this can be estimated by an intravenous pyelogram which on the 'postmicturition' film will show an outline of the residual urine.

## 3. EXAMINATION OF THE URINE

This will include a search for the presence of red blood corpuscles, pus, and organisms, as well as abnormal chemical constituents such as albumin and sugar.

*Clinitest.* In addition to the ordinary tests using reagents and heat, the Clinitest is now an approved method of testing. All the reagents are compressed into a single tablet and there is no need for external heat.

## 4. BLOOD UREA

The normal is 2·50–6·67 mmol per litre (15 to 40 mg per cent). A more accurate test, because it is uninfluenced by diet or the state of hydration, is the serum creatinine normal value 53–106 $\mu$mol per litre or 0·6–1·2 mg per 100 ml in conventional units.

## 5. X-RAY EXAMINATION

Straight, or direct, X-ray examination will in 90 per cent of cases reveal the presence of stones.

An intravenous pyelogram (a urogram) will reveal most abnormalities of the kidneys and, in addition, is a valuable test of renal function. A damaged kidney will not secrete the dye in sufficient strength to give a radiographic shadow.

In preparation for X-ray examination of the renal tract, the bowels should be emptied by the administration of vegetable aperient on each of the two previous nights. The passage of a

flatus tube will reduce gas shadows, which so frequently interfere with a good film of the kidneys. The bladder is emptied
and the patient is encouraged to walk around the ward before
X-ray.

On the morning of the examination no fluid or food
is given. Films are taken at five, ten, and 30 minutes or
longer after the injection of 20 ml of 50 per cent solution of a
medium containing an iodine compound. A small amount of
leakage outside the vein in the arm is very painful, and
if it should occur a hot fomentation is applied.

Many patients complain of pain from the abdominal
compression used in the examination to demonstrate the
ureters more adequately.

### 6. CYSTOGRAPHY

The bladder may be visualised when the dye injected for a
pyelogram reaches the bladder, or alternatively a more adequate picture of the bladder may be obtained by passing a
catheter and filling the bladder with dye. An X-ray taken
when the patient is micturating—micturating cystourethro-
gram—will reveal whether there is reflux of urine into the
ureters from the bladder.

### 7. CYSTOSCOPY

Examination of the interior of the bladder by means of a
cystoscope is a valuable method of investigation. In most

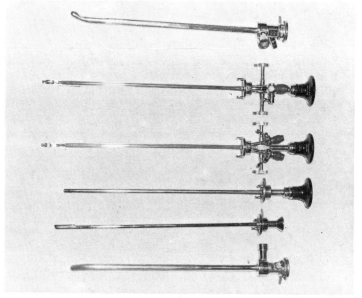

FIG. 41.4   Cystoscope, before assembly.

cases it will be performed at the end of investigation of the case, for it is a good working rule to defer, until it is absolutely necessary, any method of examination which may upset the patient. If the patient is actually bleeding, cystoscopy is frequently performed at once because should the haemorrhage cease, the opportunity to determine its source may be lost. However, a heavy loss may obscure an adequate view.

*Preparation of a patient for cystoscopy.*

(a) The suprapubic area need not be shaved in the male unless the examination is likely to be followed by open operation. It is advisable to shave female patients.

(b) The patient should be encouraged to drink freely so that the secretion of urine can be observed from each ureteric orifice. There is no objection to the patient consuming plenty of fluid up to three hours before the anaesthetic unless the anaesthetist gives further instructions.

(c) The patient should attend for the examination with the bladder fairly full, so that the surgeon is able to examine the gross appearance of the urine as it flows from the bladder. In the male, phimosis is sometimes present, and a dorsal slit may be necessary before the cystoscope is passed.

(d) Morphia (15 mg) and atropine (0·6 mg) are usually given by hypodermic injection but some other suitable premedication may be prescribed.

(e) Radiographs and notes must be available in the theatre.

(f) For every cystoscopic examination urethral dilators should be sterilised and at hand in case the condition should turn out to be complicated by a urethral stricture. Similarly, in case there is a pinhole meatus, meatotomy may be necessary, and the instruments for this operation should always be to hand. The indigo-carmine test is sometimes of value in estimating renal function: 5 ml of indigo-carmine (0·4 per cent) is injected intravenously and the time of its appearance in the bladder is noted and each ureteric flow is seen separately.

8. URETERIC CATHETERISATION AND RETROGRADE PYELOGRAPHY

A ureteric catheter may be passed up the ureter of either kidney to collect a specimen of urine from one kidney. To ensure that the label on the specimen is correct it should be written out at once and care must be taken of the specimen, since damage or loss necessitates a repetition of the whole procedure.

If a retrograde pyelogram is to be performed the catheter is left in position and the patient is taken to the X-ray department, unless a special cystoscopy room equipped with X-ray apparatus is available. The radio-opaque medium is passed up the ureteric catheter with a syringe and the kidney and ureter X-rayed.

Instructions may be given for the catheter to be left in position until it falls out spontaneously. This procedure is frequently of value in aiding the patient to pass a small stone from the kidney or ureter. Two millilitres of sterile liquid paraffin may be injected into the catheter two-hourly for twelve hours to aid the passage of a stone. After the catheter has been removed the patient is usually encouraged to get up and walk about. All specimens of urine which are voided must be retained for straining and examination in case a stone has been passed.

Patients on whom a ureteric catheter has been passed are encouraged to drink freely, and alkaline urinary antiseptics are prescribed routinely.

### 9. Aortography

The renal arteries are visualised by injecting the radio-opaque medium directly into the aorta. This helps to distinguish a cyst from a neoplasm and would help to identify an aberrant renal artery.

### 10. Renal biopsy

May be occasionally performed.

### 11. Radioisotope studies

Radioisotope studies of the kidney may be undertaken to determine further information about renal blood flow, function or the presence of a lesion obstructing a portion of the kidney.

## RENAL FAILURE

Failure of the kidneys to clear the blood of waste products may be due to inadequate blood flow, damage to the kidneys or obstruction to the outflow of urine from the renal pelvis, from the ureters or from the lower urinary tract. It may occur suddenly or it may be the result of long-standing and progressive destructive disease. Uncontrolled, the patient will die.

Renal failure, whatever the cause, is aggravated by:

1. Incorrect fluid balance which causes waterlogging of the tissues.
2. Infection which causes tissue breakdown.
3. Ingestion of protein.
4. Excessive breakdown of protein such as occurs in starvation.
5. Potassium imbalance.

## ACUTE RENAL FAILURE

*Causes*

1. Prerenal hypotension which will recover as circulatory failure is treated.

2. Renal tubular obstruction by:

   (a) Mismatched blood transfusion. The tubules are obstructed by agglutinated (clumped) red blood cells.

   (b) Myohaemoglobin produced in muscles which have been severely crushed (the crush syndrome).

   (c) Precipitation of drugs such as crystals of sulphonamides.

   (d) Bile pigments, particularly when associated with a fall in blood pressure such as following operations on patients with obstructive jaundice (the hepatorenal syndrome).

3. Tubular necrosis.

   (a) Following operation and concealed accidental haemorrhage.

   (b) Certain metallic poisons.

   (c) From acute pyelonephritis.

   (d) Bacteraemic shock.

4. Post-renal or obstructive, for example a stone or other lesion blocking the ureter of the only functioning kidney which the patient possesses.

*Clinical picture*

The patient may remain well for several days. The striking feature is oliguria (300 ml or less), leading to complete anuria. The blood urea and the serum potassium rise each day. After about six to ten days vomiting, breathlessness and increasing acidosis are evident. Before death, twitching and convulsions may occur.

*Management*

For low blood pressure the appropriate treatment to overcome these conditions is instituted. An obstructive lesion is relieved.

If the patient is anuric the most important nursing features are:

1. To stop all fluids until a satisfactory regime is instituted.

2. To stop all antibiotics and drugs because many of them are not now being excreted and cumulative effects are liable to arise.

3. All foods should be forbidden.

The patient may be kept alive for a very long time and the longer the time he is kept alive the greater is the chance that the kidneys may regenerate provided the correct treatment is undertaken. Basically this consists of the fluid intake being limited to the amount lost by sweating and respiration. This amounts to 1 litre a day, but the body produces 500 ml of water which accumulates. Therefore the total amount of fluid which can be given to the anuric patient is 500 ml. To prevent the breakdown of body protein a high carbohydrate diet is essential and must contain about 2000 calories and should be mineral-free. The fluid and carbohydrates are best combined in a solution in 500 ml of Hycal (a flavoured liquid dextrose concentrate) which provides 2100 calories. This can be administered by drinking or by a nasogastric tube into the stomach. If the patient is unable to tolerate either method 500 ml of 50 per cent dextrose is administered every 24 hours by a polythene catheter into the inferior vena cava.

VITAMINS. Because the patient's diet is lacking in vitamins these can be administered as a supplement.

When a diuresis occurs a volume of fluid equal to the amount of urine secreted plus 500 ml is given as potassium-rich fruit juice. The precise amount of fluid and its nature should be determined over 24 hours following blood and urine electrolyte estimations at least once daily.

In all cases of oliguria or anuria of sudden onset, mannitol (p. 140), 50 g in 500 ml of 5 per cent dextrose, is given in 30 minutes. If there is a response by diuresis, intravenous fluid and mannitol up to 100 g daily are given. A careful watch on the serum sodium is kept as mannitol tends to depress it. If there is no response to mannitol, structural damage has occurred and a modified Bull's regime is instituted. If this fails, peritoneal dialysis may be undertaken.

### CHRONIC RENAL FAILURE

*Causes*

1. Chronic nephritis.
2. Polycystic disease of the kidneys.
3. Kidneys destroyed by calculi.
4. Hypertensive kidney disease.
5. Bilateral hydronephrosis.

The onset of disease is gradual, the patient is anaemic, the skin dry and retinitis is usually present. Vomiting, nausea and terminal intermittent respiration occur. The treatment is a low protein diet and dialysis. A renal transplant may be undertaken.

*Dialysis*

## 1. PERITONEAL DIALYSIS

Dialysis means the transfer of solutes across a semipermeable membrane. Substances in solution pass from areas of high concentration to areas of low concentration by diffusion.

During peritoneal dialysis, fluid of a known concentration is introduced into the peritoneal cavity. Blood vessels and the fluid in the cavity are separated by peritoneum which acts as a semipermeable membrane. The concentration of certain solutes in the dialysing fluid is lower than that in the blood and, therefore, salts for excretion diffuse into the peritoneal cavity.

Dialysing fluids contain a mixture of the normal plasma electrolytes in a 1·36 per cent solution of dextrose. A hypertonic solution (6·36 per cent dextrose) may be used to withdraw fluid. Heparin and antibiotics may be added as prescribed by the doctor.

The danger of infection makes sterility during any part of the process essential. Prior to the procedure the bladder must be emptied as there is a possibility of perforation. The abdomen is shaved and cleaned with an antiseptic. A local anaesthetic is given. A catheter is then inserted into the peritoneal cavity and connected by tubing to two bags of dialysing fluid. The fluid is allowed to flow rapidly into the peritoneal cavity (1–2 litres in 10–15 minutes), it remains there for 20–30 minutes and is then allowed to drain.

It is essential that accurate fluid balance records are maintained as the amount of fluid introduced and that drained should correspond approximately. Patients should be weighed daily and observations of temperature, pulse and blood pressure maintained. Blood for urea and electrolyte estimations and dialysis fluid for culture and sensitivity are sent daily to the laboratory.

## 2. HAEMODIALYSIS

The artificial or mechanical kidney is basically a semipermeable membrane of Cellophane.

(a) On one side of the membrane is a bath of fluid. The composition of the fluid is such that the substances which it is desired to attract into the bath are absent or of lower concentration than in the blood.

(b) On the other side is the patient's blood.

The process is one of dialysis. The essential ions are kept in the blood by maintaining an identical concentration in the bath. The substances which it is particularly desirable to attract from the blood, in cases in which this is used, are urea and potassium ($K^+$).

The patient is connected to the machine by canalising an artery and vein. The blood passes along one side of the Cellophane and is returned to the previously filled reservoir of venous blood before being returned to the body by a vein.

The machine requires the undivided attention of a team—including a biochemist.

*Renal transplantation*

Renal transplantation has been discussed in Chapter 27.

*Anabolic hormones*

Breakdown of protein tissue (catabolism) increases the amount of nitrogenous and potassium products in the blood. Synthesis or building up of lean tissue is known as anabolism. Occasionally these hormones (Deca-Durabolin is one) are of value, particularly in:

1. Some cases of acute renal failure, by depressing the formation of nitrogenous and potassium end products.
2. To counter the protein breakdown (catabolic) phase following acute illness, trauma, or major surgical interference.

## DISEASES OF THE KIDNEYS AND URETERS
### CONGENITAL ABNORMALITIES

Congenital abnormalities of the urinary tract are legion. The commonest are:

Polycystic disease of the kidneys
Horse-shoe kidney
Absence of one kidney
Ectopic kidney.

1. **Polycystic kidney** (congenital cystic kidney). This condition is probably due to failure of complete fusion of the cortex of the kidney with the medulla. Clinically, the disease is usually seen about the age of 40. Both kidneys are enlarged and irregular. The patient's symptoms are those of incipient renal failure from which, at a later date, he will die unless a renal transplant is successful.

2. **Horseshoe kidney.** The kidneys are joined together across the midline, usually at their lower poles. The importance of the condition lies in the necessity for recognising it prior to operation. A horseshoe kidney is liable to all the diseases which may occur in an anatomically normal organ.

3. **Absence of one kidney.** This may occur as a result of failure to develop. Such knowledge is vital in cases of disease of the only kidney which is present.

4. **Ectopic kidney.** The kidney may be situated in the pelvis instead of in its usual position in the loin.

## INJURIES TO THE KIDNEYS

Injuries to the kidney may occur as a result of a fall or kick, usually taking the form of rupture of the organ. If the peritoneum in front of the organ is torn, peritonitis may occur. In some cases the condition is one of bruising.

*Clinical features*
Following a severe rupture of the kidney there is obvious haematuria, swelling, and pain in the loin combined with the general signs and symptoms of internal haemorrhage.

*Treatment*
In severe cases exploration of the kidney is carried out. When the condition is one of bruising, healing usually occurs if the patient rests in bed. All urine voided is kept and the time of evacuation marked on the label so that the amount of blood in each specimen can be compared.

## SURGICAL DISEASES OF THE KIDNEYS

The various surgical lesions of the kidneys are a source of great confusion to the nurse. Their names are complicated and sometimes bewildering. Very simply:

*Glomerulonephritis*, which is a medical condition and often not a true bacterial infection, is a disease which affects the more intimate parts of the nephron.

*Pyelonephritis* is an infection of the renal pelvis and of the solid or parenchymatous portion of the kidney, often with small abscesses which destroy its substance.

*Hydronephrosis* (pyelectasis) is a condition in which the renal pelvis is distended due to partial obstruction, usually at the expense of the parenchyma of the kidney which, in extreme cases, is no more than a thin sac and the number of functioning renal units may be very small indeed.

*Pyonephrosis* is a condition in which a hydronephrotic kidney has become infected, and the kidney may be no more than a bag of pus.

### HYDRONEPHROSIS

Hydronephrosis is a condition of dilatation of the renal pelvis. In an extreme case the kidney is simply a sac of clear fluid. The condition develops as a result of intermittent obstruction to the outflow of urine. Complete obstruction results in atrophy of the kidney.

The obstruction is sometimes caused by failure of nervous co-ordination in the ureter, but most cases are secondary to some other condition. If the primary cause is unilateral, one kidney is affected. If the cause is bilateral, both kidneys may be affected. The term pyelectasis is gradually replacing hydronephrosis in common usage and the affection of the ureter inaccurately described as dilatation is known as ureterectasis.

### Conditions causing unilateral hydronephrosis

1. A stone in the ureter.
2. The pressure of tumours on the ureter.
3. Kinking of the ureter from bands or aberrant blood vessels.
4. Nervous inco-ordination at the junction of the renal pelvis with the ureter.

### Conditions causing bilateral hydronephrosis

1. Senile enlargement of the prostate.
2. Urethral stricture and congenital urethral valves.
3. Phimosis.
4. Carcinoma of the cervix uteri.
5. Bilateral renal or ureteric calculi.
6. Retroperitoneal fibrosis.

*Treatment*

Treatment of most cases will be that of the primary cause. In severe unilateral cases a plastic operation or even nephrectomy may be necessary.

### Complications

1. Renal failure (particularly in bilateral cases).
2. Infection (pyonephrosis).

## INFECTION OF THE KIDNEY AND URINARY STONES

### PYELONEPHRITIS

Acute pyelonephritis is a pyogenic infection of the renal pelvis and the kidney surrounding it. Unless treated seriously and with great care chronic pyelonephritis will occur. The causal organisms are *Escherichia coli* or any of the common pyogenic organisms.

Pyelonephritis may occur in pregnancy and is due to progestin causing interference with the muscular contraction of the ureter rather than the effect of pressure of the uterus.

*Clinical features*

1. *Pain in the loin and in the lower abdomen*. The pain may re-

semble that of acute appendicitis. In addition there is usually frequency of micturition with scalding pain.

2. *Pyrexia* of the order of 39° C. (103 °F) is usually present. A rigor may be the presenting symptom.

3. *Vomiting* and the signs of a general febrile condition may be marked. On examination there is tenderness on the affected side of the abdomen. The urine contains pus and organisms.

*Treatment*

The causal organism is isolated and its sensitivity determined. While this is in progress the reaction of the urine to litmus must be determined. If it is acid an alkaline mixture is given, e.g. mist. potassium citrate. Antibacterial therapy is commenced and when the laboratory sensitivities are to hand any change of preparation which is indicated is made. Three litres of fluid must be taken daily. The dosage of antibacterial substances is based on an intake of 3 l of water.

When the acute stage has subsided full investigation of the

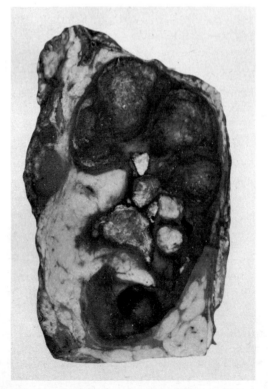

Fig. 41.5   Pyonephrosis. The substance of the kidney, which contains several stones, has been destroyed.

urinary tract must be carried out to determine any causal condition for the inflammation. The urine should be repeatedly examined for organisms when there has been apparent cure, otherwise chronic pyelonephritis will occur.

Chronic pyelonephritis is frequently a distressing condition which is often slow in responding to treatment. Many cases of chronic pyelonephritis in adults have had their origin in repeated urinary infection in infancy and childhood. Children who have had more than one attack of urinary infection should be investigated. Many will be found to have congenital anomalies of the renal tract. Some have neurological disturbances of the bladder leading to urinary retention and infection, while others will have anomalies of the junction of the ureter and bladder which allow reflux to occur up the ureters when the bladder contracts. This reflux can be minimised by instructing the patient in the art of double micturition—the child micturates, waits for a few minutes until the ureters drain into the bladder and then empties the bladder again. Reflux can be cured by a plastic operation in which the new valvular mechanism is constructed at the junction of the ureter and bladder.

*Treatment*

Treatment is on the usual lines of a urinary infection. The appropriate antibiotic or sulphonamide drug is prescribed. Repeated examination of the urine must be made until all organisms have been eliminated.

### PYONEPHROSIS

Pyonephrosis is a condition of inflammation of the kidney and renal pelvis in which the renal susbstance has been almost completely replaced by a bag of pus. The patient complains of severe pain in the loin, which is swollen and tender. Rigors may be present and the temperature is often elevated to 39° C (103° F).

*Treatment*

Drainage of the abscess by nephrostomy or removal of the kidney will be necessary. Nursing treatment is similar to that of acute pyelonephritis.

### KIDNEY STONES

Most stones are secondary to infection (recurrent pyelonephritis), but parathyroid overactivity may be shown to play an increasingly important part in their formation. Due to the concentration of the urine, the condition is said to be commoner in tropical climates. Patients who excrete abundant calcium in the urine, for example patients suffering from tuberculous arthritis of the spine with marked decalcification, are more likely to form a stone. Excessive intake of calcium and vitamin D also increases the likelihood of stone formation. Its formation can, to a large extent, be prevented by regular change in the position of the frame to which the patient is secured. The consumption of abundant fluid is a further preventive measure which may be undertaken in these cases.

**Types of stone**
Renal stones may be:

1. Solitary.
2. Multiple.

They may be composed of:

(a) Oxalates.
(b) Phosphates.
(c) Uric acid.
(d) Urates.
(e) Fibrin.
(f) Cystine.

*Symptoms and signs*
Small stones give rise to prominent symptoms. A large stone may form quietly, but cause greater damage to the kidney.

1. *Pain.* Typical ureteric colic is extremely painful. The pain in the loin is sharp and biting and radiates with greater severity to the testicle in the male or to the labia in the female. The patient writhes about in pain and may vomit.

2. *Strangury.* There is a great urge to pass urine every few minutes, but only a drop or two is voided.

3. *Haematuria.* The urine may be tinted with blood or there may be frank haemorrhage.

A small stone may be passed by the patient as a termination of the violent pain with considerable relief. When large fixed stones are present the pain is a more constant dull ache in the loin. Occasional bouts of pyrexia occur as a result of infection.

Investigations should be full and complete and may include a calcium balance, which may reveal the presence of hyperparathyroidism.

*Treatment*
1. TREATMENT OF THE ACUTE ATTACK. This consists of rest in bed and the relief of pain by the injection of pethidine.
2. IN THE QUIESCENT STAGE. Antispasmodics are prescribed

and the patient is advised to walk about. The passage of a ureteric catheter may aid the passage of the stone. If the stone fails to pass, its removal from the kidney (nephrolithotomy) or ureter (ureterolithotomy) will be undertaken, and if the damage to the kidney has been severe, removal of the organ may be necessary.

## PERINEPHRIC ABSCESS

A perinephric abscess is an infection beneath the fatty capsule surrounding the kidney. The infection may arise as a result of the rupture of a small abscess in the kidney, but more usually it is blood-borne from a boil, carbuncle, or septic finger.

*Symptoms and signs*
   The patient who has recently recovered from a staphylococcal infection runs a temperature for which no obvious cause can be found. There may be a dull ache in the loin. Later, the pain increases in severity and the loin becomes swollen and bulging.

*Treatment*
   Incision of the abscess and drainage is usually required. The drainage tube will be left in position for at least a week, and in most cases a little longer. Antibiotics are usually unnecessary.

## TUBERCULOSIS OF THE KIDNEY

The kidney may be infected with tubercle bacilli from the blood stream or from a tuberculous lesion in some other portion of the genito-urinary tract. Unchecked, the disease is disseminated into the ureters, the bladder, and the opposite kidney.

*Symptoms and signs*
   1. Frequency of micturition is the outstanding symptom.
   2. Pain may be present in the loin, or true ureteric colic and haematuria may occur, due to small portions of granulation tissue passing down the ureter.
   3. Painless haematuria.
   4. The symptoms and signs of tuberculosis may be present elsewhere.

*Investigation*
   Intravenous pyelogram may reveal distortion of the renal pelvis, and the typical cystoscopic appearance is a 'golf' hole appearance of the ureteric orifice.

URINE. The urine is acid in reaction, contains pus and is sterile on routine culture. Tubercle bacilli may be found on examination of the urine, early morning specimens being sent on three successive days or only after culture on special media.

*Treatment*

Streptomycin 1 g, INAH 400 mg and PAS 12 to 15 g daily for six months after the urine has been shown to be sterile is the usual chemotherapy. If resolution is not complete on chemotherapy, partial or total nephrectomy may be undertaken provided the disease is now limited to one kidney. Where there is gross contraction of the bladder, bladder drill is commenced. This consists of persuading the patient to avoid micturating as long as he possibly can, so that contraction of the bladder is delayed. In addition, the general measures for the care of tuberculosis must be instituted—good food and sanatorium conditions and screening of the family for tuberculosis.

### NEW GROWTHS OF THE KIDNEY

Simple tumours, although they do occur, are not very common. Malignant new growths are the nephroblastoma (Wilms tumour) which is seen in infants and the hypernephroma (carcinoma of the kidney) of the adult. Both tumours are extremely malignant, and blood-borne metastases to other organs are early and extensive.

Carcinoma of the renal pelvis may occur in association with carcinoma of the ureter or bladder.

*Symptoms and signs*

Painless haematuria is the commonest symptom. In addition, there may be pain in the region of the affected kidney. Intravenous pyelogram is essential in localising the disease. More refined techniques include angiography, isotope scans and ultrasonic detection.

*Treatment*

Removal of the kidney is the treatment of choice, but the end results are poor, since spread by the blood stream, particularly to the bones, occurs at an early stage in the disease. Radiotherapy may be given postoperatively and chemotherapy using actinomycin is also used.

## THE CARE OF PATIENTS FOR OPERATION ON THE KIDNEY

Operations on the kidney consist of:

1. Nephrolithotomy, that is, removal of a stone.

2. Pyeloplasty to correct hydronephrosis.
3. Nephrostomy. (Insertion of a tube into the kidney.)
4. Nephrectomy. (Partial or total removal of the kidney.)
5. Correction of stenosis of the renal artery.

*Preoperative care*

Locally, sepsis should be reduced as far as possible by the administration of antibacterial drugs according to the results of the sensitivity tests. The urinary function must be at the highest possible level, and the blood urea reading is a fairly satisfactory rough guide. In most cases a figure of under 40 mg per cent is desirable.

PREPARATION OF THE SKIN

The loin, back, abdomen, and chest are shaved in the usual way. A large cross may be made on the leg with a skin pencil by the doctor to indicate the side of the operation. Preoperative drugs are given as prescribed and the bladder is emptied. The bowel is emptied with suppositories the night previous to surgery.

Radiographs and notes must be brought to the theatre and arrangements are made for an X-ray to be taken on the theatre table during the operation if this proves to be necessary. In cases of stone the patient is X-rayed immediately before going to theatre as the stones are sometimes passed 'silently' or change their position in the urinary tract while awaiting operation. Most cases will be operated on lying on the opposite side with the lower leg flexed, the upper leg straight, and the trunk secured to the table by a strap and maintained by sandbags or rubber cushions.

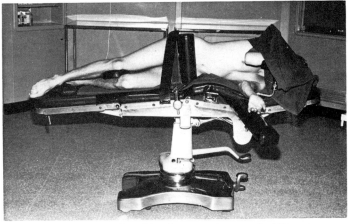

FIG. 41.6  Usual position for operations on the kidney.

*Postoperative care*

On return to bed the patient should be laid flat on the affected side. Later, he should be propped up to encourage drainage from the kidney down the ureter to the bladder. A careful watch must be kept for haemorrhage. A high fluid intake is encouraged.

The signs and symptoms of renal failure must be carefully watched for, and, in addition, the supervention of chest complications. Urinary antiseptics must be continued.

THE DIET should be rich in fluids and vitamins.

PAIN must be relieved by analgesics.

URINE. The amount of urine, the presence of blood, or the onset of retention must be carefully noted. A fluid balance chart is essential.

THE WOUND. Some degree of sepsis is almost inevitable if the wound has been drained. The sutures are removed when the wound has healed, usually the eighth to tenth day.

MANAGEMENT OF THE TUBE. The tube left in the perinephric space is usually removed on the third day, but if a tube has been inserted into the renal pelvis it is left until it loosens itself—about the tenth day. It should be connected to a Bardic bag outside the bed.

PERIOD IN BED. This varies from two to three days in most cases.

## Complications

1. *Haemorrhage.* After an exploration of the kidney or the removal of a stone the urine is blood-stained for 24 to 36 hours. Clots sometimes give rise to ureteric colic. There is also some discharge of blood in the loin. If this is excessive or if the pulse rate is rising, medical aid must be summoned at once. Greater care is necessary after partial nephrectomy because haemorrhage is a more likely complication, since there is a raw surface on the kidney, while in the case of total nephrectomy the vessels have been cleanly ligatured.

2. *Acute circulatory failure.* This is more common after a nephrectomy, particularly if the operation has been difficult because of extensive adhesions.

3. *Renal failure.* Careful observation for the onset of the symptoms of renal failure is important. It is particularly liable to develop if acute circulatory failure has been severe, since a low blood pressure prevents the kidneys excreting freely. The treatment of this condition has been described (p. 450).

4. *Peritonitis.* Peritonitis may occur if the peritoneum has been opened inadvertently at operation.

5. *Pulmonary collapse.* All operations on the kidney necessitate manipulation below the last rib or even excision of the rib with subsequent risk to the pleura and lung above.

## THE URETER

The only condition which requires special consideration is the presence of a stone in the ureter. If the stone fails to pass spontaneously, or after the passage of a ureteric catheter, the stone may have to be removed by operation. The preparation and aftertreatment are similar to that of an operation on the kidney. The only special points of importance are:

1. SKIN PREPARATION. The whole abdomen should be prepared on both sides, as well as the usual kidney area, since a ureteric stone may be removed through a lower midline incision.

2. X-RAY immediately before the operation is essential and the patient must not be allowed to stand up or walk about after it has been taken. A stone which was in one portion of the ureter may have changed its position since the previous X-ray.

3. THE TUBE. The wound usually seeps urine for several days, and special care is necessary to control infection in the urine and in the wound.

### URINARY DIVERSION

*Transplantation of the ureters*

This operation may be performed for carcinoma of the bladder, after severe crush injuries, or for a severely contracted tuberculous bladder. An occasional indication is an ectopic bladder, a condition in which the pubic bones fail to fuse and

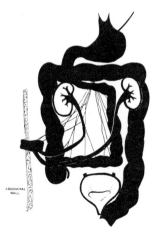

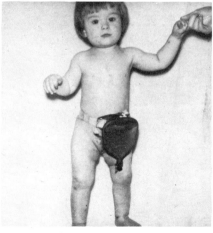

FIG. 41.7   Transplantation of ureters into an isolated segment of ileum.

FIG. 41.8   Child wearing urinal.

the bladder mucous membrane lies on the abdominal wall, dribbling urine continuously from the exposed ureteric orifices. The ureters may be transplanted into:

1. The pelvic colon and the patient passes urine by the rectum. This operation carries the risk of ascending urinary infection and also of excessive reabsorption of chloride ions from the rectal mucosa.
2. An isolated loop of ileum. This avoids both complications of colonic transplants.

Before operation the rectal sphincter should be examined for continence.

A common indication in children for transplantation of the ureters into an ileal loop is a paralysed bladder with a myelomeningocele. The operation may be necessary to gain continence or to prevent renal deterioration in the chronically infected neurogenic bladder. Transplantation into an ileal loop rather than the colon has the advantage of less electrolyte disturbance, less infection and of course is essential if the anal sphincters are paralysed. The main disadvantage is the need of a urinal bag (Fig. 41.8).

PREPARATION AND AFTERCARE

The mental preparation of the patient who is to undergo ureteric transplant either to the pelvic colon or into an isolated loop of ileum is extremely important. The change in habit following surgery must be fully explained to the patient.

Electrolyte balance and kidney function are corrected as far as possible. Antibiotics and chemotherapy are given routinely for both urinary and bowel preparations. The bowel is further prepared by enemas and colonic washouts.

POSTOPERATIVE CARE. The care is that of any patient returning to the ward following major surgery.

Points applicable to ureteric transplant to the pelvic colon:

1. Rectal tube *in situ*. Continuous drainage into a Bardic or Aldon bag should be set up. This tube is inserted while the patient is in theatre and should be watched very carefully postoperatively to ensure that drainage is constant. Should drainage be negligible this should be immediately reported to the medical staff.
2. A nasogastric tube is aspirated hourly as required.
3. Intravenous fluids should be given and correct fluid balance is very important.
4. Sedation.
5. There may be a urethral catheter *in situ* but this is only acting as a drain. There may also be a wound drain.

6. Aperients and enemas postoperatively are withheld as for any other type of intestinal surgery.

7. Dietary modifications may be necessary depending on electrolyte and blood urea levels both in the postoperative and convalescent stages. Table salt is avoided and sodium bicarbonate 1 g and potassium bicarbonate 1 g daily are given to counteract acidosis and hyperchloraemia.

For ileal loop transplant the immediate aftercare is similar.

The main difference is that the patient now passes urine straight on to the skin surface and has no sphincter control. It is necessary that the patient be given a urinating appliance. Immediate provision for this is made by the use of disposable ileostomy bags for collecting the urine. Once the patient is ambulant a proper appliance is fitted and the patient taught the method and care of application.

Patients who have had an ileal loop transplant have less rigid dietary restrictions.


## RETROPERITONEAL FIBROSIS

Retroperitoneal fibrosis is a rare condition, sometimes caused by drugs like methysergide. It may cause obstruction to the ureters or the inferior vena cava. Steroids may be used in treatment.

# CHAPTER 42

# Diseases of the Bladder, the Prostate, and the Male Genital Organs

The normal bladder has a capacity of about 360 ml.

## ACUTE RETENTION OF URINE

The patient is unable to pass urine and he complains of severe pain. The cause may be:

1. *Reflex.* Postoperative retention is very common. Following operations on the rectum and anus great difficulty with micturition, if not actual retention, is usual.

2. *Organic nervous diseases.* Lesions of the central nervous system may affect the bladder centre in the spinal cord.

   (a) Fractures of the spine with damage to the spinal cord.

   (b) Tabes dorsalis, disseminated sclerosis, and other diseases of the central nervous system.

   (c) Children with myelomeningocele.

3. *Mechanical causes.*

   (a) Rupture of the urethra.

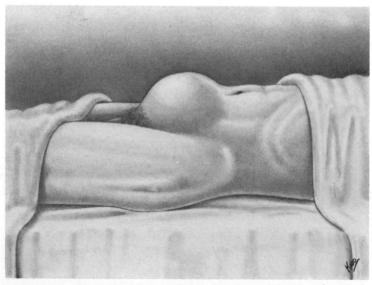

FIG. 42.1   Distended bladder in acute retention of urine.

(b)  Enlargement of the prostate.
(c)  Urethral stricture and urethritis.
(d)  A stone, a foreign body, or a growth obstructing the neck of the bladder or urethra.
(e)  A retroverted gravid uterus.
(f)  Phimosis.

*Clinical presentation*
1. *Sudden acute retention* may occur in men with no previous history of urological disorder. The causes include drunkenness and hysteria.
2. *Retention* as a culmination of previous dysuria increasing frequency and voiding a decreasing volume of urine. The attack is precipitated by cold or being unable to empty the bladder at a convenient moment.
In both types the patient is in severe pain and a firm, distended bladder is easily palpable.
3. *Acute-on-chronic retention.* This is the most dangerous form. The patient has had long-standing urinary symptoms and his general health has deteriorated because of renal failure. There is usually no complaint of pain and a complete unawareness of the severity of his condition. The large atonic bladder is painless.

*Treatment and nursing care*
The patient must never be catheterised and sent home forthwith. He should always be admitted to hospital, and the following measures are instituted:
1. ANALGESICS AND REST. The patient is in pain and anxious. Morphia (15 mg) is prescribed.

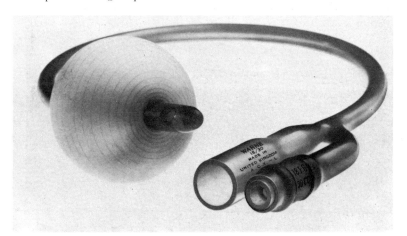

FIG. 42.2   Foley's catheter showing balloon inflated.

2. ATTEMPTED MICTURITION. This is attempted when the pain has been relieved. A dose of mist. potassium. citrate. (15 ml), a hot pack to the abdomen, or a hot bath into which the patient can pass urine, should all be tried. If these fail the retention must be relieved.

3. MECHANICAL RELIEF. Mechanical relief is given by:

(a) Urethral catheterisation is the usual method which is employed. It is a common and important surgical procedure and will be considered in detail.

(b) Suprapubic catheterisation, by open method or by puncture with a trocar and cannula, will be performed only when it is impossible to pass a catheter by the urethra.

(c) Suprapubic needle puncture of the bladder. This is generally undesirable, but it may be the only method if catheterisation has failed and surgical aid is not available.

4. THE MAINTENANCE OF THE EXCRETION OF URINE BY THE KIDNEYS is provided for by the administration of liberal quantities of fluids.

5. INVESTIGATION OF THE CAUSE includes examination of the urine, the blood, and an intravenous pyelogram is undertaken as soon as possible.

### CATHETERISATION

Catheterisation can be mechanically simple, but on occasions it is extremely difficult or impossible. The management of the catheterised patient and the prevention of infection are always difficult and require great care and patience. The problems which arise from catheterisation may be summarised according to the anatomical site which is affected in the urinary tract.

1. **The urethra.**

(a) Trauma. The catheter may tear the delicate lining of the urethra and this is more likely to occur the more frequently the catheter has to be passed. A water-soluble lubricant is used. The more rigid the catheter the greater the trauma.

(b) The wider the catheter the greater is the pressure against the cells of the lining wall.

A large catheter is more traumatic, but a small catheter once passed is more readily blocked by blood clot or debris.

Urethritis is more likely to develop from catheterisation and infect the bladder causing cystitis, and the kidney causing pyelonephritis.

## 2. The penis.

(a) Meatal stricture is liable to develop from the combined effects of a large catheter made of irritating material and from infection.

(b) Balanitis and meatal ulceration. If the prepuce cannot be retracted a dorsal slit will have to be performed to avoid balanitis. Strapping the catheter to the glans penis may cause irritation. It is preferable to use a self-retaining catheter.

## 3. The bladder. The bladder may be infected by:

(a) Careless catheterisation including neglect of asepsis.

(b) Infection creeping up the lumen of the catheter and, in this connection, air bubbles are particularly important as a source of infection. Closed drainage using an Aldon bag prevents airborne infection.

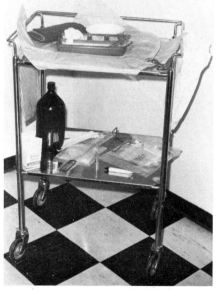

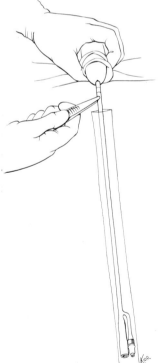

FIG. 42.3　Catheterisation trolley.
Upper shelf: Basic pack
Lower shelf: Catheters
　　　　　　Aldon bag and holder
　　　　　　Local anaesthetic and lubricant
　　　　　　Savlon
　　　　　　Specimen bottles
　　　　　　Sterile face masks
　　　Disposable bag on side of trolley.

FIG. 42.4　Method of passing catheter.

**4. The kidneys.** The kidneys are particularly easily infected in cases of long-standing chronic retention of urine in which hydronephrosis has developed and the ureteric orifice mechanism in the bladder is no longer adequate to prevent regurgitation back into the ureters.

The choice of catheter will be determined by consideration of all the factors which have been mentioned above together with consideration of the cause of retention.

The 'Portex' Gibbon catheter constituted a major advance because:

1. It is easy and safe to pass.
2. It eliminates urethritis by its small size and non-irritant nature.
3. It requires the minimum of attention since changing and washouts are usually unnecessary; its main disadvantage is that it does not accommodate a bladder washout if one is required.

The catheter is supplied pre-sterilised by gamma rays.

In a case of suspected rupture of the urethra or bladder a catheter must never be passed in the ward.

Catheterisation can be an extremely dangerous operation.

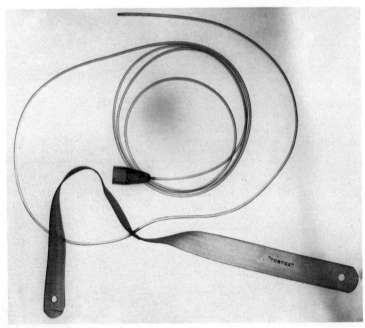

FIG. 42.5    Gibbon catheter.

Force must not be used and unless full asepsis is maintained the patient may lose his life.

Many of these patients are agitated, in pain and dirty, so that the initial treatment consists of morphine or pethidine intramuscularly and giving the patient a hot bath. He may pass urine into the bath, obviating the need for a catheter. The majority do not, so catheterisation has to be undertaken.

A good light, an assistant and all the equipment necessary, including at least a second catheter (in case one is dropped) should be available.

1. The genitalia are washed.
2. After masking, a full scrub-up is undertaken and sterile gloves are put on.
3. The genitalia are cleansed with 0·25 per cent chlorhexidine.
4. The patient is draped with sterile towels.
5. A whole tube of gel containing lignocaine 1 per cent and chlorhexidine 0·25 per cent is injected into the urethra, the tube being previously immersed in an alcoholic solution of chlorhexidine solution for 10 minutes.
6. A penile clamp is attached to keep the gel in the urethra. About 3 minutes is necessary to produce adequate analgesia.
7. A catheter is passed using a no-touch technique (Fig. 42.4).
8. The catheter is connected at once to an Aldon bag (Fig. 42.7).

If the catheter is to be left indwelling it should be connected at once to an Aldon bag which must be kept lower than the bladder at all times. A specimen of urine is taken as soon as the bladder is entered. Further specimens are taken by inserting a needle low down in the connecting tube before it enters the bag so that the seal is not broken. At a similar point the connecting tube is clamped off when the bottle is changed. This prevents the ascent of air bubbles carrying possible infection into the bladder.

On the very rare occasion when it is impossible to withdraw fluid from the balloon of a Foley's catheter, chloroform should be injected through the side tube.

*Suprapubic cystotomy*

This procedure consists of opening the bladder by an incision in the lower abdomen. It may be performed for acute retention of urine if it is impossible to pass a urethral catheter or if there is gross infection of the urine.

A self-retaining catheter (Fig. 42.2) may be inserted through a bladder perforator in certain cases of retention.

# DISEASES OF THE BLADDER

## RUPTURE OF THE BLADDER

A blow on the lower abdomen, especially if the bladder is full, is the commonest cause of rupture. Through the tear, urine seeps into the peritoneum (intraperitoneal rupture). As a complication of a fracture of the pelvis the bladder may also be ruptured, but the tear is extraperitoneal and in this variety there is no danger of peritonitis.

Both injuries are severe. Untreated, the patient with an intraperitoneal rupture develops peritonitis, while the patient with an extraperitoneal rupture develops extensive fulminating cellulitis as a result of extravasation of urine over the tissues of the abdominal wall and the perineum.

*Clinical features*

1. The patient is usually in a state of acute circulatory failure.
2. The lower abdomen is tender and rigid.
3. No urine has been, or can be, passed. The patient should be discouraged from attempting to pass urine because it flows through the rupture.
4. Catheterisation (which should be performed in an operating theatre) recovers only a small quantity of bloodstained urine.

*Treatment*

Acute circulatory failure is treated and a laparotomy performed. The bladder is sutured and the peritoneum may be drained if the rupture has been intraperitoneal.

A urethral catheter or occasionally a suprapubic catheter is inserted to keep the bladder empty during healing as well as a tube in the retropubic space.

## CYSTITIS

Cystitis is a condition in which the bladder mucosa is inflamed. Many patients, particularly women, attribute any symptom, such as dysuria or scalding pain on micturition, to 'cystitis'. In many instances pyelography and examination of mid-stream specimens of urine reveal no abnormality. Only an initial specimen of urine or a urethral swab will contain pus and organisms.

Acute cystitis may be part of a general urinary infection.

Chronic cystitis is usually associated with obstruction to the outflow of urine. The presence of a foreign body, such as a stone passed from the kidney, or an abnormality of the bladder, e.g. a diverticulum or cystocele predisposes to infection.

Infection may pass down the ureter from a diseased kidney and give rise to a similar type of infection in the bladder. The organisms may be pyogenic or tuberculous. Ascending infection from the urethra is a common cause of cystitis, as are:

1. Catheterisation.
2. Gonorrhoea.

Urethral stricture and enlargement of the prostate as well as spinal injuries, all of which interfere with the effective drainage of the bladder, predispose to infection.

*Symptoms and signs*
The principal symptoms are:

1. Suprapubic pain.
2. Scalding pain on passing urine.
3. Frequency of micturition.
4. Haematuria may be present if the inflammation is severe.

In some cases an underlying neoplasm gives rise to the superficial symptoms of cystitis. Examination of the urine reveals the presence of pus, organisms, and possibly red blood corpuscles.

*Treatment*
The most important single factor in treatment is to encourage the patient to empty the bladder completely. In acute cases the patient has to be in bed, and consume 3 litres of fluid daily. The reaction of the urine is changed by giving mist. potassium. citrate. Antibiotics are prescribed only after bacteriological examination and sensitivity tests. Personal hygiene and care of the general health are important in overcoming the condition. When the symptoms subside a full investigation, particularly to discover any cause of defective bladder emptying which can be remedied, is undertaken.

Bladder washouts (lavage) are not usually performed unless specially ordered. Fluid must not be forced into the bladder under pressure, and bladder washouts should be of the correct temperature: 37° C (100° F). Normally 180 to 210 ml of fluid are instilled, but if the patient complains of pain before this volume has been used no attempt should be made to force a further quantity into the bladder. The common solutions used are:

Silver nitrate 1/15,000 to 1/5000.
Acetic acid 0·5 per cent.
Hibitane 1/5000, in pure aqueous solution—not the form in which it is sent for ward stock.
Noxyflex 1 per cent for continuous irrigation.
        2·5 per cent for instillation.

BLADDER LAVAGE: IRRIGATION
Bladder washout (irrigation) may be ordered for:

Chronic cystitis
Haematuria with clot formation as the presenting sign of disease
Haematuria following operation on the bladder or prostate.

The fluid usually used is saline 0·9 per cent, sterile, and at room temperature.

1. CONTINUOUS LAVAGE—OR CLOSED SYSTEM. The irrigating fluid is suspended from a drip stand, passes down a giving set, and enters the bladder through one arm of a three-way catheter. Together with the urine it drains out of the bladder via the other arm of the catheter into an Aldon drainage bag. The rate of the flow of the irrigating fluid is prescribed by the doctor, e.g. immediately after operation it may be free-flowing, or 1½-litre in one hour.

Before putting up a fresh container of irrigating fluid the drainage bag is allowed to empty into a jug, then respigotted or reconnected and the contents are measured. The nurse washes and dries her hands. The litre of fluid is checked and put up, and the flow regulated as prescribed. The amount of irrigating fluid and of drainage is recorded/charted. Whilst the irrigation is in progress, the nurse observes:

–that the fluid is flowing into the bladder at the prescribed rate
–that it is draining out of the bladder into the drainage bag
–whether any bleeding is increasing or decreasing
–the presence of any clots
–any distension of or discomfort in the bladder or abdomen
–the amount flowing in as compared with the amount draining out
–the condition of the suprapubic wound and its dressing.

The irrigation continues until the urine is clear—usually, for not less than 48 hours and for three to four days. The drainage system is changed as necessary. When the continuous irrigation is to cease, the patient is informed and made ready by being given privacy and by having personal and bedclothing rearranged.

The flow of the irrigating fluid is stopped, the giving set disconnected and the catheter arm spigotted—sterility being maintained—leaving continuous drainage of urine via the catheter and drainage tubing and bag. A note is made on the fluid chart to this effect, i.e. irrigation ceased. The patient is repositioned, encouraged to drink fluids in abundance, and all intake and output carefully measured and recorded. Used equipment is disposed of in the soiled dressing bag.

If requested, 24 hours after discontinuation, a catheter specimen of urine is collected and sent to the laboratory.

2. HAND IRRIGATION. A basic dressing trolley is prepared, with the addition of a 50 ml catheter-tip syringe, irrigating fluid, bowl, receiver, spigot.

The patient is informed of what is going to happen and his co-operation obtained. The trolley is taken to the bedside, privacy is ensured, and the patient is placed in a comfortable position with his legs apart.

Using the aseptic technique, the dressing packet is opened and prepared. Outer packs are opened, the contents are placed on the sterifield. Some irrigating fluid is poured into the bowl. A towel is placed under the catheter, the receiver is placed between the legs. The spigot is removed and discarded, or the drainage bag is disconnected and its end covered with a sterile swab.

Using gentle pressure on a syringe 30 ml of fluid is instilled and then sucked back, noting the amount, colour, presence of clots, etc. It is repeated as necessary until no clots return.

A clean spigot is put in, or the drainage bag is reconnected. The receiver is removed.

N.B. If after instillation of the first 30 ml no fluid is drawn back, the medical officer is notified at once, no attempt being made to introduce more fluid at this stage.

The meatus and nearby catheter are swabbed. The patient is dried and made comfortable. The trolley and its contents are removed. A report/record is made of the result.

### STONES IN THE BLADDER

Bladder stones develop as a result of infection.

The stone may form in the bladder or may enlarge in the bladder after being passed from the kidney. The main symptoms are pain, frequency of micturition by day, haematuria and strangury.

X-ray reveals the presence of the stone, which is removed by the introduction of a crushing instrument *per urethram*, or, if too large and very hard, by the suprapubic route. Very occasionally a stone is not opaque and can be diagnosed only on cystoscopic examination.

## NEW GROWTHS OF THE BLADDER

A new growth in the bladder may be malignant from the beginning. If it is simple (papilloma) there is a strong tendency to recur in spite of treatment, and eventually to become malignant. Because of this the condition is now usually called papillomatous disease of the urinary tract. The disease is multicentric in origin so that even a small lesion confined to the mucous membrane is to be regarded as the first manifestation of the disease. Because lesions may erupt and may invade the bladder wall a patient suffering from the disease must be cystoscoped at regular intervals for the remainder of his life.

Workers in certain industries of which rubber manufacture is an example should be screened for disease by cytological examination of the urine at regular intervals.

*Symptoms and signs*

1. Painless haematuria is the most constant symptom. At the end of micturition almost pure blood may be passed.

2. Frequency and scalding on micturition develop if secondary infection occurs.

3. Pain may be intolerable in the late stages of carcinoma, and frequently takes the form of severe sciatica from infiltration of the sacral plexus.

4. Bimanual examination of the bladder, with the finger in the rectum and the hand on the abdominal wall, may reveal a swelling.

*Treatment*

In addition to a full urinary investigation, cystoscopy is performed to confirm the diagnosis and a biopsy may be taken. Cystodiathermy, i.e. burning the growth by means of the diathermy electrode, or endoscopic resection if possible is performed. More extensive lesions are treated by:

1. Megavoltage radiotherapy.
2. Partial cystectomy.
3. Total cystectomy with urinary diversion (p. 463).

## DIVERTICULUM OF THE BLADDER

A diverticulum may occur in the bladder secondary to obstruction in the urethra or as a result of inherent weakness of the musculature of the bladder. The condition is frequently complicated by sepsis, stone formation, and the occurrence of a new growth.

The treatment is that of the causal condition combined, if necessary, with excision of the diverticulum.

## DISEASES OF THE PROSTATE

The prostate is a gland about the size of a walnut, situated in the proximal portion of the male urethra.

The commonest lesion is prostatic obstruction. This results in increasing urinary disturbance and damage to the kidneys. The bladder is never completely emptied, so that back pressure causes hydronephrosis. The patients are usually advanced in years, 60 or over being the usual age. Disturbance of the patient's general health may be very great.

*Causes*

1. *Simple (benign) enlargement.* This is the commonest type.
2. *Prostatic fibrosis* in which the internal meatus is almost closed by narrowing.
3. *Carcinoma of the prostate.*

*Symptoms and signs*

1. *Increased frequency and difficulty of micturition* are prominent complaints. The patient's sleep is disturbed. The general health and well-being deteriorate from lack of sleep.
2. *Haematuria* may occur in some cases as a result of congestion.

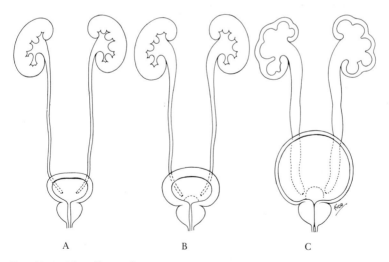

FIG. 42.6   The effects of prostatism. A, Normal. B, Moderate enlargement, hydronephrosis and hypertrophy of the bladder. C, Gross enlargement, extensive hydronephrosis, hydroureter and atonic distended bladder.

3. *Pain and scalding on micturition* develop from infection of the residual urine.

4. *Acute retention of urine* may develop. About 1 in 10 patients present with acute retention. In a neglected case renal failure will set in, and the patient may be admitted to hospital in coma or in a semicomatosed state.

5. The gland may be felt to be enlarged on rectal examination.

*Treatment*

If at all possible prostatectomy in some form, or even in stages, is carried out. If the patient's condition is too poor then an indwelling catheter may be all that is possible and a Foley catheter, preferably made of inert silastic material, would seem to be the one of choice. Occasionally a permanent suprapubic catheter has to be left in place. The precise method of treatment will depend on:

1. *The nature of the obstruction* (p. 477).
2. *The effect it produces.* Most important are those on:
   (a) The kidneys.
   (b) The bladder.

Stone formation, infection or diverticulum formation may be extensive.

3. *General health of the patient.* Many patients have associated disease like coronary insufficiency or chronic bronchitis.

Choice of operations

TRANSURETHRAL RESECTION OF PROSTATE. Gland resected *per uretheram* by resectoscope. No abdominal wound.

RETROPUBIC (MILLIN). The prostate is removed by operation in the space between the back of the pubis and the bladder (which is not opened).

SUPRAPUBIC-TRANSVESICAL (Freyer, Harris, Wilson-Hay). The bladder is opened and the prostate enucleated. Freyer's original type—Wilson-Hay—improved haemostasis.

PERINEAL approach rarely used.

Preparation for operation

The preparation and aftercare of all types of operations for the relief of prostatic obstruction are basically similar. It is the details which confuse the nurse. Consideration of the two basic troubles serves to show the lines along which treatment should be directed. They are:

1. *The maintenance of adequate renal function.* The best general test of renal function is the level of the blood urea—normal

2·50–6·67 $\mu$mol per litre (15 to 40 mg per cent). Whatever the level it will be raised by:

(a) Blood loss which is sufficient to lower the blood pressure because the kidneys fail to excrete in conditions of hypotension.
(b) Infection which prevents the kidneys from functioning satisfactorily.

It will be lowered by:

(a) Control of infection.
(b) Free drainage of the bladder which also means that the kidneys can work without back pressure.
(c) A large intake of fluids resulting in a correspondingly large output of urine.

2. *Postoperative bleeding.* It is impossible by any method of prostatectomy to stop all the bleeding in the theatre and, for this reason, the nurse has a very special responsiblity in the postoperative care of these patients. There are two dangers:

(a) Haemorrhage may increase on return to the ward and
(b) The blood lost may form clots in the bladder, causing bladder distension. This in turn prevents retraction of the blood vessels and increases further the amount of bleeding. The clots may block the drainage tube or catheters and the patient is in severe pain. To aggravate matters already bad the consequent hypotension causes diminution or cessation of renal excretion and increases the likelihood of renal failure.

For all these reasons the following lessons emerge:

1. Renal function should be as good as possible as measured by the blood urea or blood creatinine. Preferably it should be normal and the higher it is above normal the greater the risk of operation.
2. The patient should be in the best possible general condition and have a haemoglobin reading of 12 g per dl.
3. Postoperatively all measures should be taken to prevent clot formation.

GENERAL CARE

1. *Renal function* is improved if necessary by catheter drainage and by urinary antiseptics, and bladder washouts are given if the urine is grossly infected.
2. *Large fluid intake encouraged.* Tea, coffee, lemonade, cocoa, or other drinks to which glucose has been added may be given. A jug of fluid should be available on the top of the patient's bedside locker and the nurse must encourage the

patient to drink with unrelenting persistence. Sufficient fluid must be taken to keep the patient's tongue moist and a careful fluid balance chart must be kept.

3. *A specimen of urine* is sent to the laboratory for examination and the blood urea and blood creatinine are estimated.

4. *The scrotum* is supported on a broad piece of Elastoplast strapped across the thighs. This simple procedure diminishes the risk of epididymo-orchitis, which is a not uncommon complication in these cases.

5. *Breathing exercises* are important, since they improve the patient's general condition and diminish the risk of postoperative pulmonary complications.

6. *The pressure areas* require meticulous care. Faulty junctions of the drainage apparatus result in a wet bed, and every effort must be made to keep the patient dry.

7. *The blood pressure* is estimated.

The patient is fit for operation when the blood urea is about 6·67 $\mu$mol per litre (40 mg per cent) or below, and the urine is almost free of pus.

The general condition of the patient must, of course, be considered in assessing fitness for an operation.

POSTOPERATIVE CARE

The aftercare of a case of prostatectomy is of the greatest importance. The outstanding complications are:

1. Haemorrhage.
2. Infection.
3. Renal failure.

Other complications which are liable to occur are:

1. Pulmonary complications.
2. Epididymo-orchitis.
3. Obstruction of the bladder neck.

Careful and thorough preliminary treatment considerably reduces the risk of postoperative complications. However, prostatectomy is a severe undertaking, the majority of patients being men of advanced years.

ON RETURN FROM THE THEATRE the patient is positioned recumbent in bed. The foot of the bed should be elevated and a slow transfusion of blood is continued if necessary. Fluids of a diuretic nature such as mannitol may be given intravenously.

There must be a careful check on the respiratory movement and oxygen administered if necessary. If the patient is collapsed the blood transfusion is usually speeded up by the house surgeon until the blood pressure is satisfactory. Bacteraemia as a cause of hypotension should be excluded.

The patient is usually nursed on a siliconised mattress. He

is moved frequently in bed to prevent the onset of chest complications, and is propped up in bed and allowed to sit out of bed on the second or third day.

CARE OF THE DRAINAGE TUBES

Two tubes are usually in position at the end of the operation:

1. A small corrugated drain in the retropubic space which is removed in 48 hours.
    2. Either:

    (a) A urethral catheter—closed prostatectomy.
    or
    (b) A large tube in the bladder through which urine and
        blood will drain—open prostatectomy.

In either type of operation it is important to ensure that there is free drainage.

CLOSED. In the closed method of prostatectomy a three-way Foley catheter with continuous irrigation is left in the bladder and connected to a closed system of drainage. Special care

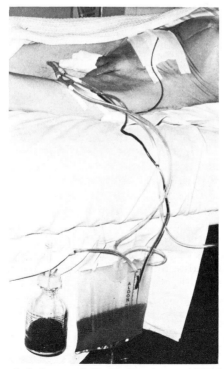

FIG. 42.7   Closed drainage of the bladder by a urethral catheter to an Aldon bag.

must be taken to make sure that blood-stained urine is flowing freely and not allowed to stop initially between the theatre
and the ward. Some surgeons maintain a continuous irrigation
of the bladder by using a three-way Foley's catheter or a polythene tube with a small irrigating side tube. Instead of sodium
citrate normal saline may be used.

*Removal of the catheter.* The catheter is removed at a varying
period between three and 10 days. After removal of the catheter the patient should pass urine every hour so that the bladder does not become distended and stretch the healing
wound. On the first night after removal he should be woken
every 2 hours to pass urine.

OPEN. The suprapubic tube is usually a Marion's tube and a
continuous irrigation of sterile water is run into the side tube.
Urine and blood may be sucked from the centre tube or a
closed drainage system may be instituted. If the tube becomes
blocked with clots these can be easily removed with sponge
forceps. Epsilon-aminocaproic acid 0·5 g may be given for 12
hours intravenously (it is a potent antagonist of urokinase
which is a fibrinolytic enzyme which increases bleeding following prostatectomy). After 24 hours the urine should be a light
pink and in two or three days it should be normal in appearance. An alternative method is to fix a small suction plate to
the wound. Each day the bladder has to be washed out and
on about the fourteenth day the patient passes urine and the
wound heals.

In all forms of prostatectomy:

*The scrotum* must be carefully supported if the risk of epididymo-orchitis is to be diminished. Sometimes the vas deferens
is tied through two small incisions in the groin or within the
pelvis as a preliminary measure to avoid this complication.

*The fluid intake* must be abundant and the consumption of
fluids must be encouraged by the nurse. The blood urea always rises after the operation, since prostatectomy 'upsets'
the kidney functions temporarily, and if fluid is not supplied
these patients become uraemic, have no pain, are sleepy, and
lie quite still as they die gradually from renal failure. Urinary
antiseptics, including antibiotics, are of the greatest value in
controlling infection and thereby diminishing the risk of renal
failure.

*The sutures.* The superficial sutures are removed about the
eight to tenth day.

Most patients are fit for discharge about two weeks after the
operation, provided no complication has arisen.

## Complications

1. *Clot retention.* If clot retention occurs the bladder should
be irrigated gently with 3.8 per cent sodium citrate by means

of a large glass syringe. *Epsilon* aminocaproic acid (p. 482) may be used to diminish bleeding. If the patient develops a clot retention which it is impossible to clear by mechanical means the bladder may have to be reopened.

2. *The patient pulls out the catheter.* This will have to be re-inserted, sometimes under a further anaesthetic.

3. *Circulatory collapse* is prevented by adequate blood transfusion and keeping the drainage tubes free so that clot retention does not occur.

4. *Infection and septicaemia.*

5. *Suprapubic leakage* may occur after the catheter has been removed. It usually clears up after three or four days further catheter drainage. Intermittent drainage should be instituted before removal of the catheter.

6. *Epididymo-orchitis* is usually prevented by bilateral ligation of the vas deferens at operation. The scrotum, however, should always be well supported.

7. *Secondary haemorrhage* is an occasional complication about 8 days postoperatively and requires bladder washouts, free drainage and antibiotics.

8. *Stricture formation* may cause a diminishing stream of urine and bougies may have to be passed.

9. *Incontinence.* Some incontinence is very likely to be present in the early days after removal of the catheter. It is prevented and diminished by urethral exercises. The patient is instructed to commence passing urine and then to stop and start again three or four times during the day. This promotes tone in the sphincter muscle.

10. *Persistent pyuria* is common after the operation and is not significantly diminished by operating under an antibiotic umbrella. Antibacterial substances are only given if there is evidence of gross infection.

## CARCINOMA OF THE PROSTATE GLAND

Carcinoma of the prostate is not uncommon. An established malignant prostate is usually too fixed to be removed.

The signs and symptoms are similar to those of senile enlargement, but pain is more prominent. Spread of the growth to the bones occurs early in the disease and the serum acid phophatase is elevated.

*Treatment*

Stilboestrol (5 mg t.d.s. is the usual dose although some authorities advise 100 mg daily) or dienoestrol by mouth are the preparations most commonly used and are given indefinitely. Some patients, however, complain of painful breasts. Stilboestrol is not without risk, and carcinoma of both male breasts has been seen as a complication of its use. Thrombosis is a calculated risk of oestrogen therapy but is worth taking in view of the gravity of the condition. Stilboestrol diphosphate (Honvan) or Tace may be prescribed if stilboestrol is ineffective. Occasionally bilateral orchidectomy may be performed.

Endoscopic resection is frequently performed for temporary relief in this condition. A channel is cut by means of a resectoscope, using diathermy coagulation.

After the operation a catheter is left in the urethra for three days.

### PROSTATIC CALCULI

Prostatic calculi may occur as a result of infection or small abscess formation and usually require no treatment.

## THE PENIS AND URETHRA

### CIRCUMCISION

This operation is usually performed for phimosis. If balantis (infection under the prepuce) is present the prepuce is slit on its dorsal surface, since circumcision in the presence of infection is likely to be followed by extensive skin sloughing. In the infant circumcision is a very minor procedure, but in the adult it is a more severe undertaking.

Many infants are referred to clinics for advice on circumcision but only in a few is it necessary. The baby's prepuce is naturally tight and it may not retract easily until he is three or four years old. A common cause of reference is the ulcerated

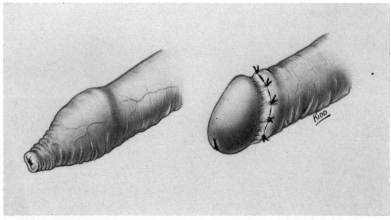

A                                      B

FIG. 42.8   A, Phimosis. B, Circumcision.

foreskin associated with ammoniacal dermatitis (napkin rash). For this condition, circumcision is strongly contra-indicated and will remove nature's protection for the glans and external urinary meatus and so allow ammonia to burn the glans. This will produce stenosis which is a complication of a meatal ulcer. Ammoniacal dermatitis is caused by bacteria from faeces fermenting the urea in wet napkins, with the production of ammonia. The treatment is to allow the child to be without a napkin as much as possible.

In many cases, when the foreskin is too tight, a dorsal slit, and not circumcision, is all that is required.

### Complications of circumcision

1. Haemorrhage.
2. Infection.
3. Urethritis, particularly damage to the external urinary meatus.
4. Meatal ulcer.

*Balanitis* requires repeated antiseptic dressings such as eusol, and the provision of free drainage by dorsal slit if necessary.

*Carcinoma* of the penis occurs occasionally, and treatment necessitates removal of the organ and the lymphatic glands in the groin.

THE WOUNDS. After the extensive dissection which is necessary to remove the glands in both groins it is usually difficult to secure healing of the wounds. The skin flaps are thin and lymph accumulates beneath. Firm pressure dressings are most important. Lymph which accumulates may be aspirated, with every care taken to avoid infection. Less effective is continuous suction.

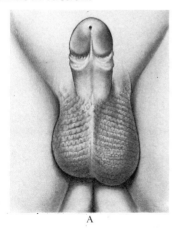

FIG. 42.9A    Pin-hole meatus.

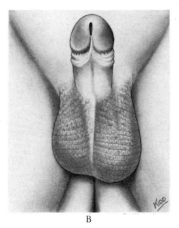

FIG. 42.9B    After meatotomy.

*Pin-hole meatus.* This condition (Fig. 42.9A) causes urinary obstruction. The treatment is enlargement of the meatus (Fig. 42.9B).

## RUPTURE OF THE URETHRA

Rupture of the urethra is a serious injury usually caused by a fall astride a spike or the sharp edge of a kerbstone. Frequently it is associated with a fracture of the pelvis.

*Clinical features*
1. Pain is present in the perineum, which is swollen and tender.
2. Bleeding occurs from the urethral orifice.
3. There is retention of urine.

*Treatment*

The patient is advised not to pass urine, because it would only flow into the tissues and add to the dangers. Morphia (15 mg) is prescribed to relieve the pain of retention until he can be taken to the theatre.

The urethra is explored by an incision in the perineum with the patient in the lithotomy position. The divided urethra is sutured and the wound is left open so that irrigation can be carried out and infection prevented. The bladder is drained suprapubically to divert the flow of urine until the urethra has healed.

In the immediate postoperative period sulphonamide drugs, urinary antiseptics, and fluids are given. As soon as healing occurs dilatation is performed, and the patient is advised to return one to two months later for further dilatation and examination. A grave complication is urethral stricture.

## URETHRAL STRICTURE

The vast majority of urethral strictures used to be due to gonorrhoea but, with the easy cure of this disease by the antibiotics, instrumentation and injury are now probably the commonest causes. The urinary stream gradually diminishes until the patient is almost unable to pass urine. Back pressure results in hydronephrosis of the kidneys and hypertrophy of the bladder. Periurethral abscess is an occasional complication.

The treatment consists of repeated dilatation with bougies. In refractory cases the stricture may have to be divided by operation. Following urethral dilatation rigors are liable to develop, due to bacteraemic shock. For this reason urethral dilatation is one of the few procedures which should be performed under the cover of a broad-spectrum antibiotic.

# DISEASES OF THE TESTICLE, THE SPERMATIC CORD AND ITS COVERINGS

## UNDESCENDED TESTIS

The testes develop near the kidneys *in utero*, and at birth both testicles are in the scrotum. The maldescent is frequently associated with a hernia and gives rise to symptoms only if recurrent nipping of the testicle occurs at the external abdominal ring.

### Treatment

The testicle should be brought down by operation before the age of 7. Hormones may be prescribed to encourage normal descent and development but their value is questionable.

If a hernia is present operation will be necessary for this condition at about the age of 4 years, and should conservative measures fail to bring about the descent of the testis operative replacement of the organ in the scrotum will usually be performed.

The nurse must take care of any special stitch or retentive apparatus which may be fitted to secure the testicle in position. The operating surgeon will give precise instructions about the postoperative care of the stitches and their date of removal.

## ACUTE EPIDIDYMO-ORCHITIS

Inflammation of the testis and epididymis is known as epididymo-orchitis.

### Aetiology

In adolescents the commonest cause is its occurrence as a complication of mumps. In the adult the commonest organism is the *E. coli*, and the condition is frequently associated with enlargement of the prostate. The gonoccocus is the second commonest cause of infection.

### Symptoms

The testicle is tender and swollen and the scrotal skin may be oedematous. In many cases the condition is combined with a urinary infection, and increased frequency and scalding of micturition may be present.

### Treatment

The patient should be confined to bed and the scrotum supported on a sling of broad strapping attached to the thighs.

Urinary antiseptics, together with a course of sulphonamide therapy, are prescribed. The urine should be examined for bacteria, antibiotic sensitivity, or other abnormal constituents.

Resolution is usual and drainage is rarely necessary. The acute stage subsides rapidly, but complete resolution takes two or three months, and recurrent attacks are not uncommon.

Ligation of the vas deferens may be advisable for recurrent attacks.

### CHRONIC EPIDIDYMO-ORCHITIS

*Causes*

1. Tuberculosis.
2. Syphilis.

**Tuberculous epididymitis** may be part of a tuberculous infection of the urinary tract, or it may occur as a solitary lesion in the genito-urinary tract.

*Treatment*

Antituberculous chemotherapy (p. 74) is commenced. In refractory cases the epididymis may be excised.

**Syphilis.** A gumma gives rise to a large painless swelling of the testicle. At puberty a congenital syphilitic may develop epididymo-orchitis. The treatment is that of syphilis.

## TORSION OF THE TESTIS

Torsion of the testis gives rise to severe pain and acute swelling. Immediate operation is desirable and, because the same condition may occur on the other side, the opposite testicle should also be fixed in the scrotum.

*Vasectomy*

Vasectomy is division of the vas deferens.

It may be undertaken for:

1. Recurrent epididymo-orchitis.
2. As a method of family planning.

The operation is usually performed under local anaesthetic without the necessity for hospital admission.

### HYDROCELE

A hydrocele is a collection of serous fluid in the tunica vaginalis or sac surrounding the testicle. The condition may be secondary to disease of the testicle, but usually develops without any obvious cause.

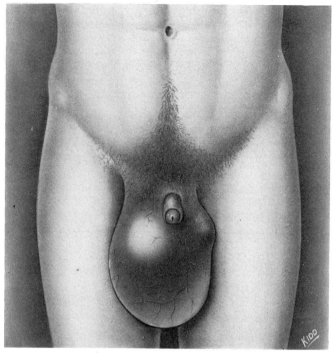

FIG. 42.10    Right hydrocele showing translucency.

## Treatment

### ASPIRATION

Aspiration by means of a needle and syringe inserted into the hydrocele under local anaesthesia.

The only preparation necessary is the cleansing of the skin with Savlon. A torch is essential to transilluminate the swelling so that the surgeon can select an area of skin between the large veins and thereby obviate the formation of a haematoma. The puncture hole in the skin is covered by collodion gauze dressings.

Tapping is only a palliative measure and the sac refills, so that the procedure will have to be repeated fairly frequently.

### RADICAL CURE

This is effected by excision of the sac or by turning the sac inside out. Diathermy is frequently used during the operation, so the nurse must remember to adjust the bandages and clothing so that a bare area of skin is easily available on the patient's thigh for the diathermy electrode.

A drain will be inserted in the scrotum for 48 hours, and

the scrotum must be supported on strapping across the thighs for ten days after the operation. This is most important if a massive haematocele is to be avoided.

### HAEMATOCELE

A haematocele is a collection of blood around the testicle. The condition is sometimes due to trauma and sometimes to a new growth. Aspiration or open drainage may be necessary.

### NEW GROWTHS OF THE TESTICLE

New growths are not common but are intensely malignant. The primary lesion rapidly results in ulceration and fungation. Secondary deposits occur high in the abdomen.

*Treatment*

The testicle is removed and megavoltage therapy is prescribed for the abdominal glands.

## THE SPERMATIC CORD

Funiculitis or inflammation of the spermatic cord may occur as a complication of epididymo-orchitis. The treatment is similar to that of infection of the testicle.

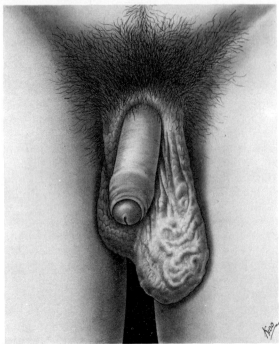

FIG. 42.11   Varicocele.

## VARICOCELE

Varicocele is a condition of varicosity of the veins in the spermatic cord, and occurs almost invariably on the left side. A slight dragging pain or, more usually, routine medical examination calls attention to the condition.

*Treatment*

The vast majority of cases require no treatment at all. A suspensory bandage is advised if the patient complains of pain. Operation may be undertaken and consists of excising the dilated veins.

## THE SCROTUM

### SEBACEOUS CYST

A sebaceous cyst is probably the commonest lesion of the scrotal skin and is excised in the usual way.

# CHAPTER 43

# Neonatal Surgery

## (The Surgery of the Newborn)

Many babies born with abnormalities which are incompatible with life can be saved by surgery. The maternity nurse or mid-wife should be aware of these conditions as so often it is as a result of her observations that prompt diagnosis and the chance to save the baby's life depend. If these babies have to be transported any distance to a neonatal surgical unit they must be accompanied by a nurse who knows how to render the appropriate first aid.

*General management*

TRANSPORT. Newborn babies travel well provided that proper arrangements have been made. Heat loss must be pre-vented, especially in the premature baby whose body tempera-ture may fall to 32° C (90° F) or less after a journey in a cold ambulance and as a result its chances of survival may be con-siderably reduced. The baby is laid flat on its side in a port-able electric incubator. If an incubator is not available the baby should be warmly but loosely wrapped and placed in a carry-cot. Hot water bottles, which are not generally recom-mended, may have to be used in this instance. The bottles should be in good condition and well protected with covers—the tightness of the stoppers should be checked by two persons. They should be placed in the carry-cot well out of any contact with the baby. Consent for operation signed by one or both parents, a specimen of 5 to 10 ml of the mother's blood in a plain tube and a written report about the preg-nancy, confinement and the baby's condition at birth should accompany the little patient.

*Aspiration* of vomit during the journey may be fatal. All

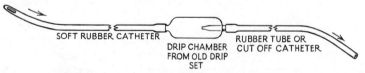

SOFT RUBBER CATHETER    RUBBER TUBE OR
CUT OFF CATHETER
DRIP CHAMBER
FROM OLD DRIP
SET

FIG. 43.1    Simple mucus extractor.

492

babies suspected of suffering from intestinal obstruction must have a soft rubber catheter (3 or 4 French gauge) passed through the nose and into the stomach. This is aspirated every ten minutes throughout the journey. If vomiting should occur the nasopharynx is aspirated with a simple mucus extractor (Fig. 43.1).

Oxygen can be administered with a plastic funnel if a portable incubator is not available. A baby with severe respiratory embarrassment, such as in diaphragmatic hernia, may not survive the journey unless an endotracheal tube is passed and positive pressure respiration carried out continuously under the supervision of a doctor who should accompany the child.

The danger of retrolental fibroplasia should be kept in mind and an atmosphere of not more than 28 per cent oxygen maintained. This should be checked with an oxygen analyser.

### Pre- and postoperative care of neonates

CONTROL OF TEMPERATURE. Tiny babies have poor control over their body temperature and must be protected from extremes. On the operating table the baby should be wrapped in wool and an electric or warm blanket used. After operation the baby is placed in a warm incubator. Full-term babies are kept at a temperature of 29·5° C (85° F) while premature babies will need the incubator at 32° C (90° F) to 35°C (95° F). An electrical rectal thermometer is of great assistance in checking temperature serially.

PROTECTION FROM INFECTION. Babies are very prone to infection, and full masking, gowning and hand-washing precautions must be taken when handling them. A positive pressure in the incubator, allowing an outward flow of air, minimises airborne infection. Staff with colds or septic skin conditions must not be allowed to attend the babies. A staphylococcal infection can be fatal. Inadequate cleansing and sterilisation of the incubator are important causes of cross infection.

GASTRIC ASPIRATION. Babies who have had gastrointestinal operations will have a nasogastric tube placed in position. This must be connected to a low-grade suction apparatus. In addition the nurse must disconnect the catheter and aspirate with a hand syringe every half or one hour, in case the tube blocks.

ATTENTION TO RESPIRATION. The baby should be nursed with the head slightly elevated to allow free excursion of the diaphragm which is the main muscle of respiration in the newborn. An oxygen concentration above 30 per cent is not usually advised because of the danger of retrolental fibroplasia, causing blindness. However, it is the concentration of oxygen in the

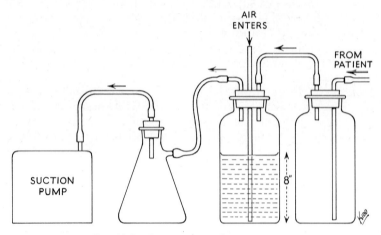

FIG. 43.2    Low-grade suction apparatus.

blood that matters and if a baby is cyanosed the oxygen concentration should be increased.

HUMIDIFICATION of the air to 80 to 100 per cent by a special humidifier will assist the baby to swallow sticky sputum. If a humidifier is not available, draping towels—which have been wrung out in warm water—in the incubator is a useful alternative.

*Aspirate of vomitus* will usually lead to collapse with cyanosis or grey pallor. The mouth and pharynx must be aspirated immediately with an efficient sucker. A tray should always be at hand with a laryngoscope, endotracheal and suction tubes.

INTRAVENOUS THERAPY. The baby may have a scalp vein needle drip held in position by strips of plaster of Paris or by a polythene cannula inserted by a 'cut-down' into a vein in the arm or leg. Whichever method is in use a three-way tap is connected to the cannula, one arm of which is attached to a 2 ml syringe and the other arm to the drip set. This syringe allows accurate administration of small amounts of fluid or rapid blood transfusion as required. A special paediatric drip set is used in which a 30 ml graduated burette is incorporated above the drip chamber (Fig. 43.3). Fluid balance charts must be kept.

Urinary output in baby boys can be measured by strapping Paul's tubing to the penis. In girls a chironseal urine collector is used.

ORAL FEEDING is commenced as soon as possible, at a time ordered by the paediatrician. At first the continuous suction is stopped and two-hourly aspirations are carried out by syringe. If less than 5 ml of colourless fluid is aspirated every two

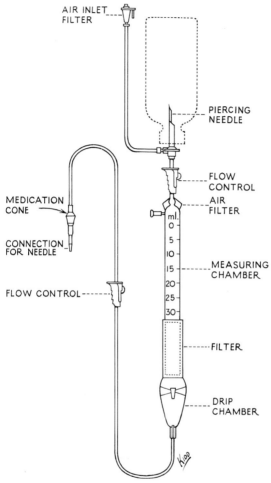

AIR INLET
FILTER

PIERCING
NEEDLE

FLOW
CONTROL

MEDICATION
CONE

AIR
FILTER

CONNECTION
FOR NEEDLE

ml.
0
5
10
15
20
25
30

MEASURING
CHAMBER

FLOW CONTROL

FILTER

DRIP
CHAMBER

FIG. 43.3   Paediatric drip set.

hours the nasogastric tube should be removed and 5 per cent
glucose water feeds given for 24 hours.

Full term babies: 30 ml at two-hourly intervals.

Premature babies: 15 to 25 ml at two-hourly intervals
according to their weight.

A nasogastric tube should be passed, left *in situ*, and aspirated before each feed. If more than 10 ml fluid is aspirated
the next two feeds should be omitted and then a smaller feed
is given. After 24 hours half-strength milk can be used in 30
to 40 ml feeds. Gastric aspirations are reduced to four-hourly
and, if all is well, are discontinued after 48 hours when full
strength milk is given three-hourly—70 ml per kilo body-

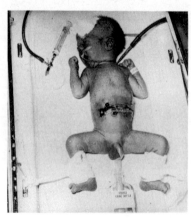

FIG. 43.4   Method of collecting urine with Paul's tubing (also illustrates nasogastric suction and intravenous scalp drip).

weight in 24 hours until the third day, up to 140 ml until the eighth day and then 165 ml during the third week.

TUBE FEEDING may be necessary in premature babies. A soft plastic tube (3 or 4 French gauge) is carefully passed via the nostril into the stomach and fixed to the nose with strapping. The barrel of a 20 ml syringe is connected to the catheter and used as a graduated funnel. The syringe must not be higher than 10 cm above the baby or the pressure produced in the stomach will be dangerous. Careful oral hygiene is necessary. If the child has a gastrostomy (for instance oesophageal atresia) the gastrostomy tube is connected as above.

### NEONATAL SURGICAL CONDITIONS

**Posterior choanal atresia.** This condition is due to the persistence of a membrane across one or both posterior nares. If bilateral, the newborn baby makes desperate efforts to inhale, goes blue and will probably die. To save his life the mouth is forced open and held open with a prop. Air will rush in and the emergency is over. The diagnosis is confirmed by attempting to pass a catheter through the nose. The membranes are perforated with an antral trocar and cannula. Polythene tubes are pushed through and left protruding from the nostrils for about half an inch. They are strapped in position and cleared with suction. The baby can now breathe with his mouth closed and will feed normally. The tubes are removed after one week and then the holes must be dilated with urethral bougies, first daily then every few days and later each month until the baby is about 1 year old.

**Retrognathia (micrognathia).** The mandible is underdeveloped and there is a cleft palate. The baby's tongue falls back

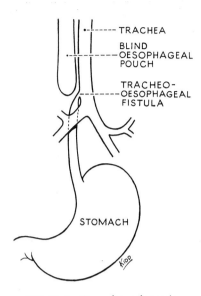

TRACHEA

BLIND
OESOPHAGEAL
POUCH

TRACHEO-
OESOPHAGEAL
FISTULA

STOMACH

FIG. 43.5   Oesophageal atresia.

and he will suffocate unless nursed face downwards and fed in
this position. The surgeon may stitch the tongue to the lower
lip or gum. The condition is recognised on sight, the tiny
lower jaw giving the baby a 'shrew mouth' appearance. Usually these tiny jaws grow normally and surgery is necessary only
for the cleft palate. Occasionally plastic operations on the jaw
may be needed.

Oesophageal atresia. The oesophagus ends blindly in the
chest. Usually the lower end communicates with the stomach
and has a fistula into the trachea (Fig. 43.5). The baby is often
born to a mother who has had hydramnios (too much liquor
amnii). The child is unable to swallow normally beyond the
oesophagus, continually dribbles mucus from its mouth and
may have cyanotic attacks. If atresia is suspected no feed
should be given. A weak child will inhale the feed and drown,
a strong child may survive but will later develop a severe inhalation pneumonia. A soft No. 8 radio-opaque catheter should
be passed into the pharynx and if it will pass no further than
four inches it is likely that the baby has an atresia. An X-ray,
with the catheter in position, confirms the diagnosis. Until
operation can be performed the baby should be nursed on its
abdomen in the head-down position, but some believe that in
order to prevent gastric juice entering the trachea the body
should be propped up and the mucus extractor should be
taken on the journey to the hospital. The nasopharynx is aspirated and no feed of any kind given. An intravenous infusion is

set up and blood cross-matched. At early operation, usually through a right thoracotomy, the fistula is closed. It may be possible to join the two ends of the oesophagus. If they are too far apart primary anastomosis may not be possible. The upper pouch is brought out into the neck to allow saliva to dribble away and the baby is nourished through a gastrostomy tube. Later, when the baby is stronger (perhaps several months old) an isolated length of transverse colon with its blood supply intact is passed up through the anterior mediastinum and is anastomosed to the oesophageal pouch above and to the stomach below.

### INTESTINAL OBSTRUCTION IN THE NEWBORN

Babies with intestinal obstruction vomit soon after birth. This becomes profuse and is almost invariably bile-stained. Later the vomit may be faeculent and contain blood due to oesophagitis and gastritis.

**Distension.** Distension of the abdomen occurs in low intestinal obstruction but may be minimal if the obstruction is high as in the duodenum. A grossly distended abdomen embarrasses respiration.

**Constipation.** The first few stools passed by a normal baby consist of a soft dark green mixture containing bile, mucus, water and desquamated epithelium from the gastrointestinal tract—this is called meconium. The first stool is passed a few hours after birth. After a few days, if a child is taking milk, the meconium will be mixed with curd—the transition stool. After four days meconium has disappeared and the pale yellow stool of infancy is passed. A baby born with intestinal obstruction may pass a little meconium, a plug of grey-white mucus or no stool at all.

DIAGNOSIS is confirmed by an anteroposterior X-ray in the upright position. This is taken with the child bandaged to a cross with the head supported to prevent it falling forwards.

*Causes*

*Duodenal obstruction.* This may be due to atresia (failure to develop a normal lumen), a diaphragm, a band of tissue, or a congenital mid-gut volvulus pressing in the duodenum. Babies with duodenal atresia are often mongols and may also suffer from congenital heart disease. Duodenal obstruction requires urgent operation. A soft gastric tube should be passed and the stomach aspirated. A cut-down drip should be started and any electrolyte disturbance corrected. Blood should be available.

*Intestinal atresia* is uncommon in the small bowel and rare in the colon. The areas of atresia may be multiple. In general, treatment consists of resection of grossly distended gut and then anastomosis of the ends. Sometimes multiple ileostomies or colostomies, with a view to later anastomosis, may be necessary.

*Meconium ileus* occurs in babies suffering from mucoviscidosis which is an abnormality of all mucus-secreting cells in the body. Fibrocystic disease of the pancreas which is also present results in no enzymes being secreted and the meconium is therefore thick and sticky and blocks the intestines. An enterostomy is performed, through which an effort is made to dissolve the sticky mass with daily washouts of 15 per cent pancreatic solution. Often the distal distended ileum is resected. When feeding is re-established, 1 g of pancreatic granules are added to each feed. The prognosis is poor, many children die of respiratory infection which is associated with viscid mucus in the bronchial tree.

*Peritonitis* in the newborn may be bacterial due to a perforation of a peptic ulcer or a gangrenous patch of bowel secondary to strangulation or obstruction.

*Meconium peritonitis* is due to a perforation before the baby is born, causing a chemical irritation. Treatment is by urgent laparotomy.

*Strangulated inguinal hernia* is seen quite frequently in the neonatal period. It is important to examine both groins of a baby who has vomited. An irreducible lump demands urgent operation.

*Rectal atresia.* The rectum may end blindly at the level of the levator ani muscles or in the less severe case just deep to the skin. The nurse bathing the baby for the first time will notice that there is no anal opening. A straight X-ray taken after holding the baby upside down will help to determine the level of a high atresia. Occasionally there is a fistula from the blind rectum into the urethra. Treatment consists of bringing the blind rectum down to the perineum and stitching it there. Frequent digital or bougie dilatation of the rectum may be necessary during the follow-up care.

*Omphalocele* (*exomphalos*). Between the seventh and tenth weeks of foetal life part of the gut normally lies in the umbilical cord. If this fails to return to the abdomen the baby is born with some of the abdominal viscera in a transparent sac at the base of the umbilical cord. In severe cases most of the intestines, perhaps the liver, the spleen and even the kidneys, may be outside the abdomen, whilst in the milder cases only coils of small bowel may be in the sac. Great care should be taken to avoid rupture of the sac before the operation is performed. Aspiration with a nasogastric tube will prevent swallowed air distending the intestines, making reduction into the abdomen easier. The surgeon usually finds that there is an associated malrotation of the intestine and often a band of tissue obstructing the duodenum (Ladd's band). This is divided.

*Diaphragmatic hernia.* Severe hernia occurs most commonly on the left side if the diaphragm is not properly formed. The abdominal viscera herniate into the chest, the left lung cannot expand and the mediastinum is pushed over to press on the right lung. The child is born with respiratory distress, which may be so severe that, unless an endochtracheal tube is passed immediately and positive respiration with oxygen commenced, the baby will die. Oxygen should not be given through a mask as the stomach may become blown up, causing further pressure on the lungs and killing the child. Operation is performed urgently to reduce the herniated abdominal viscera back into the abdomen and to close the defect in the diaphragm.

## HIRSCHSPRUNG'S DISEASE

This is a congenital lesion, probably genetic in origin, due to the absence of ganglion cells of the myenteric nerve plexuses (of Auerbach and Meissner) in the rectum and colon. The bowel is paralysed, peristalsis does not occur and the contents of the gut cannot move. The normal bowel proximal to the paralysed section becomes very distended with gas and faeces. The baby's abdomen is distended, he passes little or no meconium and soon vomits. If a little finger is passed into the rectum the baby may deflate and be well for a few days before the symptoms recur.

### Treatment

Treatment depends on the severity of the obstruction. Babies with only a short length of abnormal colon may be treated by the frequent passage of a soft rectal tube or small saline washouts. Then diagnosis can then be confirmed by a radio-opaque enema and rectal biopsy. Babies with a long segment require an emergency laparotomy and a colostomy is performed in the normal colon. Once the wound has healed and feeding established, the child can go home. There is no urgency to proceed to the next stage of treatment, which should be deferred until the baby weighs about 11·4 kg. He is then readmitted for the operation of rectosigmoidectomy.

## TALIPES DEFORMITIES

**Club foot (talipes equino-varus).** The cause of this condition is unknown. There is usually no bone deformity and the muscles are healthy. Malposition of the foot *in utero* is sug-

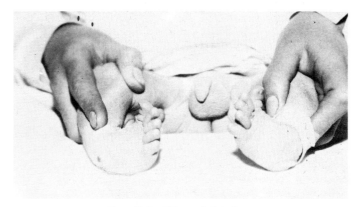

FIG. 43.6   Bilateral club foot.

gested as a probable cause of the condition. Recent research suggests that difficult cases are due to poorly developed muscles on the outer side of the leg and foot. The positional cases are easier to treat. Untreated, walking is difficult and painful corns develop on the feet.

*Treatment*

The condition is obvious at birth and treatment is instituted at once.

1. MANUAL CORRECTION. In the first 14 days of life the deformity of the foot is corrected each day by manipulating it with the hands and retaining it in position with strapping.

2. DENIS BROWNE CLUB FOOT SPLINT. This is applied on the fourteenth day and continued for 12 months. It must be removed once weekly for manipulation of the foot and not finally discarded until the foot can be held actively in the normal position.

3. SOFT TISSUE OPERATIONS:

(a) Lengthening of the tendo achillis.
(b) Release of structures on the medial foot.

4. Manipulation with a Thomas' wrench and immobilisation in plaster is necessary in late and neglected cases.

5. In very advanced cases improvement is effected by removing a wedge of the tarsus and fixing the foot in plaster.

Bone operations are not performed under the age of 10 to 12 because the bones are still growing.

# CHAPTER 44

# Surgical Aspects of Tropical Diseases

The management of disease endemic in tropical countries is a problem for the physician and the specialist in hygiene. Occasionally, however, surgical aid is necessary in the treatment of complications which may arise and, with increasing facilities for travel, the patient may present himself in more temperate regions with tropical disease. Most tropical diseases are caused by bacteria or parasites and in many cases there is a complex and interesting life cycle which is beyond the scope of this short chapter to discuss.

## PLAGUE

Plague is caused by the *Pasteurella pestis*. The skin is covered with petechial spots. The lymphatic glands, particularly in the groin and axilla, are enlarged and may suppurate and require incision. More severe forms known as pneumonic and septicaemic are invariably fatal.

## YAWS

This is a contagious disease due to *Treponema pertenue*. It has three stages like syphilis but the secondary stage is characterised by 'raspberry-like' papillomas. In the tertiary stage deep ulcers like gummas develop. It is not transmitted from mother to foetus and does not invade the cardiovascular or nervous systems. The administration of Terramycin is curative.

## DELHI BOIL

*Leishmania tropica*, a minute parasite, causes an indurated ulcer usually on the face. This is known as a Delhi boil. The condition can be cured by intravenous injection of 10 per cent solution of antimony tartrate.

## LEPROSY

This condition is due to invasion of the skin by the *Mycobacterium leprae*. The onset is insidious; nodules develop in the skin which may invade the peripheral nerves causing pain, and later anaesthesia and paralysis occur. The changes which follow

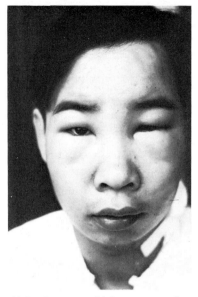

FIG. 44.1  A patient with lepromatous leprosy.

are due to loss of the nerve supply with the result that gross deformity and destruction of tissue results.

There are two clinical types:

1. Lepromatous in which there is very little resistance by the body.
2. Tuberculoid—high body resistance.

*Treatment*

Leprosy is only mildly contagious and isolation is quite unnecessary. Diaminodiphenylsulphone (DDS) is curative but must be continued for at least a year. An alternative new drug is Lampren 100–600 mg daily. Well planned plastic operations can do much to prevent or correct the hideous deformities.

## TRICHINIASIS

A small round worm which infects meat, usually pork, is carried from the alimentary tract to the muscles. There is slight aching of the affected muscles. The disease subsides harmlessly without specific treatment.

## FILARIASIS

The adult worm of the genus *Filaria sanguinis hominis* is a round worm which causes elephantiasis by obstructing the lymphatic vessels of the lower limbs. Only the microfilariae of the adult worm reach the peripheral circulation at night and they can be demonstrated by nocturnal samples of blood. Treatment is unsatisfactory.

## AMOEBIASIS

Amoebic dysentery is caused by the *Entamoeba histolytica* which attacks the colon causing symptoms of colitis, perforation of the colon, ulceration of the rectum and in the worst cases stricture. If the diagnosis is made at this stage, the patient, after treatment with metronidazole, is usually cured.

In less striking infections the diagnosis may not be made and the organism migrates to the liver where it forms an abscess by destruction of liver tissue. The abscess, which has to be drained, contains liver substance and blood which accounts for the typical 'anchovy sauce' appearance of the pus. The administration of metronidazole is curative but may damage the myocardium.

## BILHARZIA

*Schistosoma haematobium* is a trematode worm whose ova are shed in human faeces and urine. The disease is acquired by bathing in infected water. In addition to infection of the liver the ova invade the mucous membrane of the bladder or rectum causing cystitis or proctitis with bleeding and irritation. The ova can be recovered from the patient's faeces or urine. Later carcinoma of the bladder may develop. Treatment by the administration of niridazole is curative.

## MALARIA

The main surgical significance of malaria is the ease with which the enlarged soft spleen can be ruptured. Splenectomy may be indicated.

## ASIATIC CHOLANGIO-HEPATITIS

Obstruction of the common bile duct by the liver fluke is quite common in the Far East. The smaller ducts in the liver are also involved and the patient presents with pain, Charcot's biliary fever and jaundice. As soon as he is fit the duct is emptied of stones and the liver fluke—because of similar changes in the liver a wide opening in the lower end of the duct into the duodenum is effected so that inaccessible stones and flukes as well as pus can drain. The gall bladder is also removed.

# CHAPTER 45

# Injuries and Diseases of the Central Nervous System

The nervous system is composed of the central nervous system, formed by the brain and the spinal cord, and the peripheral nervous system, the constituents of which are the sensory and motor spinal nerves, together with the autonomic nerves.

The central nervous system is the centre of all vital activities, and damage to even a small area may result in loss of function over wide areas of the body. At almost all points the central nervous system is endowed with a strong bony protection—the skull and the spinal column—and while this stands it in good stead in the event of injury, it renders the diagnosis and treatment of established diseases more difficult and more complicated than those of similar lesions elsewhere.

## PREPARATION OF THE PATIENT FOR NEUROLOGICAL EXAMINATION AND INVESTIGATIONS

The diagnosis of a lesion of the nervous system may be made only after the most painstaking examination, aided by careful investigation.

1. PHYSICAL EXAMINATION

For this the patient must be undressed and in bed or on a couch, but before the examination has been completed the doctor will usually require to perform certain tests with the patient out of bed. This will include the observation of the patient's gait, and slippers should be at hand. A dressing gown is unnecessary as it hides peculiarities of gait and disorders of co-ordination.

The following instruments and equipment will be required:

(a) Percussion hammer.
(b) Tuning fork.
(c) Ophthalmoscope.

(d) Torch.
(e) Auroscope.
(f) Pins, cotton-wool, coins, and similar objects for examination of sensation.
(g) Hot and cold water in separate test tubes.
(h) Charts for testing vision.
(i) Scents for testing sense of smell.
(j) Tape measure to assess wasting of the thighs (for example in a lower motor neurone lesion).
(k) A pair of geometrical dividers to estimate two-point discrimination.

2. SPECIAL INVESTIGATIONS
These include:

(a) The blood Wassermann and Kahn reactions will almost invariably be tested.
(b) Lumbar puncture and examination of the fluid by a clinical pathologist, provided papilloedema is not present.

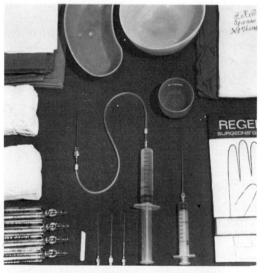

FIG. 45.1   Preparation for cerebral angiogram.

| | |
|---|---|
| Neck towels | Receiver |
| Bowl for heparinised saline | Towel, gown, gloves |
| Gallipot with cleansing lotion | Swabs |
| Radio-opaque medium | File |
| Angiogram needles—selection | |

1 × 20 ml Syringe mounted with special angiogram tubes, adaptor and needle
1 × 10 ml Syringe with filling needle.

(c)  Fields of vision.
(d)  Radiographic examination:
    (i)  Straight X-ray of skull and spine. The cervical spine as well as the skull should always be X-rayed in cases of head injury.
    (ii)  After the injection of air or carbon dioxide between the spinal cord and its coverings (pneumo-encephalogram).
    (iii)  After the injection of air or carbon dioxide into the ventricles of the brain (ventriculogram). Positive contrast ventriculograms are also performed using Myodil or a water-soluble contrast.
    (iv)  Cerebral angiogram. For safety the contrast medium is put in a 10 ml syringe and saline for irrigating the needle during X-ray in a 20 ml syringe—this is because *both* solutions are colourless.
    (v)  Myelography. Injection of oil-based contrast to outline the spinal cord. Nerve roots can be demonstrated using a water-soluble contrast (radiculogram).
(e)  Electroencephalogram (EEG).
(f)  Brain scan after introduction of a radioactive substance into the circulating blood.
(g)  Thermography.

*Lumbar puncture*

Lumbar puncture is performed for the following purposes:

1. DIAGNOSTIC, e.g. to determine the presence of pus or blood in the cerebrospinal fluid. The pressure of the fluid may be measured by a manometer, and changes in pressure are a significant finding in tumours of the brain and spinal cord. The normal range of cerebrospinal fluid (CSF) pressure is 70 to 170 mm of water. Lumbar puncture, as well as being contraindicated if papilloedema is present, is also contraindicated if a cerebral abscess or other space-occupying lesion is suspected. This is because 'coning' can follow lumbar puncture when the intracranial pressure is raised, even in the absence of papilloedema. After a lumbar puncture air is sometimes injected and a radiograph taken. This is known as a pneumo-encephalogram.

2. THERAPEUTIC. Chloromycetin and cephaloridine are examples of drugs that can be given intrathecally.

3. ANAESTHETIC. The anaesthetic solution is injected through the lumbar puncture needle by means of a syringe.

PREPARATION FOR LUMBAR PUNCTURE

A wide area of the back from the upper dorsal region to the

buttock is prepared in the usual way. A series of sterilised lumbar puncture needles, serum and hypodermic needles, as well as syringes and a manometer are required. A tiny area is anaesthetised with a local anaesthetic.

The nurse opens the outer wrapping of the basic dressing pack, and of other packs as required. She supports the patient whilst the doctor performs the lumbar puncture. As required she may assist the doctor by holding specimen jars, the manometer, or by compressing the jugular vein for Queckenstedt's test.

On completion of the procedure the doctor withdraws the needle and seals the puncture.

The patient is made comfortable with one pillow and advised to rest. Observations are made on the patient.

The trolley is covered and removed. The LP needles and manometer are rinsed, placed in the appropriate container and returned to CSSD. Any specimens are sent to the laboratory.

When the lumbar puncture needle has been inserted into the subarachnoid space, CSF, which is normally clear and colourless, will be released. If the puncture has been traumatic, the CSF will be bloodstained, but the fluid rapidly clears if allowed to drain into separate bottles. All specimens are then sent for microscopy, culture, and measurement of their protein, glucose and chloride content.

POSITION OF THE PATIENT. The puncture may be performed with the patient:

1. Sitting upright with his legs over the side of the bed.
2. Lying in the left lateral position.

Whichever position is used it is important to have the spine well flexed, so that the bony spaces through which the lumbar puncture needle enters the spine are as wide open as possible.

*Aftercare.* Headache is common after lumbar puncture, and is thought to result from lowered intracranial pressure. If distressed, the patient should lie flat for 24 hours.


## HEAD INJURIES

Head injuries are exceedingly common, and the majority are so trivial as never to be seen in hospital. Nevertheless there are over 100,000 hospital admissions for head injury each year, and most of these are treated in general surgical wards. Only a small minority require transfer to neurosurgical centres for specialised care and treatment of complications.

The brain is a soft organ with the consistency of porridge, enclosed in a rigid skull. Damage to the brain in a head injury may be local at the site of impact, and/or distant on the opposite side. If the moving head strikes an unyielding object such as a road, movement of the skull ceases abruptly but the brain undergoes a slower deceleration and so becomes compressed at the site of impact. There follows a recoil movement of the brain which then strikes the opposite side of the skull thereby sustaining a second injury (*contrecoup* phenomenon).

Damage to the brain may be obvious to the naked eye (*contusion* and *laceration*), or only microscopic (*diffuse neuronal damage*). The severity of the lesion does not necessarily correlate with the patient's clinical condition: patients may be fully conscious and orientated with contused or lacerated brain, yet there may be prolonged unconsciousness with no macroscopic injury.

Further damage may be inflicted on the brain as a result of the initial injury. Swelling from *oedema* is a normal sequel to damage to any part of the body, and is part of the inflammatory response. Such swelling leads to raised intracranial pressure because of the unyielding nature of the skull. Pressure may be further raised by *intracranial haemorrhage* from vessels torn at the time of injury. Both oedema and haemorrhage can lead to serious *cerebral compression*. Because of this high pressure state, the brain tends to be thrust down (i.e. herniate) through the opening at the base of the skull (the foramen magnum) compressing vital centres of the brain controlling the heart and respiration. This herniation is known as *coning* and may occur rapidly, demanding prompt treatment if the patient is to survive. If the signs of cerebral compression are to be picked up at the earliest possible moment, patients with head injuries require careful and continual observation by the nurse.

### ASSESSMENT OF HEAD INJURIES

This relies on observing the sequence of events following a head injury. We seek to chart the patient's *progress* with carefully repeated observations, and it must be emphasised that isolated observations are valueless.

1. **Level of consciousness.** This is really the level of responsiveness. It is the most important fact to know about a head injury. The patient's level of consciousness should be described in simple words, e.g. 'alert, orientated in time and space, obeys commands and answers questions appropriately' or 'restless and unco-operative, abusive and ignoring commands'. Words like 'coma' and 'stupor' should be banished for ever, as they are ill-defined and have different meanings for different people.

The level of consciousness should be recorded at the time

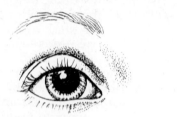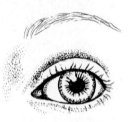

FIG. 45.2 Unequal pupils in cerebral compression. The right pupil is dilated and does not react.

of admission, so that a base-line is drawn to appreciate subsequent changes. Cerebral compression produces progressive deterioration in a patient's level of consciousness.

Very frequently patients cannot remember events immediately preceding the accident (*retrograde amnesia*) or following the accident (*post-traumatic amnesia—PTA*). An estimate of these periods of amnesia should be made, for severity of the head injury appears to correlate with the duration of the PTA.

2. **Pupillary changes.** The size, equality and reaction of pupils to light must be recorded. In cases of cerebral compression, the pupils are occasionally constricted in the early stages, but this observation may easily be missed. As the compression increases, the pupil on the side of the lesion dilates and becomes less responsive to light (Fig. 45.2). The opposite pupil follows a similar pattern until ultimately both pupils are fully dilated and unresponsive (i.e. fixed) to light.

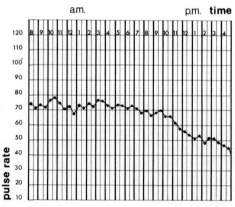

FIG. 45.3 The pulse chart in cerebral compression showing bradycardia.

Pupil inequality by itself, as an isolated finding, is quite meaningless. The important point is the *progression* of pupillary signs, combined with the overall assessment of the patient.

3. **Pulse rate.** Cerebral compression characteristically produces a slow bounding pulse (Fig. 45.3).

4. **Blood pressure.** Raised intracranial pressure would normally drive blood out of the brain, so to ensure its adequate perfusion and nutrition, there is a compensatory rise in the blood pressure.

5. **Respiratory rate.** Usually the respiratory rate slows and breathing becomes deeper in the presence of cerebral compression.

6. **Temperature.** Blood in the subarachnoid space produces a moderate pyrexia. Temperatures in excess of 40° C may occur where there is damage to the hypothalamus or midbrain.

The vast majority of head injuries admitted to hospital are conscious on arrival and make an uneventful recovery, returning home after 24 hours. Observation for this period is mandatory for patients who lost consciousness from their injury, to ensure that any complications that might arise are quickly discovered and promptly treated.

## INJURIES TO THE SKULL AND SCALP

Before considering in detail the treatment of head injuries, we must describe briefly the injuries to the skull and scalp of which the cerebral damage may be only a part.

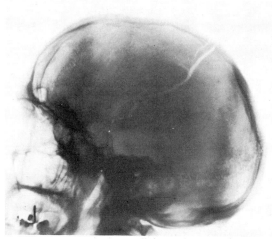

FIG. 45.4    Radiograph of fissure fractured skull.

## SCALP WOUNDS

Haemorrhage is profuse, but easily controlled by pressure on the edges of the wound as a first-aid measure and later by suture. If it is to be sutured an adequate area of skin around the wound has to be shaved. The patient with a scalp wound, however trivial, must be given penicillin antitetanic serum or tetanus toxoid as appropriate, and all cases should be seen by a doctor in case there is deeper damage. Healing, because of the abundant blood supply, is always rapid.

## INJURIES TO THE SKULL

Fractures of the skull may be simple or compound. They may affect the vault, or the base, or both.

**Fractures of the vault.** These may be:

1. Fissured, i.e. a crack.
2. Depressed, i.e. a portion of the skull is driven into the cranial cavity.

Vault fractures are usually diagnosed by careful examination of appropriate skull X-rays.

**Fractures of the base** may damage the cranial nerves with resulting impairment of function. Thus there may be weakness (*paresis*) or complete paralysis of muscles supplied by the cranial nerves (e.g. ocular muscles, facial muscles), and impairment or loss of sensation (e.g. smell, sight, hearing).

*Symptoms and signs*

1. **Anterior fossa fractures**

   (a) Epistaxis (bleeding from the nose).
   (b) The escape of cerebrospinal fluid down the nose (CSF rhinorrhoea).
   (c) The presence of bright red blood under the conjunctiva of the eye. It is bright red because oxygen from the air passes through the thin conjunctiva. No posterior border to this subconjunctival haemorrhage can be seen.

2. **Middle fossa fractures**

   (a) Bleeding and the escape of cerebrospinal fluid from the external auditory meatus. (Otorrhoea.)
   (b) The occurrence of deafness or facial paresis following the accident.

3. **Posterior fossa fractures**

   (a) Swelling of the occiput due to the escape of blood under the scalp.

(b) Signs of cerebellar inco-ordination.

**4. Head injuries of the newborn.** The skull may be fractured at birth. The infant skull may bend rather than fracture, and a pond-shaped depression of the vault is not uncommon.

## THE TREATMENT OF HEAD INJURIES

The principles of treatment are:

1. To effect recovery in the acute stage.
2. To ensure that a constant watch is kept for any change in the patient's condition which may call for operative interference.
3. To prevent and treat infection.
4. To prevent, as far as possible, residual chronic disability.

*General nursing care of head injuries*

All patients with an open wound must receive penicillin and tetanus toxoid if not already actively immunised. Tetanus antitoxin may be given if there is a specially high risk of tetanus, but patients should *always* be tested for hypersensitivity before receiving the full dose.

Observations should be constant and always written down clearly, indicating right from left when this is relevant. Staff must be able to detect the normal from the abnormal and minute to minute changes in the signs.

1. THE PROVISION OF A FREE AIRWAY is essential to the maintenance of life. An obstructed airway not only deprives the brain of oxygen, but the resulting congestion increases intracranial haemorrhage, oedema and intracranial pressure. A tongue falling back in the deeply unconscious patient, blood trickling down the trachea, or secretions in the mouth are all possible causes of obstruction and must be dealt with accordingly.

If breathing is still unsatisfactory an endotracheal tube is passed and assisted respiration commenced, but if unconsciousness lasts more than a few hours and is not improved, a tracheostomy should be considered and all the measures outlined in Chapter 18 instituted without delay.

2. POSITION IN BED AND THE AVOIDANCE OF FURTHER INJURY TO THE UNCONSCIOUS PATIENT. The best position in which to maintain a satisfactory airway is semiprone. A pillow is placed under the chest to prevent the patient rolling onto his face. Another is placed between the knees with the upper leg drawn up. This keeps the patient stable and prevents the appearance of pressure sores. There is no need for a pillow under the head.

If the patient is restless, he is liable to fall out of bed. Padded cot-sides may be needed. Restlessness may be marked, making nursing care difficult and causing distress to other patients. Only when a patient is totally unmanageable should he be sedated. In such cases, Valium is the drug of choice; paraldehyde should be avoided.

3. RECORDS. A head injury chart should be started immediately a patient is admitted to hospital. It should record:

(a) An estimate of the patient's level of consciousness (i.e. level of responsiveness).
(b) The size, equality, and reaction of the pupils to light.
(c) The pulse rate, blood pressure, respiratory rate, and temperature. Temperature is taken in the axilla (or rectum in unconscious patients).
(d) The movement of limbs.
(e) The frequency and nature of any fits.

The frequency of these observations depends on the patient's condition and is decided by the doctor-in-charge. If the patient is shocked, he should consider the possibility of injuries elsewhere in the body.

4. THE CARE OF THE INCONTINENT. Frequent changing of bed linen, careful washing, drying and powdering, together with special care of the pressure areas, must be carried out. The patient's position in bed should be changed every two hours. It is important to ensure that incontinence is not retention with overflow and that the patient is not restless from a full bladder. A Foley catheter may be inserted into the bladder.

5. MEASURES TO REDUCE SWELLING OF THE BRAIN include intravenous administration of:

(a) Frusemide (Lasix).
(b) Mannitol (10 or 20 per cent).
(c) Hypertonic urea, 90 g in 200 ml of invert sugar. This means is less popular than formerly, and is contra-indicated unless:
  (i) The blood urea is normal.
  (ii) There is no bleeding.
  (iii) The cardiovascular system is normal.
(d) Dextrose (50 per cent).

Hyperventilation using a ventilator also reduces swelling of the brain.

Dexamethasone damps down the inflammatory response. Suitable dosage is 12 mg stat i.m. or i.v. and continue with 4 mg i.m. six-hourly for a few days, and then reduce. Its usefulness in the treatment of head injuries is not universally accepted.

6. HYPOTHERMIA may be advisable when the temperature regulating centre is damaged or there is hyperpyrexia which in any case increases the brain's demands for oxygen. A temperature of 32° C is usually sufficient and this may be obtained by the usual hypothermic drugs, e.g. Largactil, removal of the bedclothes and the use of a fan. Ice packs to the body may be necessary. Hypothermia in itself reduces cerebral swelling.

7. MAINTENANCE OF NUTRITION. While dehydration therapy may result in rapid improvement in the first day or two its continuance tends to produce electrolyte disturbance and by the third day at least two litres of fluid must be given daily. An intragastric drip is the usual method if the patient is unconscious and sufficient calories can be added in the form of glucose, milk and eggs.

8. PREVENTION OF INFECTION at the site of injury and in the lungs is attempted by the administration of antibiotics. The role of prophylactic antibiotics remains controversial, but it would seem reasonable to give such antibiotics (e.g. penicillin and sulphadimidine) to patients with compound fractures of the skull.

9. CONVALESCENCE. As soon as the patient is conscious, he may have a pillow. After a few days, depending on his progress, he should be encouraged to take part in the general ward activities. This diminishes the psychological effects and increases the rate of recovery. For this reason the patient is always better nursed in an open ward rather than a side ward.

*Local treatment*

1. *Wounds* are cleansed and sutured. Care is taken to examine for complications like a depressed fracture which may need elevation and middle meningeal haemorrhage which will require a craniotomy.

2. *Bleeding from the ear or nose.* The nose and ear must not be packed, since infection may be driven into the meninges and a cerebral abscess or meningitis may develop. A bleeding ear should be covered with a sterile dressing secured with a bandage. A bleeding nose should be allowed to drip until the bleeding stops. Systemic antibiotics may be given to prevent infection, and a lumbar puncture will frequently be performed to assist in the diagnosis and sometimes to effect relief of a severe headache. Persistent rhinorrhoea— that is, escape of cerebrospinal fluid through the nose—may call for operation. A fascial graft closes the tear in the dura. If rhinorrhoea occurs the patient is instructed not to sniff, to blow the nose or to smoke. Observation should be made as to which nostril leaks cerebrospinal fluid and a specimen of the discharging

fluid is tested for sugar.

If there are discharges from the nose the intravenous route should be used for feeding an unconscious patient.

## COMPLICATIONS OF HEAD INJURIES

1. **Complications of the unconscious state**

    (a) Early: Airway obstruction by vomit, blood, secretions

    Shock from other injuries.

    (b) Late: Infection of the lungs and urinary tract.

    Pressure sores.

    Weight loss.

2. **Intracranial haemorrhage**

    (a) Extradural.

    (b) Subdural

    (i) Acute—first 48 hours

    (ii) Subacute—2nd to 14th day

    (iii) Chronic—after 14th day.

    (c) Subarachnoid.

    (d) Intracerebral.

3. **Infection**

    (a) Meningitis.

    (b) Abscess.

4. **CSF leak**

    From (a) nose (rhinorrhoea)

    (b) ear (otorrhoea).

5. **Epilepsy**

    (a) Early onset—during first week after head injury.

    (b) Late onset—after first week.

**Residual disability**

A. *Physical disability*. From damage to:

1. Cerebral hemispheres

    (a) Dysphasia

    (b) Hemiparesis.

2. Cranial nerves

    (a) Anosmia

    (b) Visual field defects

    (c) Squints

    (d) Facial weakness

    (e) Deafness and vertigo.

B. *Mental disability*. There may be alteration of personality, and impairment of intellect and memory. Headache, dizziness, fatigue, irritability, and pain at the site of injury are common features of the normal recovery process following a head injury. When properly managed, they are short-lived, but they may persist for weeks or months after the injury (*post-concussional syndrome*).

*Advice to patients on leaving hospital*

The patient must be reassured that he will probably make a complete recovery, and he can help this by taking part in normal physical and mental activities. He may find that his previous occupation is now too worrying, and it may be necessary to advise him about alternative employment. Recovery may be slow and gradual.

## DISEASES OF THE BRAIN

Localised abscesses and primary new growths are the main diseases amenable to surgical treatment. Some intracranial aneurysms and forms of hydrocephalus are treated surgically. Parkinson's disease may be controlled or very noticeably ameliorated by pallidotomy or the related operation of thalamotomy.

### CEREBRAL ABSCESS

It may result from extension of infection from the middle ear or from a frontal sinus. Occasionally the infection is bloodborne. The clinical picture is similar to that of a cerebral tumour.

*Treatment*

This consists of drainage of the abscess by aspiration

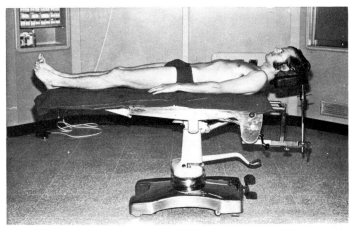

FIG. 45.5   Position for craniotomy.

through a needle and injection of the appropriate antibiotics together with injection of radio-opaque medium to outline the size of the abscess cavity. Craniotomy is occasionally necessary at a later date to excise the abscess wall.

## CEREBRAL TUMOUR

A cerebral tumour may be a simple tumour, commonly a meningioma, or it may be a malignant tumour of the cerebral tissues. Tumours of the pituitary gland are also included in the term 'cerebral tumours'.

The principal symptoms and signs are:

1. Vomiting, unrelated to food.
2. Severe headaches.
3. Papilloedema (swelling of the optic disc due to increased intracranial tension).
4. The localising signs vary with the site of the tumour and consist of sensory and motor changes in various portions of the body.

*Treatment*

If possible, excision is undertaken; but a palliative decompression may be all that can be offered. Radiotherapy is

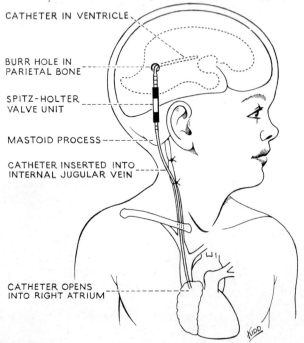

CATHETER IN VENTRICLE

BURR HOLE IN PARIETAL BONE

SPITZ-HOLTER VALVE UNIT

MASTOID PROCESS

CATHETER INSERTED INTO INTERNAL JUGULAR VEIN

CATHETER OPENS INTO RIGHT ATRIUM

FIG. 45.6 Plastic catheter from ventricle to internal jugular vein guarded by Spitz-Holter valve.

another means of treating malignant cerebral lesions, often after confirmation by burr hole biopsy.

## HYDROCEPHALUS

Some cases of hydrocephalus undergo spontaneous resolution. Others are progressive and a chart kept of the size of the head shows an abnormal increase in size and down-turning of the eyes. These cases may be improved by a drainage operation from the ventricles either to the right atrium or to the pleural or peritoneal cavities. A catheter is inserted in the ventricle and is passed via the internal jugular vein to the right atrium below. This entry into the vein is guarded by a Spitz-Holter valve which prevents blood flowing back.

The Spitz-Holter valve is a device which allows fluid to pass through it in one direction only. It lies subcutaneously behind the right ear. The nurse should always keep a careful watch that the valve is functioning properly. In the baby the fontanelles will bulge, the eyes will turn down and there may be convulsions and head retraction if this is not functioning correctly. The older child may complain of headache. Vomiting, drowsiness and a slow pulse may demand urgent operation.

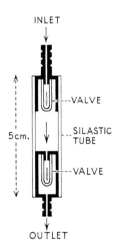

INLET

VALVE

SILASTIC
TUBE

5 cm.

VALVE

OUTLET

Fig. 45.7   Spitz-Holter valve.

The valve itself can normally be compressed easily with the finger and is felt to refill promptly. If it is not functioning correctly it may feel hard, incompressible and fail to refill after emptying. Sometimes a child with an urgently raised pressure can be tided over by pumping the valve (that is pressing it against the skull with the fingers several times an hour).

Other operations for hydrocephalus:

1. A direct attack on the site of the block.
2. Short circuiting the block, for example Torkildsen's operation (lateral ventricle connected to cisterna magna).
3. Thecoperitoneal shunt used only for communicating hydrocephalus (from lumbar theca to peritoneal cavity).

### PARKINSON'S DISEASE

The tremors and rigidity in Parkinson's disease may be relieved by the operation of thalamotomy which involves making a lesion in the ventro-lateral nucleus of the thalamus. This is performed with mathematical precision by a technique in which full craniotomy is not performed. If results are unsatisfactory, a further lesion in the pallidum (pallidotomy) may be considered. Administration of the drug L-Dopa may reduce the need for stereotaxic surgery.

## THE CARE OF A CASE OF CRANIOTOMY
### (An operation in which the skull is opened)

It may be necessary to open the skull for:

1. An injury causing depression of the bone or haemorrhage from a middle meningeal artery.
2. A tumour of the brain or meninges or of the pituitary gland. Surgical treatment is now advised early in acromegaly before optic tract pressure occurs.
3. To control an aneurysm by clipping it at its neck, isolating it by clipping the vessels on either side or investing it in muscle wrapping.
4. An abscess of the brain or meninges.
5. To divide an intracranial nerve root, e.g. division of the sensory root of the fifth for trigeminal neuralgia.
6. Hypophysectomy for carcinoma of the breast.
7. To perform a ventriculogram. This consists of the injection of air into the ventricles after cerebrospinal fluid has been withdrawn.
8. Hydrocephalus.

*Preoperative care*

This will vary considerably from case to case. It will have to be modified if the indications for craniotomy are urgent, and the operation has to be performed almost at once. It will also vary a little with the type of lesion and the degree of consciousness or unconsciousness of the patient. The following is the main outline of the general nursing of these cases:

1. MAINTENANCE OF HEALTH IN ALL OTHER ORGANS IS ESSENTIAL. The patient's limbs may be paralysed, therefore physiotherapy must be provided to prevent permanent deformity.

Insensitive skin areas must be kept clean, free from pressure, and protected from any object such as a hot-water bottle or a cigarette, which may cause a painless burn.

2. FEEDING. The conscious, lucid patient will present no difficulty in feeding unless he has a paralysis of the palate, mouth, or tongue. In the latter case, or if the patient is unconscious, feeding by an intragastric drip will be necessary. The nurse must not attempt to pour fluid into the mouth of an unconscious or semi-conscious patient. Aspiration of food into the lungs is bound to occur with disastrous consequences.

3. THE MOUTH. The mouth will require frequent moistening and cleansing. The danger of parotitis is considerable if the patient is not drinking.

4. PREPARATION OF THE SCALP. This is left until the patient is under anaesthesia. The hair is shaved at this stage for two reasons:

(a) Psychological benefit of the patient.
(b) It is said to produce cleaner skin than if it is done in the ward.

5. DRUGS. Preoperative drugs will be administered as prescribed.

*Postoperative care*

This will vary according to the nature of the operation performed. Careful attention is necessary, and the nurse must be in constant attendance. As with head injuries, an observation chart is vital and should record:

(a) Level of consciousness (i.e. responsiveness).
(b) Pupillary size, equality, and reaction to light.
(c) Pulse rate, blood pressure, respiratory rate, and temperature.
(d) Movement of limbs.
(e) Frequency and nature of fits.

Abnormal signs must be noted and reported at once. At all times the nurse must make a special note of the level of consciousness.

POSITION IN BED. Most cases will be nursed propped up as soon as possible. Special care must be taken to see that the patient does not damage the area of his head on which the operation has been performed. The hands of a restless patient must be secured in light splints so that he does not 'pick off' the dressings.

FEEDING. Feeding must be carefully supervised as indicated in the preoperative treatment.

THE BLADDER. Many patients after major craniotomy operations require catheterisation. Restlessness may simply be due to urinary retention and quickly subsides once urinary flow is restored.

THE DRESSING. Drainage is not usually performed, and unless there are special indications, for example, the onset of pyrexia, or pain, the dressing is not taken down for three days, when half the sutures are removed, and the remainder on the fifth day, when the wound is usually healed. Occasionally there may be a discharge of blood or cerebrospinal fluid, but this requires no special treatment beyond redressing. A Redivac drain is placed under the flap for 24 to 48 hours.

General attention to the bowels and skin areas is important.

THE CARE OF THE EYES is important after section of the trigeminal nerve, because the cornea is insensitive and grit or dust will cause considerable damage to its surface. Sometimes the lids are sewn together (tarsorrhaphy) to protect the cornea. In other cases the eye is protected with a Buller's shield or a celluloid cup, and later replaced by spectacles to which is fitted a special extension to protect the eyeball entirely from the air.

MENTAL REST must be secured. Visitors must be reduced to a minimum and all worry, as far as possible, must be avoided.

## OTHER DISEASES OF THE HEAD

**The scalp.** Sebaceous cysts are common. Osteomas occur occasionally. The scalp area is a favourite site for blood vessel tumours, e.g. haemangiomas.

## INJURIES OF THE SPINE AND SPINAL CORD

Injuries to the spine and spinal cord are of the greatest importance. If the cord is damaged the segments of the body below the level of the injury may be completely cut off from the central nervous system. The muscles are paralysed and the skin and other organs are insensitive.

The nursing care of these patients calls for skill of a very high order.

### FRACTURES OF THE SPINE

The commonest injury in this area is a fracture; much rarer is a fracture-dislocation of the spine.

They may be:

*Incomplete.* Those which do not interfere with the continuity of the spinal column, for example fractures of the spinous or transverse processes.

*Complete fractures* are those which interrupt the continuity of the column and consist of fracture-dislocation of the spine and are most common at C5 to C7 and L3 to L5.

### SPINAL CORD INJURIES

Fracture-dislocations in particular are very frequently associated with injury to the spinal cord. Damage to the cord may be of two types.

1. *Recoverable.* This is due to—
   (a) Spinal shock.
   (b) Bruising, oedema, or pressure of haemorrhage into its coverings. (N.B. injury to the cord itself is permanent and irrecoverable.)
2. *Irrecoverable.* This is due to damage inflicted on the cord and includes transection (tearing).

The clinical features of both types of injury may be the same in the very early stages, and the only method of absolute differentiation is that, in time, spinal shock and oedema will recover, while a transection is an irreversible condition. However, if there is no sign of recovery in 24 or 48 hours the chances of useful function below the level of the lesion are negligible.

In the acute stage the site of damage is vital. The higher in the cord the site of injury the greater is the extent of paralysis and the area of anaesthesia.

*Spinal shock* is a transient condition and, in time, full restoration of function will occur. Similarly, oedema will usually resolve with very little, if any, residual disability.

*Transection* terminates fatally sooner or later, but if the site of injury is very low, recovery with considerable disability may occur.

Above the level of the fourth cervical segment complete lesions are fatal, since respiratory paralysis occurs at once. There is little that can be achieved by surgical operation apart from reduction of the fracture or fracture-dislocation of the spine. The treatment is confined entirely to the nursing care, which aims at the maintenance of health in the paralysed tissues so that, if recovery of nervous function results, the tissues are in good condition to resume their duty. Fracture-dislocations of the cervical spine may be treated by skull traction.

*Symptoms and signs*

Most cases are associated with a fracture or fracture-dislocation of the spinal column. There will be a history of a severe injury. Below the damaged area all the tissues are paralysed. For example, a fracture-dislocation of the mid-thoracic spine may result in the following symptoms:

1. Paralysis of the muscles of the legs and the abdomen. Initially the legs are flaccid, becoming spastic as spinal shock gradually subsides.
2. Absence of all sensation in the skin below the costal margin. The patient is unaware of the position of his legs, the condition of his bladder, and, of course, is unable to feel pain, heat, or cold.
3. The reflexes may be absent in the lower limbs initially but become exaggerated as spinal shock subsides.
4. Absence of control of the bladder. After a period of urinary retention due to spinal shock, the bladder becomes automatic, emptying when the pressure within rises.
5. The patient may be in acute circulatory failure. Paralysis and loss of sensation may result in:
   (a) Wasting of the muscles.
   (b) Trophic changes (i.e. a dry withered appearance of skin and later ulceration).
   (c) Bed sores.
   (d) Urinary infection, to which a neglected patient will usually succumb. The bladder must receive the appropriate care if its function is defective. A tidal drainage system may have been applied or a Gibbon catheter inserted.
6. Hypostatic pneumonia.

*Treatment*

FIRST-AID TREATMENT. All cases suspected of a fracture of the spine should be carried in the prone position, and kept in this position until the fracture has been reduced. There is however no great objection to carrying them supine provided a pillow is placed in the small of the back to keep the spine extended.

FRACTURE OF THE SPINE WITHOUT PARALYSIS. The fracture is easily reduced by placing the patient in extension in bed with a pillow under the small of the back. Extension exercises are practised and in two weeks the patient is discharged wearing a posterior spinal support.

FRACTURE OF THE SPINE WITH PARALYSIS. Most cases are nursed on a sorbo bed with a pillow behind the dorsolumbar spine. A ripple bed or Stryker frame may be of value. All cord injuries suffer from urinary retention for days or years or perhaps permanently and much of the mortality of spinal injuries is due to urinary infection causing pyelonephritis, the infection initially having been introduced by catheterisation. Many surgeons advise scrupulously aseptic intermittent catheterisation in the first instance. An indwelling Gibbon catheter should be inserted as soon as it seems that long-standing retention is inevitable. If infection supervenes suprapubic cystotomy may be necessary.

## CARE OF THE PARALYSED LIMBS

*Skin and pressure areas.* These must be kept dry and clean, since many patients are incontinent of faeces as well as urine. The buttocks and sacral areas require the greatest care. The patient must be turned every two hours or as frequently as possible. Hot-water bottles are not allowed. A suitable sorbo bed and the careful use of air rings and rubber cushions will minimise risks. The arms should be nursed outside the bedclothes and the elbows slightly flexed. The fingers should be curved around a small ball or a piece of sorbo rubber. The legs are supported by sorbo wedges to guard against footdrop. One limb should never lie over the other and a bed cradle is used to relieve the weight of the bedclothes.

*Muscles.* The muscles waste rapidly and contractures are liable to develop. All the joints should be put through a normal range of movement each day, and the physiotherapist must attend to give massage in the early stages and to encourage exercises as recovery takes place. Splintage is inadvisable.

*Meteorism* (i.e. distension due to gas in the intestinal tract). this must be relieved by the passage of a flatus tube. If the patient is in plaster it may be necessary to cut an abdominal window in the plaster to give relief.

*Hypostatic pneumonia.* Hypostatic pneumonia is particularly liable to occur in these cases, and is best prevented by frequent movement of the patient, antibiotics and deep breathing exercises.

*Sign of recovery.* The return of sensation followed by twitching of the muscles of the paralysed limb are the first signs of recovery. Recovery of finer sensation follows.

Electrical reactions are performed as a guide to recovery. The absence of signs after a few days usually indicates a complete transection of the cord, and leaves no doubt about the permanency of the damage.

*Rehabilitation.* Suitable cases will require rehabilitation including occupational therapy. It is very easy for the patient to develop a neurosis if he is allowed to think his back has been split in two!

If some muscle groups are damaged and others intact, exercises and re-education are an important part of treatment at this stage if the patient is to secure the best possible functional result. The arm and trunk muscles of the patient should be used in his own nursing care, so that they are kept healthy and increased in power if possible.

## DISEASES OF THE SPINE AND SPINAL CORD

### CONGENITAL

Spina bifida
Meningocele
Myelomeningocele

These conditions are due to a failure of fusion of the laminae of the vertebra, particularly in the lower portion of the spine.

1. **Spina bifida.** Spina bifida is a condition in which the spinal cord is covered only by skin or muscle instead of by bone. In mild cases there are no symptoms or signs, and the condition is diagnosed as an accidental finding on X-rays. In other cases there is evidence of flattening, and the overlying skin is covered with a soft tuft of hair. There may be partial paralysis of the feet due to traction on the nerves supplying the feet as these nerves emerge from the spinal cord. Club foot deformities may occur.

An operation may have to be undertaken to separate the nerves in the cord from the skin, and deformity of the feet will require correction.

2. **Meningocele.** The membranes of the cord (the meninges) bulge on to the skin, and the appearances are those of a large bluish cyst, which becomes more tense as the baby

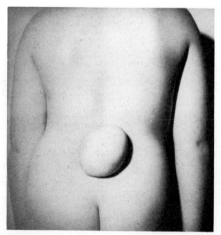

FIG. 45.8   Meningocele.

coughs or cries. The spinal cord itself is not involved. The condition is noticed at birth.

Unless the greatest care is taken the coverings rupture, with the escape of cerebrospinal fluid. Infection sets in and the infant dies of meningitis.

*Treatment*

If the skin overlying the bulging is healthy there is no urgency to operate. It is essential that the skin be very carefully protected—maceration from wet napkins leading to ulceration must be avoided. Wool or lint may be used to pad the swelling which should be washed, dried and powdered at each napkin change. Most of these children will grow up to be normal adults after closure of the defect, although some will have minor neurological defects in the legs or difficulty with the anal or bladder sphincters.

3. **Myelomeningocele.** This is a condition in which nervous tissue bulges through the bony defect and the spinal cord is exposed on the surface as a flat ribbon. It is usually associated with some paralysis below the level of the lesion. Paralysis may be minor or in the most severe cases complete paraplegia may exist. In addition, there may be deformities of the lower limbs, deformities of the vertebral column, dribbling incontinence, and hydrocephalus.

*Treatment*

Myelomeningocele is a condition which requires operation usually within 24 hours of birth. The baby should be handled gently to avoid rupture of the delicate sac. A moist saline pad should be placed over the lesion and lightly bandaged in position. If the bladder is paralysed suprapubic pressure will cause urine to be passed. A specimen of the mother's blood as well as details of the pregnancy and labour should be sent with the baby on transfer to another hospital for operation. The aim of surgery is to achieve satisfactory closure of the defect. Postoperatively the baby is nursed on its side in an incubator, being changed from side to side every two hours or alternatively partly suspended face downwards in elastic slings passed under the abdomen. Babies are nursed with the head low for the first few days to minimise a leak of cerebrospinal fluid. The baby should be handled as little as possible and should be fed in the incubator while lying in slings, thus avoiding any pressure on the delicate wound in the back.

As these children grow, facilities for their care and education outside the hospital have to be used.

## ACQUIRED

Tuberculosis of the spine
Tumours

**Tuberculosis of the spine.** Tuberculous disease of the spine (Pott's disease) is a blood-borne tuberculous infection which may occur at any age, but usually occurs in children. Any site may be attacked, but the dorsolumbar area is the one most commonly affected.

*Clinical features*

1. *Local pain.* Pain in the back is frequently the first symptom. The child is careful about putting his feet on the floor, because stamping them quickly may jar the spine and increase the pain. Referred pain may occur, and, if referred to the abdomen or chest, appendicitis or pleurisy may be suspected.

2. *Rigidity.* Rigidity of the spine occurs in the early stages, and is due to spasm of the spinal muscles in an attempt to restrict movements which cause pain.

3. *Deformity.* Kyphosis is the commonest deformity and if severe limits free movement of the chest.

4. *Abscess formation.* Abscess formation may be an early symptom or may appear as the disease progresses. Classically, it appears in the groin (psoas cold abscess). It is painless, and the temperature may be only very slightly raised. Incision is rarely performed.

5. *Nervous signs.* Nervous signs may appear as the disease progresses, and are due to a cold abscess pressing on the spinal cord. A complete paralysis, similar to that described under Injuries to the Cord, may appear.

*Treatment*

The principles of treatment are:

1. The improvement and restoration of the general health (antituberculosis measures, including streptomycin, PAS and INAH).

2. Local treatment aims at complete rest of the spine until the softened diseased bone has recalcified and abscesses, if present, have resolved.

In lesions of the thoracic and lumbar spine, a plaster bed will usually be employed. In the rarer cases of tuberculosis affecting the cervical spine a frame may be used or only a cervical collar may be necessary. Some cases require preliminary traction.

*Abscess formation.* In most cases anterolateral decompression is performed.

*Paraplegia.* Special care must be taken of the paralysed limbs as described on page 525. Most cases recover spontaneously if immobilisation of the spine is continued. Occasionally operative measures may have to be taken to evacuate the abscess in the spine. In a case of Pott's disease in the adult a bone graft may be undertaken to aid recovery.

*Education of the child*

Since treatment will be spread over two or three years it is desirable that the child should be treated in an institution specially equipped so that he can continue, as far as possible, a normal education.

## TUMOURS OF THE SPINE AND SPINAL CORD

Secondary malignant growths in the bony spine are common, and a sign that the disease is already far advanced. Radiotherapy may be appropriate.

**Primary tumours of the spinal meninges and the spinal cord.** Primary tumours in this area are much less common than secondary lesions in the bone. The chief symptoms and signs are those of increasing paralysis preceded by pain and later followed by anaesthesia.

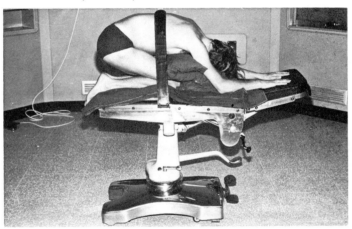

FIG. 45.9    Position for laminectomy.

Careful investigation is necessary to localise the exact site of the tumour. A lumbar puncture is performed and the pressure of the cerebrospinal fluid is measured. During the lumbar puncture, Queckenstedt's test is performed: compression of the jugular veins produces a rapid rise in the CSF pressure, and when the jugular veins are released the CSF pressure quickly falls again. A slow (or absent) rise and fall suggests a partial (or complete) block in the spinal subarachnoid space. A specimen of fluid is sent to the laboratory for examination. The protein content of the cerebrospinal fluid is raised when there is evidence of a spinal block.

The lower border of the tumour is outlined by lumbar myelography. However, if the block is complete, cisternal myelography may be considered.

*Treatment*

Laminectomy is undertaken to remove the tumour.

The usual position is the Mohammedan praying position to avoid any venous congestion due to pressure on the abdomen and therefore to reduce bleeding to a minimum. The position for this operation is shown in Figure 45.9. The laminae of several vertebrae are removed with special forceps and the strong spinal muscles retracted by a self-retaining retractor.

Nursing care is similar to that described for injuries of the spine, and the aftercare of the wound is the same as that for any other clean operative wound.

# CHAPTER 46

# The Peripheral Nerves

Lesions of the peripheral nerves include:
1. Injuries.
2. Peripheral neuritis.
3. Neuralgia.
4. Tumours.

## INJURIES TO THE PERIPHERAL NERVES

An injury to a nerve results in loss of function in the area supplied by that nerve. If the division is complete, the loss of function is complete. If it is partial, only a partial disability results. Complete division of a nerve may result in:

1. *Motor changes*, i.e., immediate loss of power and later wasting in the muscles which the nerve supplies.

2. *Sensory changes*. Pain, heat and cold cannot be appreciated in the skin area supplied by the nerve.

3. *Trophic changes*. By this is meant the curious undernourished appearance which develops in the skin. At first it is white, dry and scaly. Later the skin is shiny, then bluish in colour and painless ulceration may occur.

### TYPES OF INJURY

1. *Complete division* (the most severe injury).
2. *Partial division.*
3. *Contusion.* The nerve fibres have been bruised and fail to conduct the impulses, but usually full recovery takes place in time.
4. *Compression.* A constant source of pressure, e.g. a tumour pressing on the nerve may result in failure of conduction. Occasionally the tumour arises in the nerve sheath.

### THE TREATMENT OF NERVE INJURIES

1. *Prevention*
The nurse must take every precaution to avoid injury to the nerves. The important examples are:
(a) An unconscious patient's arm must never be allowed to

531

hang over the edge of the bed or the operating table as this may cause a radial paralysis.

(b) Intramuscular injections are given into the only safe place, i.e. the upper outer aspect of the buttock where there are no important nerves.

(c) Skin traction on a Thomas' splint or abduction frame must avoid the neck of the fibula, because the lateral popliteal nerve is very near the skin surface at this point and may be damaged.

### 2. *Treatment*

The vast majority of nerve injuries are not operated upon until the surgeon is certain that division has occurred. In many cases he will advise waiting to see if recovery takes place.

In all cases he will require that the paralysed or anaesthetic area be kept in good condition, so that when recovery takes place the tissues can take up their function again. The following general principles are fundamental:

*Paralysed muscles* must not be overstretched. For example, a drop wrist (due to radial paralysis) is placed on a cock-up splint and kept on the splint until recovery occurs. Not for one second must the wrist be allowed to drop; even when changing the splint the wrist must be *held* cocked up. Failure to do this will delay recovery several weeks. Similarly, a drop foot is splinted at the right angle and kept splinted.

Massage is valuable in maintaining the circulation. Passive exercises help to avoid contractures. Regular electrical (galvanic) stimulation is useful in maintaining circulation and movement.

*Insensitive skin* requires special care. Insensitive fingers are easily burnt quite painlessly by cigarettes. The patient must be warned of the danger, but it is wise in addition to cover the fingers or hand with a kid glove, as this increases the margin of safety.

Hot-water bottles, the ends of bed cradles, radiant heat lamps, and other ward furniture must be carefully guarded.

## PERIPHERAL NEURITIS

Although the word 'neuritis' implies inflammation of a nerve, this is not a constant feature of peripheral neuritis. The causes are numerous, and include:

Hereditary diseases, e.g. peroneal muscular atrophy
Metabolic disorders, e.g. diabetes mellitus
Nutritional deficiencies, e.g. vitamin B deficiencies
Poisons, e.g. alcohol

Infections, e.g. diphtheria
Drugs, e.g. furadantin
Malignant disease, e.g. carcinoma of the bronchus.

The symptoms are:

1. Flaccid weakness which may progress to paralysis.
2. Parasthesiae (numbness, tingling, pins and needles) spreading up the limbs in a "glove and stocking" manner. There may be great pain, and the muscles may be extremely tender.

Treatment is related to cause. Surgery has nothing to offer.

## NEURALGIA

This describes paroxysmal pain along the course of a nerve. Examples are trigeminal and glossopharyngeal neuralgia, postherpetic neuralgia, and phantom limb pain. Surgical treatment aims at dividing the sensory nerves involved. Numerous procedures are described but relief is by no means guaranteed. Occasionally phantom limb pain is relieved by electrical stimulation of the dorsal columns of the spinal cord via an electrode implant (p. 39).

## TUMOURS OF THE NERVES

Multiple fibromata may occur in the condition known as multiple neurofibromatosis (Von Recklinghausen's disease). A

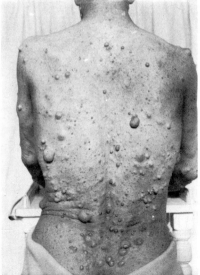

FIG. 46.1   Multiple neurofibromatosis.

solitary fibroma may occur and is a not uncommon cause of pain in the severed nerve of an amputation stump.

## LESIONS OF THE INDIVIDUAL NERVES

Only the common lesions of the peripheral nerves will be mentioned:

### THE CRANIAL NERVES

The first (olfactory) is the nerve of smell. Injury destroys the sense of smell.

The second (optic) is the nerve of vision. Injury causes blindness in the affected eye.

The third, fourth and sixth control the movements of the eyeball. If one of these nerves is damaged a squint will result.

The fifth is mainly a sensory nerve, supplying the face. Inflammation will cause pain in the affected area—trigeminal neuralgia.

The motor portion of the fifth cranial nerve supplies the muscles which control mastication, and damage will cause interference with this mechanism.

The seventh or facial nerve may be injured as a result of a fracture of the skull, at operation, or without any apparent cause (Bell's palsy). The patient dribbles from the drooping corner of his mouth and is unable to close the eyelid on the affected side (Fig. 46.2).

The eighth is the auditory nerve. Injury to this nerve will cause deafness and labyrinthine disturbance.

The ninth or glossopharyngeal supplies the palate, and par-

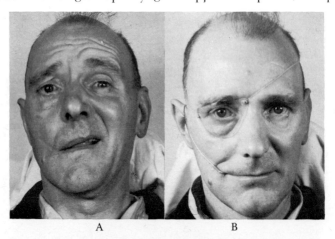

A                                    B

FIG. 46.2  A, Facial paralysis. B, Paralysis splinted. A plastic eye-shade protects the cornea from dust.

alysis results in difficulty in swallowing. It may occur as a complication of diphtheria.

The tenth cranial nerve, the vagus, controls the heart rate and the movements and secretions in the gastrointestinal tract. Occasionally to reduce excessive gastric acid secretion some of its fibres are divided (p. 369).

The eleventh is the accessory nerve, injury to which results in wasting of the trapezius (shoulder) and sternomastoid muscles.

The twelfth, the hypoglossal, is the motor nerve of the tongue, and injury will cause wasting of one side of the tongue.

## THE BRACHIAL PLEXUS

1. *Birth injuries*. The brachial plexus (a nerve junction at the side of the neck and under the clavicle) may be injured by the tearing of the large nerve trunks during birth.

2. *Traumatic lesions* may be due to stretching of the shoulder girdle.

3. *Cervical rib*. This condition usually causes no trouble until the patient is about 40 years of age. The nerve roots are irritated as they pass over the rib.

Injuries to the brachial plexus may involve the whole plexus or only certain fibres. A typical Erb's paralysis is shown in Fig. 46.3. It is an injury to the upper portion of the brachial plexus.

## THE NERVES OF THE ARM

1. The axillary nerve may be damaged in injuries around the shoulder joint, and this results in wasting of the deltoid muscle.

2. Injury to the radial nerve causes wrist drop (Fig. 46.4).

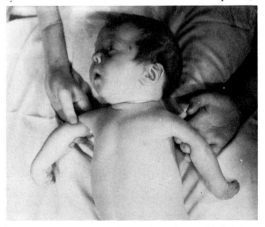

FIG. 46.3   Bilateral Erb's paralysis due to birth injury.

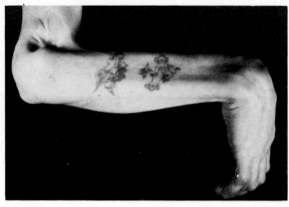

FIG. 46.4  Wrist-drop. Radial paralysis. The nerve was injured in the wound above the elbow.

3. As a result of injury to the ulnar nerve at the elbow the skin over the inner one and a half fingers of the hand is anaesthetised and there is wasting of certain forearm muscles and small muscles of the hand.

4. Injury to the median nerve causes anaesthesia over the outer three and a half fingers and also wasting of the small muscles of the thumb. The median nerve is sometimes compressed in the carpal tunnel and simple release is curative.

### THE SCIATIC AND LATERAL POPLITEAL NERVES

The sciatic nerve may be damaged as a result of dislocation of the hip, and its branches may be damaged by wounds elsewhere between the hip and knee. The main disability caused is foot drop and the loss of all muscular power below the knee.

### SCIATICA

Sciatica is a common complaint and is due to many causes:

1. An inflammatory condition of the nerve.

2. An irritative condition in the root of the nerve, such as an osteophyte, if the patient is suffering from osteoarthrosis of the spine, or a prolapsed intervertebral disc.

3. The condition may be secondary to a growth of the pelvic organs, e.g. carcinoma of the rectum or uterus infiltrating the sacral plexus or secondary deposit from more distant sites such as the bronchus.

*Clinical features*

The pain is felt in the lower back and radiates into the buttock, down the back of the thigh, often into the outer side of the calf and heel and across the outer border of the foot. It is usually made worse by movement or coughing and is eased by rest.

Most cases are associated with backache and are due to degenerative disease of the lumbar spine, that is osteoarthrosis, spondylosis, disc degeneration or prolapse of a disc due to degenerative disease or injury. The typical patient is admitted with acute back pain and sciatica and has had a sudden onset of pain following lifting a weight or rising from the bent position. He is usually in great pain with a rigid lumbar spine and has a positive straight leg raising test (that is, can only raise a straight leg to 20 or 30 degrees before pain occurs in his back). The ankle jerk may be absent and there may be anaesthesia or weakness of the muscles which dorsiflex the foot if a nerve root is being pressed upon.

*Treatment*

The patient with severe pain should be:

1. Put to bed on a mattress which does not sag.

2. Analgesics should be freely prescribed in the acute case during the first few days.

3. Skin traction to both legs for 10 to 14 days will often relieve an acute attack.

4. As the pain settles spinal extension (not flexion) exercises should be commenced.

5. A suitable belt is prescribed (e.g. Goldthwaite type) to support the lumbar spine.

6. In obstinate cases several weeks in a plaster jacket may be necessary.

7. Manipulation of the spine under anaesthesia may benefit selected cases.

8. Operative removal of the prolapsed disc may be necessary when repeated attacks of sciatica due to disc protrusions are failing to respond to conservative treatment.

*Advice to the patient*

After subsidence of the acute attack, the patient should be advised:

1. To avoid heavy lifting.

2. To sleep on a firm bed.

3. To avoid rising from a chair too suddenly.

4. To do spinal exercises regularly and to swim if at all possible.

5. A change of occupation may be necessary.

## FEMORAL NEURITIS

The pain is felt in the front of the thigh and is often extremely severe and may be associated with wasting of the quadriceps muscles and absence of the knee jerk. The causes are similar to those of sciatica with which condition it is often confused.

The patient is most comfortable sitting up with the knees and hips flexed, whilst the patient with sciatica is most comfortable when he is flat.

Treatment consists of rest, warmth and analgesics combined with the prescription of a belt for the lumbar spine. The occasional infiltration of the nerve with a local anaesthetic may be helpful.

## PREPARATION FOR OPERATION FOR THE RESUTURE OF A PERIPHERAL NERVE

When it has been decided to operate on a peripheral nerve it is vital to avoid infection.

In addition to the precautions mentioned elsewhere of splintage, massage, and the preparation of the skin, latent sepsis is sometimes discovered by provocative vigorous massage and heat to see if infection can be caused to flare up. In this case operation is deferred.

The incision made for suture of a peripheral nerve is frequently very long indeed, and the nurse must prepare a very extensive area of skin.

Postoperatively, maintenance of the correct position of the limb is secured by splints or other retentive apparatus.

CHAPTER 47

# Fractures

Fractures are very common indeed, but the fracture is only part of a complex injury. In the simplest fractures there is danger in varying degrees to the muscle, tendons and overlying skin. Perfect anatomical position and the soundest union of the fracture may be obtained, yet if some simple point in the treatment has been neglected the end result may be unsatisfactory. For example, a perfect result may be obtained in the bony injury of a Colles's fracture, but if the patient has kept her fingers absolutely immobile until the plaster or splint is removed the stiffness which is present may persist for ever.

The nurse must be aware of the common sites and the main features of a fracture. Not infrequently she is the first person to see the patient who is brought into hospital suffering from a fracture. She must take the appropriate steps to provide adequate splintage so that the fracture does not become compound, and to ensure that the patient is in the best possible position to avoid further damage as a result of his fracture. For example, a patient with a suspected fracture of the cervical spine must not flex his head.

### TYPES OF FRACTURE

There are two main types of fracture:

1. **Closed or simple fracture.** The bone is broken but protected against the risk of external infection by intact skin or mucous membrane.

2. **Open or compound fracture.** The broken bones communicate with the exterior through a wound of the skin or mucosa, and are thereby exposed to contamination by pyogenic or gas-forming bacteria.

#### ANATOMICAL VARIETIES OF FRACTURE

1. **Oblique or spiral fracture.** The fracture line runs obliquely or twists around the bone in a corkscrew-like fashion (Fig. 47.1 A and B).

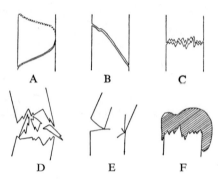

FIG. 47.1   Varieties of fracture.

2. **Transverse fracture.** The fracture runs across the bone (Fig. 47.1 c).

3. **Comminuted fracture.** The bone is divided into more than two pieces or fragments. There are three or more fragments—that is, two main fragments and some smaller ones between them (Fig. 47.1 d).

4. **Greenstick fracture.** The fracture is incomplete and does not extend across the whole diameter of the bone. This type of fracture is common in children because their bones are more elastic and tend to bend rather than to break (Fig. 47.1 e).

5. **Impacted fracture.** One fragment is driven into the other and locked in position. The result is that the abnormal mobility which is a common sign of a fracture will be absent in these cases (Fig. 47.1 f).

Any of these anatomical varieties may be simple or compound. Should a nerve, viscus or a large artery be damaged by the fracture it is known as a 'complicated fracture'.

A separated epiphysis is really a fracture through the metaphysis and not the epiphysis; uncorrected, deficient growth of the bone results.

### CAUSES OF A FRACTURE

1. *Direct violence.* A blow may cause a fracture of the bone immediately beneath the site of impact.

2. *Indirect violence.* A fall on the heel may cause a fracture of the spine, due to the transmission of the violence by the bones of the legs.

3. *Muscular violence.* Sudden strong muscular contraction may cause a fracture. Transverse fractures of the patella usually arise in this way, e.g., in jumping.

**Pathological fractures.** Pathological fractures are the result of bone disease, for example, a cyst or tumour causing preliminary softening. A pathological fracture may occur secondarily with little or no injury.

## SYMPTOMS AND SIGNS OF FRACTURE

1. *Pain* aggravated by movement is the most prominent symptom. Pain, although usually present, is by no means invariable. Impacted fractures are sometimes relatively painless.

2. *Loss of function* is usually complete but one must beware of missing an impacted fracture of the humerus or femur where the patient despite the fracture can sometimes use the limb fairly well.

3. *Swelling and bruising.*

4. *Deformity* is present if there is displacement of the fragments.

5. *Shortening* of the limb is present when overriding or impaction of the fragments occurs.

6. *Abnormal mobility.*

7. *Crepitus*, or grating, on movement of the fragments will be present. This is a sign which should never be elicited. It is painful, not without danger, and usually unnecessary.

8. *Tenderness* over the fracture line is usually present.

Radiographic examination must always be undertaken and should include two views. If possible, it is taken before the fracture is reduced, always after reduction of the fracture, and again after each change of plaster or splint.

Not all the signs detailed will be present in every case of fracture, and the pitfall in diagnosis lies in the fact that, in many cases, tenderness may be the only feature suggestive of the presence of a fracture.

## COMPLICATIONS OF FRACTURES

Complications of fractures may be general or local.

### General

1. *Acute circulatory failure.* Blood loss is usually severe in multiple fractures and in large compound fractures. It has to be treated without delay. In compound fractures the blood loss is obvious—but it is easy to overlook the considerable haemorrhage into the tissues around a simple closed fracture. In a simple fracture of the femur this amounts to at least one litre.

2. *Hypostatic pneumonia.* This is a frequent complication in a patient of advancing years and is prevented by:

(a) Allowing the patient out of bed as soon as possible.
(b) Changing the patient's position in bed as frequently as possible.
(c) Deep breathing exercises.

3. *Pulmonary embolism* is a real risk complicating fractures of

the legs or pelvis in elderly patients and in selected cases anti-coagulant therapy will reduce its incidence.

4. *Bed sores* (p. 198).

5. *Decubitus renal calculi.*

6. *Fat embolism* is very much commoner than has been suspected in the past. The clinical picture is one of deep unconsciousness, high fever, tachycardia and tachypnoea. The patient is treated by hypothermia and in addition all the measures for the management of deep coma including tracheostomy are undertaken.

**Local**

1. *Injury to blood vessels, nerves, joints, and the viscera* may occur, and is indicated in the discussion on the appropriate fracture. Adhesions or traumatic arthritis may occur if the joint is injured or if the limb is not used. Volkmann's ischaemic contracture due to loss of circulation in the muscles is another possible complication.

2. *Infection* is the great danger of compound fractures, i.e.:

(a) Anaerobic tetanus and gas gangrene may occur. All patients with open wounds are treated prophylactically according to their immunity status to prevent tetanus.

(b) Aerobic or septic infection of the soft tissues or bone may occur.

3. *Non-union.* The fracture may fail to unite. The ends of the fragments become smooth, so that there is an additional joint in the limb (Figs. 47.2 and 47.3). The commonest cause

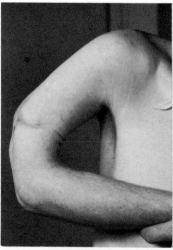 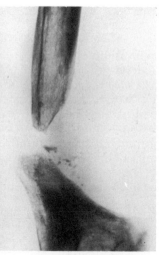

FIG. 47.2   Ununited fracture of humerus.

FIG. 47.3   Radiograph of same case showing non-union of bone.

of non-union is immobilisation for too short a period. Too frequent changing of plasters or splints will disturb the delicate healing tissues. Owing to an inadequate blood supply certain sites are more prone to non-union than others. The lower third of the tibia is a particularly common site of this complication. Infection may cause non-union; it always delays union. The inter-position of soft tissues between the fragments is an occasional cause of non-union.

4. *Mal-union.* The fragments have not been reduced, consolidation occurs in the faulty position, and deformity persists (Fig. 47.4).

## THE TREATMENT OF FRACTURES

When a patient sustains a fracture there is an exudation of blood between the fragments. This haematoma is converted into granulation tissue in the course of a few days, and calcium is deposited in its substance. This tissue is now known as callus. In time the callus is converted into bone. If the bone ends are allowed to grate on each other constantly the callus is unable to grow in strength and bone is unable to form. It is for this reason that complete immobilisation of the fragments is so important.

*The principles of treatment are:*
  1. Reduction of the fracture.
  2. Complete immobilisation until the fracture has united.
  3. Restoration of full functional activity.

### THE REDUCTION OF THE FRACTURE

The reduction or setting of the fracture is necessary only if displacement has occurred. Full reduction is not always neces-

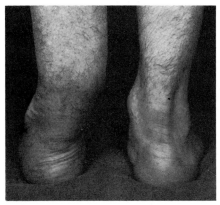

FIG. 47.4   Mal-united Pott's fracture.

sary for full restoration of function, and the surgeon will decide whether or not this has to be attempted after full consideration of the case. Reduction is usually effected by manipulation, and occasionally skeletal traction may be advisable. Sometimes it may be necessary to perform an operation to reduce the fragments and secure them in position. This is known as open reduction and can be undertaken only after the most meticulous care has been taken to prepare the skin.

### IMMOBILISATION OF THE FRACTURE

Complete immobilisation of the fragments is essential for union. Plaster of Paris, because it can be moulded around the limb to splint most fractures, is used very extensively. In certain sites splints may be the treatment of choice, e.g., a Thomas' splint for fracture of the femoral shaft. The period of immobilisation in plaster or splints cannot be definitely laid down. The correct period is until the fracture is united, and this will show considerable variation in different patients. Certain impacted fractures of the upper limb are self-immobilising and require no splintage.

With the advent of antibiotics to prevent infection, there has been a tendency to use internal fixation by screws or nails to obtain a better position in suitable cases. This has the further advantage that the joints above and below are not immobilised and do not become stiff. The screws and pins are made of vitallium or stainless steel.

### The care of the patient in plaster and splints

Plaster and splints are of the greatest value in treating fractures, but a nurse must never forget that they can be horribly destructive, and if the greatest care is not taken the patient may, overnight, have lost the whole limb because a plaster was too tight. The nurse must *never* neglect the most trivial complaint of a patient whose limb is enclosed in plaster.

The extremities, particularly the fingers and toes, are watched, and pain, coldness, discoloration, loss of movement or numbness, must be reported at once, whatever the time of the day or night. In addition, pain at any point in the limb, e.g. at the rough edges of the plaster, is carefully noted.

After the first 48 hours the presence of pyrexia, sleeplessness or the slightest deterioration in the general condition are significant and should be reported at once. These general symptoms and signs, together with the patient's complaint of pain, are the only guide to what is happening under the plaster—for example, a plaster sore.

Patients are often frightened by the fearsome-looking appearance of the saw used for removal of the plaster. In addition it makes a good deal of noise. The saw blade does not rotate but merely vibrates and the nurse can reassure the patient that it does not cut the flesh.

### APPLICATION OF PLASTER OF PARIS:
The following are required:

> Bowl of tepid water
> Pail to collect papers, ends of plaster, etc.
> Stockinette of appropriate size
> Velband 3 inches and/or 6 inches
> Plaster shears, cutters, scissors
> Plastic aprons and sheets.

### APPLICATION TO A LIMB
Stockinette is applied to the limb, reaching two inches above and below the extent to which the plaster is to be applied. The same area is covered with Velband.

The limb is held in position, the palms of the hand being used to support it. The paper wrapping is removed from the plaster of Paris bandage. About six inches of the bandage is released and the bandage immersed in the tepid water until bubbling ceases. It is lifted from the water, using two hands, and is squeezed at the ends from without inwards.

The bandage is applied to the limb commencing at the site of the fracture, then from below to above. An even steady tension is used without twisting. The stockinette is turned back and fixed by one of the layers of bandage. The plaster is polished (smoothed) and moulded to the limb. The skin above and below the plaster is cleaned and dried so as to allow observation of the parts. The colour is checked to ensure adequate circulation.

If conscious, the patient is asked if he is comfortable and told to move the fingers or toes. If an outpatient, he is given a leaflet with instructions before he goes home.

In bed, a leg is rested on a covered pillow and a cradle placed over it with the bedclothes turned back, thus allowing circulation of air and the plaster to dry. An arm is elevated, and suspended using a roller towel.

The fingers or toes are checked at least hourly for the first 24 hours for changes in colour, swelling, disturbed feeling and movement. These changes are reported if present. The patient is told to move his fingers or toes to assist the circulation.

The plaster is examined for cracks, softness and discoloration—these signs are reported when present. Any complaint by the patient of pain, tightness or discomfort *must* be reported immediately.

If a patient in a non-weightbearing leg plaster is allowed out of bed, he should use crutches when walking, instructions in using them first being given.

When removing the plaster, care must be taken not to damage the skin. Afterwards, the area is washed and dried. the application of a crêpe bandage or of Elastoplast may be ordered for support.

### RESTORATION OF FUNCTIONAL ACTIVITY

This is designed to achieve full movement of all the joints which are not immobilised, in the early stages, and later a full range of movement in the joints which have of necessity been kept at rest.

The muscles tend to waste from disuse, and active movements must be encouraged. In certain cases massage is of great advantage, but used indiscriminately it may produce the opposite effect to that desired. Rehabilitation and graduated exercises are all-important when union has occurred.

Most patients have a very long way to go after the plaster has been removed. Left to their own devices, their condition becomes stationary and they are mentally dispirited. Physiotherapy, such as massage, radiant heat, wax baths and remedial exercises, precede courses of organised games or occupations in the correction of gait and posture.

## THE TREATMENT OF COMPOUND FRACTURES

As an urgent operation the wound is cleansed, foreign matter and dead tissues are excised, and the skin sutured if possible. If this is not possible, early healing is encouraged by the provision of free drainage and minimising infection. Under suitable conditions a large skin defect may be closed by skin graft. The fracture is reduced and immobilised.

The principles of treatment of a compound fracture are the same as those for treatment of a simple fracture; in fact, the underlying principle is to convert them into closed fractures at the earliest opportunity.

### GENERAL AND FIRST AID TREATMENT

1. The limb must be lightly but firmly splinted.
2. Haemorrhage may be severe, and must be controlled.
3. Human tetanus antitoxin may be prescribed as a prophylactic measure unless the patient has already been immunised by tetanus toxoid.

## LOCAL TREATMENT

When the patient's condition has improved sufficiently he is taken to the operating theatre and anaesthetised. In many cases the removal of the clothing is not completed until he has been anaesthetised. The limb is shaved, washed and painted with Savlon (1 : 100). The wound is then cleansed with saline, foreign bodies removed, and dead tissue cut away. Bleeding is controlled. The skin is sutured if possible. If this is not possible, or the time since the injury is more than 12 hours, the wound is left open. The fracture is reduced and the limb encased in plaster without cutting a window. Systemic antibacterial substances are of the greatest value in preventing and diminishing infection.

*Postoperative care*

In many cases a low-grade pyrexia occurs for some days and then subsides. The plaster is changed in two or three weeks and the patient is radiographed when a new plaster has been applied.

A swinging temperature may occur, due to inadequate drainage. The fingers or toes, as the case may be, are carefully inspected after the application of plaster, and any of the symptoms enumerated on page 544 must be reported at once.

Some haemorrhage always occurs, due to oozing from small blood vessels, and the plaster will usually be blood-stained to some extent. Later, secondary haemorrhage may occur as a result of extensive infection. Gas gangrene may develop under the plaster, and its onset is heralded by intense pain and rapid deterioration in the patient's general condition, a rapid pulse and toxic appearance, and possibly by a foul smell (p. 72).

*Diet.* In the first two days the diet should consist of plenty of fluids, but as soon as the patient feels like it a normal diet is given, rich in calcium and vitamin D and including 600 ml of fresh milk daily.


## FRACTURES OF THE UPPER LIMB

### FRACTURES OF THE CLAVICLE

Fractures of the clavicle are fairly common, and usually occur in the middle third of the bone as a result of a fall on the outstretched hand. Pain is present over the bone and is more severe on movement of the arm. Deformity is usually obvious. A figure-of-eight bandage is applied after large pads of gamgee have been placed in front of the shoulders and in the axillae. The shoulders are held well backwards by the bandage, so maintaining reduction of the fracture. Bandages will require tightening every two or three days. A sling is used on the affected side to elevate the shoulder.

Perfect anatomical union is rarely regained and some deformity persists, but the functional end result is good. The nurse must encourage the patient to use the fingers, the wrist and the elbow joint as much as possible. Tingling or blueness of the fingers must be reported.

If it is essential to obtain union of a fractured clavicle without any deformity, for cosmetic reasons, then the best method is to nurse the patient flat on her back with a small pillow between the shoulder blades for two or three weeks. This degree of perfection is seldom necessary however.

### FRACTURES OF THE SCAPULA

Fractures of the scapula are not very common, and the majority require only a short period of rest in a sling. If the neck of the bone is damaged as part of a shoulder joint injury the restoration of movement may be slow.

### FRACTURES OF THE HUMERUS

The humerus may be fractured in the area of the surgical neck, in the shaft, or just above the elbow (supracondylar fracture).

1. **Fractures of the neck of the humerus.** Fractures of the neck of the humerus are common in old people, and, if impacted, require only a sling for one or two weeks and early shoulder movements. There is always considerable swelling, and as soon as this has completely subsided active shoulder movements must be commenced. The importance of movement in the other joints cannot be overstressed.

In younger subjects an abduction frame may be necessary after the reduction of the fracture to secure a satisfactory result.

Stiffness of the shoulder due to adhesion formation is very common following injuries. Active movements are the only method of restoration of function, and the most important movement is external rotation. Passive stretching and massage only increase the degree of disability. After external rotation has been recovered other exercises, such as 'crawling up the wall with the fingers', are of value. When the range of movement is no longer increasing or the joint is painful, a manipulation may be necessary to break down adhesions.

2. **Fractures of the shaft of the humerus.** These fractures are common, and are always associated with considerable swelling and bruising. They may be complicated by paralysis of the radial nerve, with resultant drop wrist and inability to

extend the fingers. This fracture is usually treated by a U slab of plaster of Paris or a hanging cuff. The arm is allowed to hang by its own weight in order that the fracture be reduced.

If a radial nerve paralysis is present, a cock-up splint is applied to the wrist, and is removed only when the patient is able to raise his wrist and fingers off a Linty finger splint.

Fractures of the shaft of the humerus usually require five to six weeks' immobilisation.

3. **Supracondylar fractures.** Supracondylar fractures and injuries to the epiphyses around the elbow joints are common in children. These fractures are associated with extensive bruising and oedema of the tissues around the joint. As soon as possible the fracture is reduced under an anaesthetic and maintained by flexing the elbow and applying a collar and cuff sling. Sometimes a posterior plaster cast is carefully applied.

The greatest care must be taken to observe the circulation in the fingers, and the radial pulse should be recorded hourly for 24 hours after reduction. Should the patient complain of pain or numbness, the degree of flexion must be reduced at once, otherwise a Volkmann's ischaemic contracture may develop. This is a condition of vascular spasm or occlusion resulting in fibrosis of the flexor muscles of the forearm and fingers. The median and ulnar nerves may be damaged as a complication of fractures in this area.

### OTHER FRACTURES AROUND THE ELBOW JOINT

Fractures of any of the bony processes around the elbow joint may occur. The commonest fractures are those of the olecranon process, the external condyle of the humerus, and the head of the radius. Any of these fractures may be treated, varying with their severity, by conservative methods or by open operation.

Massage around the elbow joint usually diminishes rather than increases the degree of movement. Carrying buckets and weights also has a dangerous effect. The only safe method of regaining movement is by the patient's active movements and the nurse should encourage him unceasingly once movements are ordered by the surgeon.

*Myositis ossificans.* A calcified mass sometimes forms in the intramuscular haematoma as a result of a fracture in this area. With rest the calcified mass usually disappears.

### FRACTURES OF THE SHAFT OF THE RADIUS AND ULNA

Both bones of the forearm may be fractured as a result of direct violence, or one bone alone may be fractured. After reduction of the fracture a plaster cast is applied from just below the shoulder to the knuckles. The limb is replastered in three weeks, when the swelling has subsided and an X-ray is taken. If satisfactory the fracture is usually united in a further five to six weeks. Volkmann's ischaemic contracture is also a danger in these fractures, and great care must be taken after the application of plaster.

Operative treatment may be necessary to reduce the fracture or to correct non-union. A bone graft or plating operation may be found necessary.

### COLLES'S FRACTURE

Colles's fracture is a fracture of the radius 2·5 cm above the wrist joint with backward and outward displacement of the wrist. It is one of the commonest fractures in the body, and is due to a fall on the outstretched hand. The general signs of fracture are present, and the typical deformity is the 'dinner fork' appearance of the wrist.

The fracture is reduced under a general anaesthetic and a plaster cast applied from the knuckles to just below the elbow. The hand is lightly strapped to the dorsal cast, but free movements are allowed in the finger joints. Active movements of the shoulder joint and the use of the fingers whilst the patient's arm is in plaster are of the greatest importance. Immobilisation is necessary for about five weeks.

### FRACTURES OF THE CARPAL BONES

The most important fracture of the carpus is that of the scaphoid bone. Too frequently a patient considers that he has sprained his wrist and neglects to seek advice. Continuous immobilisation, until union is complete, is necessary. Failure to unite or neglect of treatment results in severe arthritis of the wrist joint.

### FRACTURES OF THE METACARPALS AND PHALANGES

Whereas fractures of the shafts of the metacarpals do not usually require reduction, fractures through the neck with forward displacement require both reduction and fixation in flexion of the finger.

### FRACTURES OF THE RIBS AND SPINE

These fractures have been considered already under Diseases of the Lungs and Thorax (Chapter 31) and Central Nervous System (Chapter 45).

### FRACTURES OF THE PELVIS

A fracture of the true pelvis is a serious injury, since visceral damage, such as rupture of the bladder and urethra (p. 472), may have occurred, and demands immediate repair. Isolated crack fractures, for example, injury to the anterior superior spine, also occur, and require rest for six to eight weeks in bed after the application of slings.

## FRACTURES OF THE LOWER LIMB

### FRACTURES OF THE FEMUR

**Fractures of the neck of the femur.** Fractures of the neck of the femur occur in elderly people as a result of a relatively trivial injury, such as a twist of the limb, because the neck of the femur is brittle in patients of advanced years. There is sudden pain, the limb is usually but not always powerless, and the foot is rotated outwards.

Making an elderly patient bedfast risks thrombosis, chest infection and bladder failure from prostatic obstruction which the patient may have been just able to overcome while he was ambulant.

From the point of view of treatment, the site of injury is very important. High or intracapsular fractures are prone to non-union and require fixation with a Smith-Peterson nail, but this can be undertaken only if the condition of the patient is good. Alternatively replacement of the femoral head is sometimes indicated using a Thompson metal prosthesis.

Low or extracapsular fractures may be treated with a McLaughlin pin-plate. If the general condition of the patient is poor, the ideal treatment is not possible. The patient is encouraged to sit up and move about in bed as much as possible.

*Preoperative preparation of the patient for Smith-Petersen nail or pin and plate*

Most of these patients are old and often have associated chest and heart disease. Not infrequently they have been lying at home for some hours, often alone and unable to move following their fracture. On admission they may be in a state of acute circulatory failure, in pain and frequently dehydrated.

Pain is relieved with drugs and by supporting the limb comfortably with pillows. Breathing exercises and the expectoration of sputum should be encouraged. Congestive cardiac failure and cardiac arrhythmias may require treatment with drugs preoperatively. The haemoglobin, blood urea and the blood group are determined.

The patient who is to have a simple nailing will not usually require a blood transfusion, but those who require a pin and plate will nearly always need one or two units of blood during

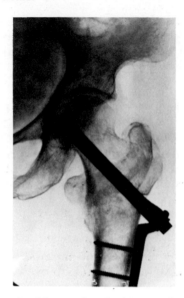

FIG. 47.5 Radiograph of fractured neck of femur after reduction and fixation with a Smith-Petersen nail and plate.

operation. Most of the bleeding comes from bone and it is not easily controlled by the surgeon. The skin preparation should extend from the lower chest to the toes, attention being paid to the skin creases of the groin and around the genitalia. The whole area is cleansed with Cetavlon but no shaving is necessary.

*Postoperative care*

The patient may usually sit out in a chair within a day or two of operation but *no weight bearing* on the injured limb must be allowed for several weeks. The pin is merely a form of internal splintage to hold the bone together until it is united and is not intended to take the patient's weight. The patient can begin active hip and knee exercises within a few days of operation. A slipper with a cross bar is sometimes prescribed to prevent external rotation but is not usually necessary if the reduction is good and the pin firmly in position. It has the disadvantage of causing sore heels and many surgeons avoid its use.

**Fractures of the shaft of the femur**

*Birth fractures* are usually treated by suspension of the legs on a gallows frame.

*Fractures of the shaft in the adult.* Fractures of the femoral shaft are common injuries. There are several methods of treat-

ing a fracture of the shaft of the femur. The use of a Thomas'
splint after manual reduction is the simplest and most generally applicable. Alternatively the limb may be slung from a
Balkan beam and a system of balanced weight traction
employed. Skeletal traction may be used.

APPLICATION OF SKIN EXTENSION:
  Extension materials used are:

| | |
|---|---|
| Traction kit (Elastoplast), | e.g. for acute back conditions and for fractured femur treated in casualty |
| Ventfoam, | e.g. for short-term extension and when the patient is allergic to strapping |
| Extension plaster, | e.g. for fractures treated in the wards. |

When necessary a broad band of at least three inches wide
is shaved down each side of the leg using a razor and a dry
talc. powder. The area shaved is then covered with one layer
of 'Rikospray' (Tinc. Benz. Co.).

When using Extension plaster, two rolls are prepared by
stitching 30 inches of traction tape over a V-shaped arrangement of the plaster. Velband 3 inch width is wrapped
round the ankle to protect the malleoli.

Two people are required, one to hold the leg, whilst the
other applies the plaster. The plaster is applied starting just
above the malleoli, and using even pressure, passing up the
leg. Vents are cut out as required to allow the plaster to
mould to the shape of the leg. It is then cut from the roll.

When both lengths of plaster have been applied, the whole
plaster is covered by 3 inch crêpe bandages commencing just
above the malleoli and bandaging up the leg. If a Thomas'
splint is to be used it is threaded on to the leg. Otherwise a
trough pillow is placed under the leg to support it. A spreader
is inserted into position, the traction tapes being tied to the
outside holes. Extension cord is tied to the centre hole of the
spreader, passed over the Buck's extension (pram handles) or
pulley at the foot of the bed, and a weight-holder is attached
to it. The appropriate weight is applied, e.g. 5 lb or as
ordered. The foot of the bed is elevated.

Each day the extension is inspected, particular attention being paid to the bandages, the plaster, the junction of the tape
and the plaster, the skin for plaster reaction or swelling, and
the weights themselves that they are correct and safely positioned and suspended. The patient is encouraged to move the
toes and foot, and to carry out quadriceps exercises and to
move about.

## APPLICATION OF THOMAS' SPLINT

The size of the Thomas' splint required is first ascertained. Using a tape measure, the circumference of the thigh is measured at an angle following the line of the groin. This measurement plus one inch indicates the size of the ring required. Splints are sized according to the measurement of the inner aspect of the ring. The length of the splint should not be less than four inches, and not more than six inches longer than the length of the leg.

The patient is asked if he is allergic to leather, and if so, the ring is covered with a cotton bandage.

Four slings of 6 inch calico are placed on the splint, each being fixed in position by two safety pins at the outer side.

In some instances, e.g. fracture, a back splint might first be applied, padded in the approved manner, with a fold of splint wool under the knee and a pad of it under the fracture. At least two people are required when threading the Thomas' splint over the leg.

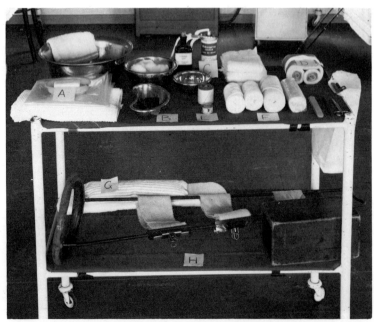

FIG. 47.6    Preparation for application of Thomas' splint.

A, Towel, disposable polythene sheet, soap
B, Razor
C, Rikospray
D, Extension tapes

E, Tape measure, needle and cotton
F, Bandages
G, Sandbag and back splint
H, Thomas' splint with sling applied. Wooden block

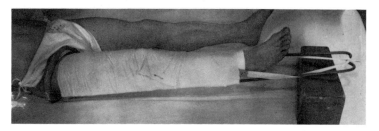

FIG. 47.7   Correctly applied Thomas' splint. Two-thirds of limb above level of bars of splint. Long gutter back splint with pad behind knee and pad beneath site of fracture to preserve slight flexion in knee and normal anterior bow of femoral shaft. Ring fitting right into groin and taking pressure on ischial tuberosity.

The splint is held in position by the application of a 6 inch crêpe bandage. The splint is elevated on the special blocks provided. Whilst the splint is in position the area under the ring is cared for by movement of the skin and application of powder; the patient himself can be instructed to carry this out.

The position of the splint and the condition of the bandage are checked daily.

When the splint is removed, it is cleaned and sent to the splint room.

*Quadriceps drill* must be encouraged to prevent wasting of the quadriceps muscles.

If perfect anatomical position has not been secured, especially in transverse fractures, operation may be advised, and a Küntscher intramedullary nail inserted for fixation.

*Pressure sores* are avoided and routine care of the skin over the back and the malleoli is particularly essential.

After ten or twelve weeks an X-ray examination usually shows satisfactory union, and walking in a caliper is allowed, most of the body weight being taken by the caliper ring and so relieving strain on the fracture site. The patient removes the caliper to exercise his knee. After a further two or three months the caliper is discarded and by this time knee movements are usually almost full, but a manipulation may be necessary.

For transverse fractures of the femoral shaft, internal nail fixation is being used to an increasing degree so that the knee is not immobilised and the patient is walking sooner.

## FRACTURES OF THE PATELLA

Fractures of the patella result in a large bloodstained effusion into the knee joint and the surrounding tissues. Transverse fractures with separation of the fragments require operative reduction and suture of the bone. When the bone is extensively comminuted it is better excised. After drainage primary closure of the wound is usually possible under antibiotic cover. All patients must practise quadriceps drill while in plaster, and when removed active movements of the joint are commenced.

### FRACTURES OF THE TIBIA

Because of its subcutaneous site the tibia is frequently fractured. Most fractures can be reduced by manipulation under an anaesthetic, and a plaster is applied from the toes to the mid-thigh. If displacement is gross and the reduction unstable, open reduction and internal fixation are used. Early movements of the toes and quadriceps drill are important, and after removal of the plaster a crêpe bandage or elastic stocking from the toes to the knees may be applied to prevent reactionary oedema.

The tibia is one of the sites where non-union may occur particularly in the lower third and a bone graft may be necessary.

### POTT'S FRACTURE DISLOCATION OF THE ANKLE

This is a common result of a twisting injury to the ankle. The fibula is snapped in its lower 5 cm, the internal malleolus of the tibia is fractured, and the foot may be dislocated outwards, inwards or backwards. Complete reduction, and immobilisation in plaster for 10 to 12 weeks are necessary. Internal fixation is often necessary and probably preferable. After about five weeks the patient is usually allowed to walk on a sorbo heel which is fitted to the plaster.

After removal of the plaster a crêpe bandage is necessary to control oedema of the soft tissues.

### FRACTURES OF THE FOOT

Fracture of the os calcis is the commonest tarsal fracture, and results from a fall from a height on to the heel. Methods to reduce the fracture are varied, but in spite of these severe stiffness of the foot is common. Early movement without weight-bearing for three months is advised in some cases.

Many cases result in considerable crippling in spite of treatment, and operative fusion of the subtaloid joint is sometimes necessary to relieve pain.

Metatarsal fractures are usually treated by a plaster cast. Fractures of the phalanges are immobilised in Elastoplast.

# CHAPTER 48

# Diseases of Bone

## ACUTE OSTEOMYELITIS

Acute osteomyelitis is an acute inflammatory process of bone. The infection may be:

1. *Blood-borne* (haematogenous). Previous infections, particularly boils and carbuncles, are not uncommon. Slight trauma to the bone usually precedes the immediate onset of the disease.
2. *Air-borne* (exogenous). Gunshot wounds and compound fractures are the commonest examples of osteomyelitis arising by this route.

*Sites of the disease.* The most common sites are the lower end of the femur and the upper end of the tibia.

*Modification of the process of inflammation in bone.* The inflammatory process is the same as in any other tissue, but dead bone can separate only very slowly. 'Sloughs' may form if resolution does not occur, and the dead bone, or slough, is known as a sequestrum.

### Symptoms and signs

#### GENERAL

The patient is extremely ill, has a toxic flush of the face, and is dehydrated. Vomiting and delirium may be present. The temperature is high, 39·5° to 40° C (103° to 104° F), and the pulse rate is rapid.

#### LOCAL

1. *Pain.* Pain is extreme over the infected area of bone. It is a continuous gnawing, throbbing pain. The child will shriek and cry incessantly. Lack of sleep and infection result in rapid deterioration of the general condition.
2. *Localised swelling* and redness will appear because pus forms under the periosteum.
3. *Tenderness* is very marked over the affected site.

4. *Pseudoparalysis and muscle spasm* are present. The child keeps the affected limb at rest to avoid increasing pain.

*Treatment and nursing care*

GENERAL MEASURES. The patient must be confined to bed and the blood haemoglobin raised by blood transfusion if it is shown to be deficient. An ESR and a blood culture are also performed.

Pain is relieved by analgesics.

CHEMOTHERAPY. Most cases of osteomyelitis are due to *Staphylococcus pyogenes*, but the organism must be isolated and the appropriate antibiotic prescribed.

LOCAL TREATMENT

1. IMMOBILISATION of the limb by a plaster cast or other adequate splinting is essential, even in mild cases, because softening of the bone often leads to a pathological fracture.

2. DRAINAGE will be necessary if a subperiosteal abscess is present or if pus is present in the medullary cavity. This may necessitate drilling of the bone.

*The wound* is covered with sulphathiazole powder and left open. Secondary suture is usually possible two or three weeks later. If the patient has been neglected, the infection very virulent, or the organisms insensitive to antibiotics, more prolonged treatment is necessary.

*Separated dead bone* (sequestrum) may be discharged, or may have to be removed from the wound.

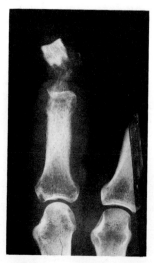

FIG. 48.1    Sequestrum of phalanx. Healing will not occur until it is extruded.

## CHRONIC OSTEOMYELITIS

This condition may follow acute infective osteomyelitis, a compound fracture or a gunshot wound. A sinus persists, heals for a time and breaks down again.

Treatment consists of rest, chemotherapy, and occasionally removal of the sequestra, bone drilling or excision of scar tissue.

*Amyloid disease.* Prolonged suppuration resulting in hypoproteinaemia may cause a dangerous degenerative condition in the connective tissue of many important organs known as amyloid disease. The liver, the kidney and the spleen are particularly liable to be affected. Its appearance may be suggested by the presence of proteinuria and polyuria and further investigation may be necessary to confirm its presence.

## BONE TUMOURS

Bone tumours may be innocent or malignant.

### 1. Innocent tumours

(a) *Osteoma.* Osteomas may occur in the skull or in long bones near the epiphyses. Very frequently a bursa develops on their surface. These tumours may cause symptoms by interference with the tendons or nerves passing over their surfaces.

Treatment consists of excision.

(b) *Chondromas* are innocent tumours arising from cartilage. Occasionally they grow into the medulla of the bones and are known as enchondromas.

Treatment consists of excision if superficial, or curettage if situated deep in the bone.

### 2. Malignant tumours

*Secondary malignant tumours* are common as a result of carcinoma of the breast, the prostate, the kidney, the bronchus and the thyroid gland.

*Primary malignant tumours* in the bone are not very common but are extremely malignant. The most frequent is an osteogenic sarcoma, and, as is characteristic of sarcomas, spread by the blood stream is early and rapid. The lungs are invaded at a very early stage.

*Symptoms and signs*

The patients are usually in the age group 10 to 20 years, but no age is exempt.

1. *Pain.* Pain is the earliest symptom. It increases in severity and in the terminal stages is extreme.

2. *Swelling* appears some time after the onset of pain. At first it is firm and bone-like in character, but later becomes softer, and a spontaneous fracture may occur. The subcutaneous veins over the swelling are dilated.

3. *Cough and haemoptysis* are very suggestive of invasion of the lungs by secondary deposits.

INVESTIGATIONS

X-ray may show the typical sun-ray appearance and destruction of the bone.

Investigations which may be undertaken include scans with strontium-90, and estimation of the serum calcium and the acid and alkaline phosphatase.

*Treatment*

Amputation of the limb holds out the only hope of cure, but the chances of complete cure are very slender. Radiotherapy in hyperbaric oxygen may be undertaken as a pre-operative measure. The relief of pain is most important.

## RARER DISEASES OF BONE

There are many rare and obscure diseases of bone. The bones form a large portion of the human body, and it is not surprising that many and varied changes occur in their substance as a result of disease at other sites in the body. Many patients with obscure bone disease die in renal failure.

### PAGET'S DISEASE

Paget's disease (osteitis deformans) may involve a single bone or be widespread throughout the skeleton. Its cause is unknown. It is fairly common in elderly patients. The affected bones slowly enlarge, become deformed and brittle.

A                                    B

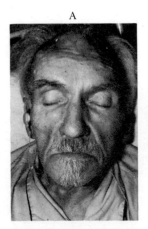
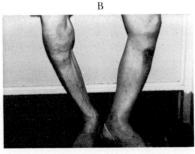

FIG. 48.2   Paget's disease.
A, The enlarged skull.
B, The legs.

*Symptoms and signs*
1.  Pain may occur in the bones or in the joints.
2.  The patient's head enlarges if the skull is involved. He complains that his hat is becoming 'too small'.
3.  A pathological fracture (p. 540) may occur.
4.  The spine becomes kyphotic.
5.  The legs are bowed and the feet become flat.
6.  X-ray changes are typical.
7.  Congestive cardiac failure may occur due to the extra strain imposed on the heart by arteriovenous shunts which occur in the involved bone.
8.  Osteogenic sarcoma may occur as a complication.

*Treatment*
There is no known cure, but treatment may be needed for pain. In mild cases aspirin or other analgesics may be all that is necessary. Pain in active disease can often be relieved by a new hormone, calcitonin, derived from the thyroid.

## OSTEITIS FIBROSA CYSTICA

Multiple cysts form in the bones. Spontaneous fractures may occur, and in severe cases deformity develops. The disease is due to an adenoma of a parathyroid gland. Removal of the adenoma results in cure.

# CHAPTER 49

# Diseases of the Joints

## SPRAINS

A sprain is a tearing of the fibres of the capsule and the ligaments around the joint. The ankle and the knee joints are those most commonly sprained. There may be an effusion of fluid into the joint, and the subcutaneous tissues may be suffused with blood.

Pain may be very severe. Swelling appears within an hour if there is a haemorrhagic effusion and within 24 hours if it is serous in type. There is restriction of movement of the joint.

*Treatment*

A sprain may cause fainting as soon as it has been sustained. Rest and cooling compresses give considerable relief in the first few minutes, but as soon as possible the joint is bound firmly with a crêpe bandage or strapping to prevent swelling. In the case of the lower limb, weight-bearing should not be allowed. Active exercises are undertaken as soon as the pain eases (about the fourth day), otherwise oedema will increase and adhesions, which give rise to stiffness later, will develop.

In all patients, but particularly in elderly people, an elastic stocking is applied before the patient gets out of bed, otherwise oedema will occur. It is worn for two weeks after the patient has commenced to walk.

## DISLOCATIONS

A dislocation is the displacement of the articular surfaces of the bones which normally enter into the formation of the joint. Subluxation is a condition of incomplete dislocation.

*Causes*

1. Trauma is the commonest cause.
2. Pathological dislocation is due to paralysis of the surrounding muscle, distension of the joint by effusion, and bony destruction.
3. Congenital—particularly dislocation of the hip.

## TRAUMATIC DISLOCATION

The greater the range of movement of the joint, the easier it is to produce a dislocation by trauma.

The shoulder joint is the most commonly dislocated joint in the body. Dislocation of the elbow is fairly common.

*Symptoms and signs of a dislocation*

1. Pain in the area of the joint is usual. If large nerve trunks are damaged, pain may be referred down the limb.

2. Swelling and bruising occur in the neighbourhood of the joint.

3. There is loss of normal movement.

4. Deformity is always present. The bones may be at an abnormal angle or the limb may be shortened.

*Treatment*

1. The displaced bone should be reduced as soon as possible. An anaesthetic is usually necessary.

2. The joint is immobilised until the swelling and oedema have subsided and the tear in the capsule has healed.

3. Function is then regained by intensive active exercises. Massage is sometimes of value, but must never be used in the region of the elbow joint, because it increases stiffness.

## DISLOCATION AT SPECIAL SITES

**The shoulder joint.** The dislocation will be reduced under an anaesthetic in most cases and the result checked by X-ray. The arm is strapped to the side for two or three weeks and then active movements are commenced. The elbow, wrist,

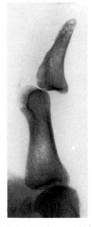

FIG. 49.1   Dislocated thumb.

and fingers must be kept in constant use. Recurrent dislocation is common in the shoulder joint, and an open operation such as Bankarts or Putti-Platt may be necessary to keep the head of the humerus in position.

**The hip joint.** Traumatic dislocation is rare because the hip is a stable joint, but it may occur as a result of severe violence.

Prolonged rest is necessary because the blood supply to the femoral head is damaged.

Congenital dislocation of the hip is the commonest of all congenital dislocations. The cause is not genetic but is probably acquired in conditions occurring in the last few weeks of pregnancy. The incidence is higher in the female than in the male. The abnormality should be discovered at birth. The infant is examined lying flat in its cot. In a normal hip the femur and pelvis move together. When the femoral head is slowly moved backwards the pelvis rotates with it because the hip is in the acetabulum and sits in the acetabulum. In a dislocated hip the femoral head is clearly seen to be moving backwards and forwards on the side of the pelvis–the pelvis does not rotate with it. Splints, such as the Malmo, are applied at birth and worn constantly during the first three months of life to maintain 90 degrees flexion and full abduction. The infant is seen at weekly intervals for adjustment of the splint.


## INJURIES TO JOINTS

### TRAUMATIC SYNOVITIS

Injury to a joint results in swelling of the synovial membrane and the formation of a serous effusion (fluid in the joint). The joint is tender, painful, and movement is limited.

*Treatment*

1. Rest on a splint, after the application of a firm bandage to prevent increase in the amount of effusion, is essential.

2. The muscles around the joint must be contracted statically while the limb is in the splint, and as soon as the splint is discarded intensive active movements are commenced. Radiant heat and short-wave diathermy are valuable in cases where the joint is stiff and the restoration of movement is slow; the muscles are flabby and atonic. Faradic electrical stimulation is used.

### TORN SEMILUNAR CARTILAGE

The semilunar cartilages are two incomplete discs of fibrocartilage attached to the head of the tibia. They may be damaged by sudden rotational strains, such as are sustained in games and certain occupations, particularly mining. The internal semilunar cartilage is damaged three times as frequently as the external.

*Symptoms and signs*

The knee 'gives way' suddenly while it is in the semi-flexed position. There is severe pain in the joint, followed by an effusion. Some degree of locking is usual if extensive detachment of a fragment of the cartilage has occurred.

*Treatment*

The treatment is similar to that of synovitis in the acute stage. Firm pressure with a crêpe bandage, the application of a back-splint, and intensive quadriceps exercises are prescribed for a period of two or three weeks. Active movements are then commenced. Should a recurrence of the trouble develop, excision of the cartilage is usually advised.

THE CARE OF THE PATIENT FOR THE REMOVAL OF A CARTILAGE (MENISCECTOMY)

Incision of a sterile joint is fraught with considerable risk of infection unless the greatest care is taken in the preparation of the skin. In the presence of any skin infection, boils, etc., operation is deferred. The limb is shaved and washed with hexachlorophane soap on the morning of operation.

THE OPERATION. This is performed after a tourniquet has been applied to the limb. A no-touch technique is used to ensure absolute sterility.

POST-OPERATIVE CARE. After the operation the limb is covered with 0·5 kg of cotton-wool and a firm bandage. A back splint is usually applied. *The tourniquet is then released, and the nurse must be certain that it has been removed before the patient leaves the theatre.* On return to bed the bedclothes are supported by a cage.

*Quadriceps drill* is commenced on the day following the operation, and continued until the dressings and skin sutures are removed 10 to 14 days later. Full movement and stability of the joint are regained only after a full course of exercises and rehabilitation.

### HAMMER TOE

This condition may be due to faulty footwear.

Situated over the first interphalangeal joint is a bursa, a callosity or a corn.

*Treatment*

Treatment consists of advising the patient to obtain correct footwear. Strapping the toes straight may suffice in early cases, and the corn may be treated by painting the surface frequently with a solution of 10 per cent salicylic acid in collodion paint.

If the deformity is fixed the corn is excised and the toe straightened by arthrodesing the first interphalangeal joint.

### HALLUX VALGUS

This deformity consists of an outward displacement of the big

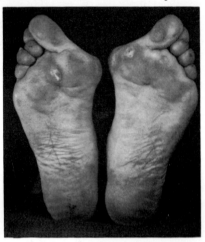

FIG. 49.2    Hallux valgus and flat foot.

toe. Over the metatarsal joint a bursa (bunion) develops as a result of irritation, and may become infected. Osteoarthritis will develop in long-standing cases from malalignment of the bones.

*Treatment*

Operative treatment is usually recommended. If the patient wishes to avoid an operation roomy footwear will give increased comfort. A septic bunion may require incision. Only when the skin has healed can a radical operation be undertaken. This consists of excision of the proximal half of the proximal phalanx of the toe and removal of the exostosis from the head of the first metatarsal (Keller's operation).

### HALLUX RIGIDUS

This is a condition of osteoarthritis of the metatarsophalangeal joint of the big toe. The operative cure is similar to that of hallux valgus.

### PERIARTHRITIS

*Frozen shoulder* is a periarthritic condition which causes considerable pain and incapacity. Locally corticosteroids are injected and a biopsy of the synovial membrane is taken.

## ACUTE INFECTIVE ARTHRITIS

Acute infective arthritis may occur as a result of the introduction of pyogenic organisms by:

1. A penetrating wound.
2. Spread from a local focus of osteomyelitis.
3. Blood-borne infection from a focus elsewhere in the body, commonly pneumonia or a septic finger. This is particularly liable to occur in the rheumatoid joint of a patient on corticosteroids.

Acute arthritis is a serious condition. There is considerable risk to life from toxaemia, and, locally, the best attainable result will be ankylosis (fixation) of the joint in the position of greatest use unless early treatment is successful.

### Symptoms and signs

There is general constitutional disturbance varying in degree with the severity of the infection. Locally there is intense pain over the joint, which is aggravated by the slightest movement. The joint is swollen, tender and hot, and the surrounding muscles are in spasm.

### Treatment

The general measures mentioned to combat infection in the treatment of osteomyelitis are employed (see p. 558).

### LOCAL TREATMENT

1. THE JOINT IS IMMOBILISED on a splint and skin extensions may be employed to separate the inflamed surfaces.
2. ASPIRATION OF THE JOINT may be performed under a general anaesthetic in an operating theatre.

If the organism is sensitive, penicillin is given into the joint as well as systemically. If it is penicillin resistant the appropriate antibiotic is used.

3. DRAINAGE (arthrotomy). Drainage, followed by immobilisation, will be required in cases which fail to respond to less drastic measures. The joint is fixed in the optimal position for ankylosis.

## ANKYLOSIS

Ankylosis or diminution of movement of a joint may be partial or complete. Complete ankylosis means that there is no movement at all. The joint may be obliterated by the formation of bone uniting two bones together, that is, bony ankylosis, or the ankylosis may be incomplete due to the presence of strong fibrous adhesions.

**Bony ankylosis.** Bony ankylosis results from septic arthritis or a tuberculous arthritis which has formed sinuses and becomes secondarily infected.

**Fibrous ankylosis.** Results from tuberculous infection in which secondary infection has not occurred. A joint in which complete ankylosis has developed is painless and stable, but one in which there is partial ankylosis may be painful, and it may be necessary to allow it to stiffen completely by immobilisation or by the performance of an operation known as an arthrodesis.

ARTHRODESIS consists of excision of the articular cartilages and then immobilising the two raw bone ends in a plaster cast so that bony union occurs, as in a fracture.


# TUBERCULOUS ARTHRITIS

Tuberculous arthritis occurs in children under the age of 5 years, although patients of any age may be affected. The most common sites are the spine, which has been described (p. 528), the hip joint and the knee.

## TUBERCULOUS ARTHRITIS OF THE HIP

*Symptoms and signs*

1. *Pain.* The pain in the joint may be associated with a limp. Later it is severe, particularly at night.

2. *Deformity and limitation of movement* occur. The hip is flexed and adducted. All movements of the joint are restricted and painful.

3. *Swelling.* The area of the joint may be swollen and thickened, and in late cases numerous discharging sinuses may be present.

4. *Pyrexia.* Pyrexia is present in the acute stage of the disease.

X-RAY reveals decalcification of the bone and destruction of the joint surfaces.


*Treatment*

ANTITUBERCULOUS CHEMOTHERAPY is commenced. The joint is rested by immobilisation on a Jones' abduction frame and skin traction is applied to effect gradual correction of the deformity. When satisfactory reduction of the deformity has been obtained, immobilisation is necessary until sound ankylosis is obtained. Operation in the form of operative fusion may be advised when recalcification occurs to prevent the deformity which sometimes occurs in tuberculosis. In the convalescent period a walking caliper is applied and active movements of the knee joint commenced.

COMPLICATIONS AND SPECIAL POINTS IN NURSING CARE

1. *Abscess formation* is not uncommon. Treatment is usually confined to careful aspiration.

2. *Multiple sinuses* are a serious complication and require meticulous care in dressing. The urine should be tested regularly once a week for the presence of albumin and casts, and a positive finding is strongly suggestive of the onset of a fatal amyloid disease. Antibiotics are of value in limiting and controlling secondary infection.

3. *Intercurrent infection* is especially dangerous in the presence of a small sinus, since secondary infection of this nature may be very virulent.

4. *Care of the skin* and pressure areas while the patient is on the frame is most important, and particularly the folds of the groin are liable to be damaged.

5. *Care of the other joints.* The child's foot and ankle joints must be put through a full range of normal movement each day, and drop foot may be guarded against by adequate splinting. A pad behind the knee prevents genu recurvatum.

6. *Static movement of the muscles*, particularly of the quadriceps, is of the greatest importance, because in the convalescent stage regaining movement of the knee will be the patient's greatest difficulty.

*Convalescence*

When the patient's limb is in a walking caliper the caliper must be removed frequently for flexion exercises of the knee. Full movement will be regained by careful rehabilitation and remedial exercises.

## TUBERCULOUS ARTHRITIS OF THE KNEE

The symptoms and signs and the course of the disease are similar to those of tuberculous disease in the hip. Fixation is best achieved by the use of the Thomas' knee splint, for which condition the splint was specially devised. Early disease confined to the synovial membrane is often suitable for synovectomy. In the adult, arthrodesis of the knee joint is frequently undertaken after a period of conservative treatment.

# SYPHILITIC DISEASE OF THE JOINTS

1. *True syphilitic synovitis* is seen only in the condition known as Clutton's joints. A bilateral painless effusion occurs in the knee joints about the age of puberty and, curiously enough, gives rise to no great disability.

2. *Charcot's joints*, or neuropathic joints, may occur as a complication of tabes dorsalis or syringomyelia. They can, of

course, arise as a complication of any condition in which the peripheral sensation is defective.

The joints are enlarged, swollen, and painless. They feel like a bag of bones, the ends of the bones crunching on one another and so 'flail' that they can be moved passively into almost any position. A knee cage or walking caliper is of some help in these cases. When successful a compression arthrodesis of the knee provides the best treatment.

## OSTEOARTHROSIS

Osteoarthrosis is a degenerative condition of the bony portion of the joint. The articular cartilage is denuded and rubbed away from the centre of the joint, while at the periphery there is abundant proliferation. The result is that movement is limited and painful. The synovial membrane is thickened, while irritation from the thickened cartilage results in a varying degree of fluid in the joint.

The condition is common in patients of advancing years, but is frequently seen in younger subjects with uncorrected deformities. The bones are out of line and the joint stresses fall unevenly at a point varying with the deformity.

*Sites of the disease.* Several small joints may be affected, but more commonly the disease attacks a single large joint, the hip, or more rarely the shoulder or the knee.

*Symptoms and signs*
  1. *Pain* is worse on commencing movement, wears off as the joint is freed, and returns again when movement is commenced after rest. Cold damp weather increases the pain.
  2. *Limitation of movement* of a varying degree is present.
  3. *Trivial injuries* increase the pain, and an effusion of fluid into the joint may occur.
  4. *Osteoarthrosis of the spine* may simulate cholecystitis, renal colic or appendicitis.
  5. *Incontinence.* This occurs because the patient cannot get to the lavatory in time.

*Treatment*
  1. Local warmth in the form of short-wave diathermy or active heat combined with exercises to maintain muscle strength and so support the joint will help mild cases. Drugs, such as indomethacin and phenylbutazone, may be used.
  2. The injection of hydrocortisone acetate suspension into the joint will often relieve pain for a considerable time. Scrupulous asepsis is essential.

3. Temporary immobilisation of a very painful joint in a splint or plaster may be necessary.

4. Surgical intervention is required to relieve pain and takes the form of:

(a) AN ARTHRODESIS.

(b) ARTHROPLASTY. Replacement by a prosthesis such as Ring or Charnley.

(c) OSTEOTOMY. Femoral osteotomy is commonly performed.

## RHEUMATOID ARTHRITIS

This is a crippling disease affecting mainly young people. It is due to degeneration of collagen tissue. Cortisone is of value, 50 per cent of patients benefit, but there are numerous side effects. The fingers are deformed most usually, but almost every joint in the body may be involved simultaneously. The disease has a subacute onset.

The treatment of the condition is essentially medical but deformities should be prevented and this must be undertaken from the commencement. Light, well-padded splints hold the joint in the optimum position. The splints are removed for active exercises to prevent adhesion formation, and physiotherapy usually consists of radiant heat, short-wave diathermy, massage, and suitable baths. The injection of hydrocortisone acetate or other steroid hormone into the arthritic joint is often very successful in the relief of pain. Some hope is offered by removal of the synovial membrane in the fingers and knees.

*Treatment of established deformities*

In a case of established deformity some form of continuous traction may be necessary to correct a flexion deformity. In advanced cases operative measures may be indicated very occasionally. Arthrodesis is still performed but arthroplasty is becoming established as being more useful.

# CHAPTER 50

# Diseases of the Ear, the Nose, and the Throat

Diseases of the ear, nose and throat are very common and the commonest of these diseases are the infections—coryza, tonsillitis, etc. Since the advent of antibiotics, surgery is now seldom needed for the control of these infections so that ear, nose and throat surgery has undergone a dramatic transformation in the past 25 years. The surgeon is now concerned mainly with operations to restore hearing and to control malignant disease, although there still remains some minor surgery such as tonsillectomy and the very occasional drainage of infected sinuses.

## SYMPTOMS OF EAR DISEASE

1. *Deafness* may be due to a variety of causes, the commonest being wax or a foreign body in the outer ear; middle ear disease, in particular chronic otitis media and otosclerosis; and diseases of the inner ear and auditory nerve. Presbyacousis, which is degeneration of the inner ear occurring normally in most people over the age of 55, is the commonest cause of deafness in the inner ear.

2. *Pain* in the ear may be caused by disease of the ear itself, or may be referred from other areas, such as the mouth and pharynx, which share their sensory nerve supply with the ear.

The commonest ear diseases causing earache are a boil or a foreign body in the outer ear, and acute otitis media. Common causes of pain referred to the ear are teething, a retained root in the lower jaw, tonsillitis, quinsy, tonsillectomy, and malignant tumours of the mouth and pharynx.

3. *Tinnitus*, or noise in the ear, is a common complaint in the elderly. The noise of which they complain is usually a high-pitched whistling noise; like presbyacousis it is due to degeneration in the inner ear and there is no treatment available for it.

4. *Discharge from the ear* is usually purulent and its common causes are otitis externa, a boil in the ear, and acute and chronic otitis media.

5. *Vertigo.* Several diseases of the inner ear are accompanied by dizziness so that the patient complains that either he or his surroundings are spinning round. There is usually also nausea and vomiting and other ear symptoms, in particular deafness and tinnitus. The commonest causes of this symptom are positional vertigo, epidemic labyrinthitis and Ménière's disease.

## DISEASES OF THE OUTER EAR

1. **Wax in the ear.** Wax is secreted by glands in the external auditory meatus and usually expels itself naturally from the ear canal. It may not do so, however, particularly if it is forced further into the ear canal by the corner of a towel pushed into the ear every morning whilst washing. Impacted wax is a common cause of deafness, particularly after bathing, because moisture causes it to swell.

*Treatment*

The wax is softened by the instillation of a few drops of warm olive oil or liquid paraffin; after 10 minutes it is syringed away with water, which must be at body temperature; if the water is not at body temperature the patient's labyrinth will be stimulated and he will feel dizzy. A mackintosh sheet is placed around the patient's neck and a receiver held under his ear. The pinna is pulled backwards and upwards to straighten the meatus and the syringe is directed upwards and backwards so that the stream of water is forced along the roof of the canal. A brisk stream of water is then directed along the external canal until the wax is extruded.

Before syringing an ear the patient should be asked if he is aware of having a perforated ear drum and has he any previous history of ear disease. After the ear has been syringed it should be inspected by a doctor to make sure that there has been no damage to the tympanic membrane.

2. **Foreign bodies.** Foreign bodies in the ear usually occur in children and consist of pencil points, beads, seeds, dried peas, etc. Treatment consists of removal of the foreign body by syringing or by the use of aural forceps.

3. **Boils.** Boils in the ear are common, particularly in diabetics, and cause a great deal of pain because the skin of the external auditory canal is closely bound down to the periosteum so that slight increase in pressure beneath it causes intense pain. If the boil causes sufficient swelling in the external canal there is also deafness and when the boil ruptures there is a purulent discharge. The patient is treated with penicillin, and incision may be necessary.

4. **Otitis externa.** Diffuse otitis externa usually affects both ears; there are many causes, but basically it is a reaction of the delicate skin of the external auditory canal. This may be caused by water being introduced during swimming, by the patient picking inside his ear with a matchstick or hair grip, or may be part of a generalised skin disease such as eczema. There is usually itching rather than pain and a thin muco-purulent discharge. The essential part of the treatment of this condition is that the external auditory canal should be cleaned out frequently, usually every day. Soothing dressings can be applied such as glycerine and ichthyol or drops containing a mixture of a steroid and an antibiotic such as hydrocortisone and neomycin.

5. **Tumours.** Apart from the outer ear, malignant disease of the ear is rare. The auricle may be the site of any of the tu-mours which attack the skin, such as basal cell carcinoma and

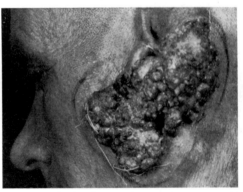

FIG. 50.1   Squamous-celled carcinoma of the pinna of the ear.

squamous cell carcinoma. The latter is considerably more common on the ear in contrast to the rest of the skin of the face where the reverse is true. These tumours, if small, are usually treated by radiotherapy, but if large are treated by ex-cision of the auricle.

## MIDDLE EAR DISEASE

### ACUTE OTITIS MEDIA

Acute otitis media arises as a result of infection passing along the Eustachian tube from the nasopharynx. The infection in the nasopharynx starts as a result of a cold, from sinusitis or because the child has enlarged adenoids. This disease almost always occurs in children and its most obvious symptom is pain in the ear. The child is also deaf. If the infection is not controlled the tympanic membrane ruptures at its centre, the ear discharges pus and the pain is then relieved.

*Course of the disease*

1. Subsidence—if the infection is brought under control by antibiotics the pain subsides and the tympanic membrane returns to normal.

2. Pus may be discharged by rupture of the tympanic membrane and healing usually follows, but if it does not the patient is left with a permanent hole in the centre of the tympanic membrane.

3. The infection may spread, causing complications, but these are now very uncommon since the advent of antibiotics. The commonest is a subperiosteal abscess over the mastoid process (commonly, but incorrectly, known as mastoiditis). This complication usually occurs about a week after the onset of acute otitis media; there is a profuse discharge from the ear and the auricle is pushed downwards and forwards by swelling behind the ear. It is treated by massive doses of penicillin and a simple mastoidectomy. Other complications of acute otitis media include meningitis, thrombosis of the lateral sinus, labyrinthitis, paralysis of the seventh cranial nerve, temporal lobe abscess and cerebellar abscess.

4. The pus in the middle ear may be drained by operation.

*Treatment*

The patient should be confined to bed and the general treatment of an acute febrile condition given. Pain in the ear is usually severe so that analgesics, including occasionally morphine, will be needed. A covered hot-water bottle or electric pad may also be given to act as a counterirritant to soothe the pain.

Antibiotics should be given, the best being penicillin. This will usually abort the attack within 24 hours and by that time the pain should be subsiding rapidly. If it has not, and the tympanic membrane is bulging because of retained pus, it should be relieved by a small incision in the tympanic membrane called a myringotomy. However, the tympanic membrane often ruptures spontaneously within a few hours of the onset of the disease. When the ear is discharging a swab should always be obtained for culture and sensitivity. Under treatment with antibiotics the discharge usually persists for two or three days, the ear then dries up and the tympanic membrane returns to normal. Treatment with antibiotics should be continued until the tympanic membrane and the hearing have returned to normal.

## CHRONIC OTITIS MEDIA

This occurs in two forms: in the first type there is a central perforation of the tympanic membrane resulting from an attack of acute otitis media in childhood, after which the tympanic membrane did not heal. The patient complains of deafness and the ear usually discharges intermittently. The discharge from his ear is due to infected secretions passing up the Eustachian tube from the nasopharynx and this is usually caused by sinusitis, enlarged adenoids or a common cold. This type of chronic ear disease does not cause spreading infection and complications do not arise. The ear should be kept dry by local toilet and by treatment of any infection in the nose, sinuses or nasopharynx. If the ear can be kept dry for six months or more, and if the patient's Eustachian tube functions normally, the hole in the tympanic membrane can be repaired, using a graft of fascia. This operation is known as a myringoplasty.

In the second type of chronic otitis media there is a perforation in the superior part of the tympanic membrane, known as the attic. The perforation is associated with a foul-smelling discharge and a cholesteatoma within the middle ear space; a cholesteatoma is a cyst lined by squamous epithelium which expands and causes erosion of the surrounding bone. Expansion of the cholesteatoma leads to infection of vital structures and the following complications may occur: labyrinthitis, paralysis of the facial nerve, temporal lobe and cerebellar abscess, meningitis and lateral sinus thrombosis. This disease must, therefore, be treated by operation. There are now several different operations for this disease but they are all based on the radical mastoid operation, the principle of which is to convert the mastoid process, the middle ear and the external auditory canal into one large cavity preventing expansion of the cholesteatoma inwards, and allowing access for toilet.

## OTOSCLEROSIS

Otosclerosis is a hereditary non-suppurative middle ear deafness. It is a very common cause of deafness in the adult population and occurs most commonly in women aged 20 to 30 years. In this condition new bone formation takes place around the stapes, one of the bones responsible for the conduction of sound, so that the bone is immobilised and sound cannot be transmitted to the inner ear. Deafness can be improved in about 80 per cent of patients by replacing the immobile stapes with a prosthesis, one of the commonest in use being made of teflon. This operation, which requires the use of an operating microscope, is called a stapedectomy. After operation antibiotics should be administered and drugs such as Stemetil may be required for dizziness.

Where the operation is contraindicated or the patient refuses, a hearing aid is a great help.

## DISEASES OF THE INNER EAR

Diseases of the inner ear cause deafness and tinnitus and, in certain cases—such as Ménière's disease—dizziness. By far the commonest lesion is presbyacousis (the deafness of old age).

Other causes of inner ear deafness are trauma, long-continued exposure to loud noises and certain drugs, particularly streptomycin, quinine and aspirin.

The deafness in these patients can be helped to a certain extent by a hearing aid.

## DISEASES OF THE THROAT

Acute infections of the throat are very common in childhood; at one time they were accompanied by severe complications, in particular rheumatic fever and acute nephritis, but these are now not often seen. Tumours of the pharynx and larynx are also important from the point of view of surgery.

### TONSILLITIS

Tonsillitis is an acute infection of the tonsils. It may be generalised (parenchymatous) or the tonsil may be covered by a white exudate in spots, that is follicular tonsillitis. About half the attacks are due to viruses and the other half to the haemolytic streptococcus; whatever the cause of the infection, the clinical features are exactly the same.

*Clinical features*
1. Sore throat.
2. Pain on swallowing.
3. Inflammation of the throat and enlargement of the tonsils.
4. Pyrexia and general constitutional malaise.
5. Halitosis.

*Treatment*
Treatment consists of rest in bed and isolation of the patient. A throat swab should be taken and the pain relieved by analgesics, particularly aspirin. The infection is often treated by antibiotics but as about half these infections are due to viruses this is often a waste of time. If antibiotics are used the best is penicillin.

### QUINSY

A quinsy is an abscess in the fascial space surrounding the tonsil, and occurs as a result of spreading infection after an attack of tonsillitis. It affects one side only, and there is gross swelling of the soft palate above and lateral to the affected tonsil, which is pushed downwards and medially. The patient complains of dysphagia, trismus and pain referred to the ear on the same side. The abscess is incised, the patient is given penicillin and six weeks later his tonsils are removed to prevent recurrence.

*Indications for tonsillectomy*

Tonsillitis and upper respiratory infection are common diseases of children, particularly at the age of 5 when the child first goes to school and is exposed to infection from other children. Nearly all children suffer to a greater or lesser extent from these infections but they almost always grow out of them in time. Bearing this in mind, the tonsils should only be removed if they are causing a great deal of trouble, so that the only common indication for tonsillectomy is repeated attacks of tonsillitis, that is at least five or six times a year, causing ill health and loss of schooling. A further, uncommon, indication for tonsillectomy is quinsy. There are now virtually no other indications for tonsillectomy, and size alone is no indication for removal of tonsils.

*Tonsillectomy*

The tonsils must not be removed when acutely inflamed. It is also important to ensure that the child has not been in contact with infectious disease immediately before operation. The usual preoperative care of the patient is also undertaken.

Tonsils nowadays are almost always removed by dissection under general anaesthetic, and removal by the tonsil guillotine has now been given up in most centres. It is also usual in children to remove the adenoids at the same time.

CARE OF THE PATIENT AFTER TONSILLECTOMY

In readiness for the patient's return from the theatre, the bed is prepared in the approved manner, with a mackintosh and towel for under the face. At hand there must be a post-anaesthetic tray and a supply of tissue wipes.

On return from the theatre the patient is placed in the semi-prone position, and to maintain this a pillow is placed at his back under the mattress. Using tissues, the face is cleaned as necessary. Observations are made on the breathing, colour, pulse and blood pressure. Any excessive swallowing is investigated, in case the tonsil bed is bleeding. Any obvious bleeding is reported.

On recovering consciousness, the patient gradually sits up. He is made comfortable. He is allowed to wash out his mouth

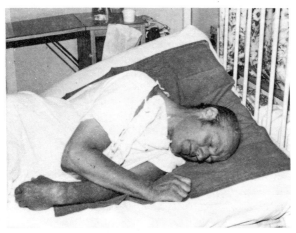

FIG. 50.2 Position after tonsillectomy. Pillows are placed behind the mattress on one side.

with glycothymoline solution. He is allowed sips of water, and as soon as he is able he is encouraged to drink and eat normally.

Observations are maintained for any bleeding. Should this occur, he is placed in a semirecumbent position, and encouraged to spit out the blood. The doctor is informed. If the bleeding point can be seen, a swab is gripped in sponge-holding or other clip forceps and pressure is applied to the patient in an attempt to control the bleeding.

POSTOPERATIVE CARE

Bleeding is the only important complication and the nurse must remember that in this case it is not only the amount of the haemorrhage which is so important as the fate of the actual blood lost. If it runs down the larynx and trachea, death may occur from suffocation or a dangerous infection may be set up in the lungs.

The patient is laid on his side and the head must be kept low by elevation of the foot of the bed or as shown in Fig. 50.2. Haemorrhage will then occur through the nose and mouth.

In every patient the pulse should be charted half-hourly for 12 to 24 hours. Until the patient has recovered his cough reflexes he must not be left alone. He can be made to sit up when conscious. The nurse should notice if he is constantly swallowing. This may be due to bleeding. If the haemorrhage is excessive, preparation must be made for immediate return to the theatre so that examination can be undertaken and further anaesthesia induced. The bleeding point is then ligated. Some patients require blood transfusion.

The throat is always sore in the postoperative phase, and an analgesic is given on the night of the operation. Aspirin emulsion and glycothymoline mouthwashes are prescribed. The tonsillar bed has a 'sloughy' appearance in the first few days. Earache is an occasional complication.

Children are usually kept in bed for three or four days and adults for one week.

## MALIGNANT TUMOURS OF THE PHARYNX AND LARYNX

Most tumours of the larynx and pharynx are malignant and are usually squamous-celled carcinomas.

A patient suffering from a laryngeal tumour presents with hoarseness and, in the early stages, may be treated by radiotherapy with preservation of the voice and a good prognosis.

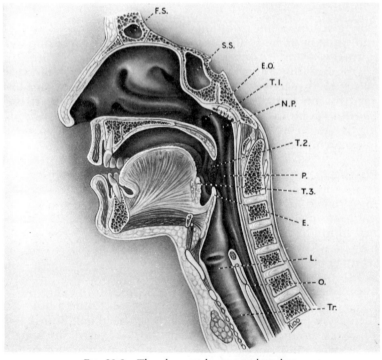

FIG. 50.3   The pharynx, larynx, and trachea.

| | |
|---|---|
| F.S., Frontal sinus | N.P., Nasopharynx |
| S.S., Sphenoidal sinus | P., Pharynx |
| E.O., Eustachian orifice | E., Epiglottis |
| T.1., Pharyngeal tonsil (the adenoid) | L., Larynx |
| T.2., Faucial tonsil | O., Oesophagus |
| T.3., Lingual tonsil | Tr., Trachea. |

In the later stages and for those tumours which recur after radiotherapy a laryngectomy is carried out.

Tumours of the pharynx present with dysphagia although they may produce no symptoms until the patient complains of a gland in the neck. Usually the larynx is invaded so that the patient becomes hoarse. These tumours fare badly with radiation so that surgical treatment is usually needed, that is excision of the tumour and the larynx as well. A block dissection of the glands of the neck is carried out at the same time.

POSTOPERATIVE CARE OF A LARYNGECTOMY

1. The care of a tracheostomy (p. 171).

2. Because these patients can no longer speak to draw attention to themselves or their needs, they should not be left unattended. If possible in the immediate postoperative period they should be provided with a bell, pencil and pad until they learn oesophageal speech or are supplied with an electric larynx.

3. Removal of the larynx entails leaving a defect in the pharynx, the edges of which are sutured. While this is healing the patient has to be fed through an intranasal nasogastric tube. The feeds may consist of a liquidised diet, milk supplemented by Complan, eggs, etc. It should be sufficient to ensure adequate hydration and nutrition; this can be assessed by the fluid balance chart and by weighing the patient.

## DISEASES OF THE NOSE

*Symptoms of nasal disease*

The common symptoms of diseases of the nose are as follows:

1. Bleeding, which is commonly called epistaxis.

2. Obstruction, which is caused by a common cold, by vasomotor rhinitis, nasal polyps, deflections of the nasal septum, a foreign body and enlarged adenoids in children.

3. Discharge, which may be thin and watery and accompanied by sneezing, when it is due to a vasomotor rhinitis, or thick and purulent when it is usually due to sinusitis.

### EPISTAXIS

Bleeding from the nose is always a symptom of a disease: in other words it is not a disease in itself. There are many causes of this symptom which may be due to a disease in the nose itself or may be a reflection of general disease. The important local causes of epistaxis are as follows:

1. Rupture of a small vessel on the anterior part of the

septum (Little's area) is common in children and is due to nose picking or the frequent upper respiratory infections to which children are prone. It is troublesome but not serious and is treated by cauterisation.

2. Rupture of a large vessel in the upper part of the nasal cavity occurs in elderly hypertensive patients and must be stopped, otherwise repeated blood loss can occur with serious effects on the brain, the heart and the kidneys. The nose is packed with gauze impregnated with petroleum jelly or paraffin. It is removed when bleeding has stopped, usually the next day. The patient should be kept in bed for several days, and after recovery may need medical treatment for his hypertension.

3. Tumours of the nose and sinuses also cause a blood-stained discharge from one side of the nose but are uncommon.

Generalised diseases causing nose bleeding include hypertension and the disorders of blood coagulation, in particular the leukemias.

## VASOMOTOR (syn. ALLERGIC) RHINITIS

This disease takes two forms, the perennial and the seasonal. In the perennial form the patient is allergic to some non-specific irritant such as house dust, whereas in the seasonal form a specific grass pollen is the cause. In both forms the patient's nose reacts badly to sudden changes in environmental conditions such as heat and cold. There is severe nasal obstruction, sneezing and a thin watery discharge from the nose. Many of these patients also suffer from asthma. In the perennial form the symptoms are present for most of the year whereas in the seasonal type the symptoms occur during the hay season, that is in June and July, being indeed often called hay fever.

*Treatment*

These patients should be investigated to see if there is any substance to which they are particularly allergic and if such is found they should be either isolated from it or desensitised to it. This is usually not practicable in the perennial form but the patient with hay fever is often helped by courses of desensitisation. Antihistamines also help a large number of these patients.

Because of the swelling and oedema of the mucous membrane in this condition nasal polyps often accompany it. These are described in the next section.

## NASAL POLYPS

Nasal polyps are collections of oedematous mucous membrane hanging by a pedicle from the lateral wall of the nose. The cause of the oedema may be either vasomotor rhinitis or infection in the sinuses. The polyps cause nasal obstruction and there is usually a nasal discharge, which is thin and watery if due to vasomotor rhinitis, or thick and purulent if due to sinusitis. If the polyps are causing symptoms they should be removed under local anaesthetic using a nasal snare. This is a minor operation which is sometimes carried out as an outpatient but it is preferable to admit the patient for one night's stay as he may bleed after operation. If this happens the nose should be packed and the packing removed the next morning.

## DEFLECTED NASAL SEPTUM

The nasal septum rarely lies strictly in the midline of the nose and is almost always slightly deflected. It may become severely deflected, however, because of trauma during birth or later during a fight or any other injury to the nose. If the septum is so severely deflected as to block almost the whole of one side of the nose, nasal obstruction will be caused. Interference with drainage of the sinuses may also be caused, leading to sinusitis. If the deflected nasal septum is causing symptoms, it should be resected. This consists of the submucosal resection of the septum, in which it is straightened by the removal of the deflected cartilage and bone under local anaesthesia.

### POSTOPERATIVE CARE

The nose is packed with gauze so that the patient must breathe through the mouth. He is propped up in bed. The packs must be removed within 24 hours. Discharge from the nose is wiped away, but the use of a handkerchief must be forbidden, tissues substituted, and antiseptic drops should be instilled into the nose.

Blood-clot and crust must not be removed, but allowed to separate. The chief complications are haemorrhage and infection, both of which may be disastrous to the success of the operation, as the occurrence of haemorrhage predisposes to sepsis. Haemorrhage is controlled by packing with gauze soaked in adrenaline (1 : 1000).

## SINUSITIS

There are four sets of paranasal air sinuses on each side of the skull: the maxillary antrum, the frontal sinuses, the ethmoid sinuses and the sphenoid sinuses. Maxillary sinusitis is common, infection of the frontal sinus is less common, infection of the ethmoid sinus is only seen in infants and infection of the sphenoid sinuses is rarely seen. All the sinuses may be infected together, however, a condition known as pansinusitis. All these sinuses are air-containing spaces within the skull; they are lined by ciliated mucous-membrane, and drain by an ostium to the nasal cavity. The maxillary sinus differs from the rest in that its ostium is almost at the top of the cavity, whereas in the other sinuses the ostium is almost at the bottom. Dependent drainage cannot occur spontaneously in the maxillary sinus, which therefore depends on the cilia to clear any infected material within it. This probably explains why maxillary sinusitis is more common.

Infections of the sinuses may be acute or chronic; acute sinusitis often follows a common cold.

**Acute maxillary sinusitis.** In addition to nasal symptoms such as obstruction and purulent discharge, there is pain which may be felt in the teeth, or may be referred to the forehead. Diagnosis is confirmed by X-rays and transillumination. The patient should be treated by penicillin after taking a nasal swab, and by systemic decongestants such as ephedrine 15 mg six-hourly. If drainage of the antrum does not occur spontaneously, it should be washed out using a trocar and cannula introduced through the lateral wall of the nose beneath the inferior turbinate under local anaesthetic.

**Acute ethmoiditis.** Acute ethmoiditis only occurs in infants whose maxillary sinuses have not developed. There is redness and swelling of the periorbital tissues. The child should be treated with penicillin and by drainage of a periorbital abscess, if it forms.

**Acute frontal sinusitis.** In this disease there is frontal headache, a purulent discharge from the affected side of the nose and swelling and redness of the forehead over the frontal sinuses. The patient has a pyrexia and may be quite ill.

*Treatment*

Patients with frontal sinusitis must be admitted to hospital and treated with large doses of penicillin, after taking a nasal swab, and with oral decongestants such as ephedrine. Because of the danger of intracranial spread of the infection, if it does not begin to respond within 24 to 48 hours the sinuses should be drained by trephining their floor.

This type of sinusitis is particularly liable to cause complications because of spread of the infection; these include osteomyelitis of the skull, frontal lobe abscess and meningitis.

### CHRONIC SINUSITIS

The only sinus which is commonly affected by chronic infection is the maxillary antrum.

Chronic infection of the maxillary antrum is associated with intermittent purulent nasal discharge and nasal obstruction, and may be a cause of headache. Because of the oedema of the mucous membrane which occurs there are also often polyps within the nose. If the symptoms from this disease are severe it is usually treated by a radical antrostomy (the Caldwell Luc operation). In this operation the antrum is exposed by an incision in the buccal mucosa after retracting the upper lip. Access to the antrum is gained by removing part of the anterior bony wall. The diseased lining of the cavities is removed with curettes and a permanent drainage hole from the lower part of the cavity into the nasal wall is made. The incision in the buccal mucosa is closed and a pack is often left in the nose. The pack must be removed the next day. It is also usual to wash out the sinuses through the freshly created antrostomy about five to seven days after operation.

# CHAPTER 51

# Diseases of the Eye

## REFRACTIVE ERRORS

In the normal eye at rest, parallel rays of light are brought to a focus on the retina, and such an eye is called emmetropic. Other eyes are abnormal in that they cannot bring parallel rays of light to a clear focus on the retina when at rest, because these eyes have an error of refraction and are therefore ametropic. Correcting spectacles will allow such an eye to achieve a clear focus when at rest. This refractive variation between eyes depends upon the length of the eye, the curvature of the cornea and, to a lesser extent, the position and refractivity of the lens in the eye. Defective or uncomfortable vision may be due solely to an error of refraction. This can be corrected by spectacles and is not regarded as a disease. The important part of the examination is to exclude defects in the eye or its associated areas of the brain which are due to disease.

Common refractive errors are:

1. *Astigmastism* in which the image focused on the retina is indistinct due to unequal refraction of the eye in different refractive planes. For example, the horizontal lines of an object may be seen clearly whereas the vertical outlines are blurred.

2. *Myopia* is a condition of short-sightedness. Near objects can be seen clearly whereas distant ones are indistinct. Myopic eyes are often large eyes, although not necessarily so.

3. *Hypermetropia*, commonly called long-sight. The distant vision is more easily achieved whereas near vision is much more difficult. The lens in the eye can to some extent be used to overcome this disability by exercising accommodation which is carried out by using the ciliary muscle of the eye to alter the curvature of the lens. The extra effort put into accommodation in this condition also leads to excessive convergence effort and may play an important part in the development of convergent squint of the accommodative type.

4. *Presbyopia* is a progressive failure of accommodative power from the age of about 14 years, when it is very large, to

the age of 70 to 80 when there is virtually no accommodative power remaining. For most people at the age of 45, the loss of accommodation is such that reading spectacles are required. The hypermetropic patient who is already using his accommodation for distance purposes will be affected by the need for reading glasses at an earlier stage, whereas a myope may be able to defer the use of reading glasses until well after his 45th birthday.

Contact lenses are lenses worn on the eye and have some advantages over the normal types of spectacles in certain cases as they can reduce the irregularity of the cornea after disease of this structure. They do not cause the large differences in the size of retinal images seen by each eye as happens with normal spectacle lenses when there is a large difference of refraction in the two eyes (anisometropia).

## THE EXAMINATION OF THE EYE

A good light is essential and a strong lens is of assistance in focusing the light. Various procedures may be adopted. A brief outline is given of what may occur, although different diseases of the eye may require different procedures for their elucidation.

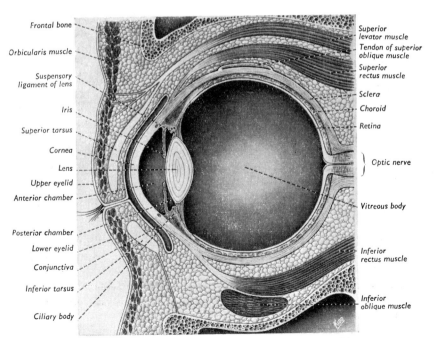

FIG. 51.1   Section of the orbit showing internal structure of the eye.

*General examination*

1. Examination of the eyelids and face may reveal diseases such as acne rosacea or herpes zoster ophthalmicus which may be associated with disease in the eye.

2. Estimation of the tension or pressure of the eye by gentle palpation with the fingers. The normal pressure is 10 to 20 mmHg.

3. The movements of the eye to elucidate different forms of squint.

4. Examination of the surface of the conjunctiva and pressure on the lacrimal sac to note any regurgitation from the sac which may indicate the tear duct being blocked.

5. The examination of the surface and transparency of the cornea. A localised abrasion may be noticed by watching for any distortion of the image reflected from a light or window on the surface of the cornea when the eye is moved in different directions. This can be shown much more readily by the use of fluorescein, which stains corneal defects green. This is best applied with sterile paper strips impregnated with sterile fluorescein, obtained in single dose dispensers and moistened with sterile saline and touched on the conjunctiva of the lower lid, or the patient's own tears may be used to release the fluorescein from the strip.

6. The depth of the anterior chamber, that is the distance between the cornea in front and the iris behind, should be noted. A deep anterior chamber may indicate the absence or dislocation of the lens. A shallow anterior chamber may indicate a leak from the anterior chamber, for instance through a small wound or leaking ulcer, or that the eye is predisposed to angle closure glaucoma.

7. The movements of the pupil and the appearance of the iris must be noted. The pupil reactions are tested first by shining a light into each eye in turn. The direct reaction is the contraction of the pupil in the eye illuminated and the indirect reaction to light is the contraction of the pupil in the other eye when one is illuminated. The reaction to convergence is the contraction of the pupils when the person looks at an object which is held close to the face.

8. Examination of the lens either by oblique illumination or by the use of the ophthalmoscope with a +12 dioptre lens in the viewing aperture when the lens may be seen against the underlying red fundus reflex. Opacities indicate cataract.

9. A rapid and useful estimation of the visual field (confrontation) can be carried out by comparing the visual field of each eye of the patient in turn with the visual field of the examiner's opposite eye.

*Instrumental examination*

1. EXAMINATION OF THE INTERIOR OF THE EYE WITH AN OPHTHALMOSCOPE. This may be made easier by dilating the pupil with a mydriatic drop. Atropine should not be used in routine examination except in children. When the pupil is dilated, a full examination of the interior of the eye is made consisting of the lens, vitreous body, and retina in turn.

2. OPTICAL EXAMINATION FOR THE ESTIMATION OF REFRACTIVE ERRORS.

3. EXAMINATION OF THE FIELDS OF VISION WITH A PERIMETER, and for a more detailed examination of the central part of the field of vision a Bjerrum screen is used.

4. DETAILED EXAMINATION OF THE EYE WITH A SLIT LAMP. In this procedure, a thin beam of light is thrown into the eye and the various structures are examined with a low power binocular microscope. The retina, the intraocular tension (applanation tonometry) and the angle of the anterior chamber (gonioscopy) may be examined by the use of extra attachments.

5. SWABBING OF THE CONJUNCTIVAL SAC IN INFECTIVE STATES to ascertain the types of organism present and their sensitivity to various antibiotics.

6. ESTIMATION OF COLOUR VISION by use of the Ishihara plates or colour lanterns.

7. TONOMETRY. Estimation of the intraocular pressure by the use of a calibrated instrument that indents the cornea (Schiotz tonometer) or by the applanation tonometer attached to a slit lamp.

## BASIC NURSING OF EYE CONDITIONS

The following general principles are of special importance in the nursing of patients suffering from disease of the eye.

1. Attention to minute detail is essential.

2. An aseptic or no-touch technique should be maintained when carrying out treatment.

3. The droppers should never touch the eye or lids, otherwise they will become contaminated, which can lead to infection within the drop bottles. Because of this, single dose dispensers are advised or, where a bottle is to be used more than once, then each patient should have his own bottle of drops and preferably the drops should be transferred from the bottle to the patient's eye with a disposable sterile dropper which is never returned a second time into the bottle.

4. The drops should be double-checked as the instillation of the wrong drops may lead to a disaster. Particularly, drops which dilate the pupil may, in certain patients, produce acute

glaucoma with serious risk of damage to the vision. Single-dose containers pose a special risk because they all look alike and the printing is very small. It is therefore most important that the name be carefully read.

5. In general, where there is a purulent discharge, the eye is not covered in order to allow the discharge to escape.

6. Where there has been an abrasion or wound of the eye either accidental or planned, as in surgery, then the eyelid may be kept closed by the fixing of a pad over the eye. If there is a large wound, then further protection may be given by using a strong shield (cartella) which fits over the pad and by abutting on the bone above and below can protect the underlying eye against an accidental knock, for instance by the patient's hand when he is sleeping.

7. The majority of patients require covering of the affected eye only. In certain circumstances, however, both eyes may be bandaged when it is essential that the eyes be kept still in order to prevent complications.

8. If the patient is totally blindfolded, then it is important not to surprise him and he should be spoken to gently as you approach and before touching him.

## DISEASES OF THE EYELIDS

**Stye** (hordeolum). A stye is a staphylococcal infection of an eyelash follicle. The pus under pressure produces pain and the lax eyelid tissues allow great surrounding swelling (oedema).

*Treatment*
Local heat. Local antibiotic treatment.

**Blepharitis.** An inflammation of the lid margins, prone to recur after cessation of treatment.

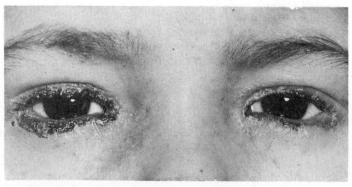

FIG. 51.2   Ulcerative blepharitis.

*Treatment*

Remove the crusts with moist swabs of saline or weak sodium bicarbonate lotion. Antibiotic ointment is rubbed into the lid margin for several weeks and reinfection excluded by vigorous personal hygiene, the use of antiseptic soap, naseptin ointment in the nose and clearing the scalp of dandruff.

**Meibomian cyst (chalazion).** This is not a true cyst but is a swelling in the lid varying from lentil to large-pea size, caused by accumulation of scavenger cells (macrophages) packed with oily material from a Meibomian gland. Normally the oil is secreted on the lid edge and thus on to the surface of the tear film covering the conjunctiva and cornea.

*Treatment*

Treatment consists of incision of the lesion and curettage under local or general anaesthesia.

**Entropion.** Entropion is a turning in of an eyelid. This causes the eyelashes to rub on the cornea, giving discomfort, but more seriously, corneal ulceration may be produced. Irritation in the eye or tight bandaging may produce spastic entropion. This is relieved by curing the primary condition or removing the bandage as appropriate. Common causes of entropion are changes in the lid due to age (senile), scarring or mechanical factors.

*Treatment*

Treatment is by surgery.

**Ectropion.** In this condition the eyelid turns outwards. The tears cannot reach the lacrimal punctum and the patient will be troubled by watering (epiphora). The exposed conjunctiva becomes inflamed and thickened, giving the more severely affected an unsightly appearance. Weakness of the lid muscle due to age or paralysis (facial palsy) may be the cause. Contracture due to skin disease or injury can readily produce this eversion.

*Treatment*

Treatment is by surgery.

**Wounds of the eyelids.** Careful repair is required to avoid complication by ectropion or entropion. The lid edge is particularly important to avoid notching and consequent watering or exposure of the cornea. Poor repair may cause trichiasis (eyelash rubbing on the eyeball) and in the inner sixth the canaliculus is liable to damage and requires skilful repair.

**Ptosis.** Ptosis of the upper eyelid is a drooping of the lid and may be due to increased weight of the lid or weakness of the muscle that elevates the upper lid. The muscle weakness may be a failure in development, may be due to acquired disease, or injury affecting the muscle, the nerve-muscle junction (myasthenia gravis), or the nerve supply which is partly from the third cranial nerve and partly from the sympathetic nervous system.

**Tumours of the eyelids.** The common malignant lesion is basal cell carcinoma (rodent ulcer), which is usually suitable for local excision but radiotherapy is effective provided the cornea, eyeball and canaliculi are shielded from damage.

## DISEASES OF THE CONJUNCTIVA

Inflammation of the conjunctiva is called conjunctivitis and this may be due to infection or allergy, or physical or chemical irritants. Infective conjunctivitis may be due to: Koch-Weeks bacillus, *Pneumococcus*, *Streptococcus*, *Staphylococcus*, *Gonococcus*, diphtheria bacillus and also various viruses.

Clinically, there is an increased redness of the conjunctiva and the eyes are uncomfortable, and, depending on the type and severity of the organism causing the condition, different types of discharge may occur from the eyes—mucoid, mucopurulent, purulent, or sanious (blood-stained). In some cases, a membrane forms on the conjunctiva and then diphtheria may be considered as a possible cause, though in recent years diphtheria has been very rare. Ophthalmia neonatorum is a conjunctivitis occurring in the newborn and is due to the infection of the eyes at birth. In a number of cases the infecting organism is the *Gonococcus*, and the condition produced is that of severe purulent conjunctivitis which, by implication of the cornea and secondary corneal ulceration, and possible infection of the interior of the eye, may lead to blindness. In parts of the world where *Gonococcus* is common, then prophylactic treatment such as sulphacetamide or penicillin may be given to the eyes at birth, but where this organism is rare, for instance here in Britain, then the eyes are swabbed clean with sterile moist swabs and only if there is any evidence of infection is a swab taken to send to the laboratory and treatment commenced with local and systemic antibiotics.

### PHLYCTENULAR CONJUNCTIVITIS

This is a disease of young people, characterised by the appearance of small grey nodules in the conjunctiva, which may easily spread on to the cornea and cause marked deterioration in vision by subsequent vascularisation and scarring of the cornea.

The conjuctivitis is often complicated by secondary infection which requires treatment in the usual way.

This disease is now thought to be a form of allergy of which tuberculous infection is one possible cause.

## TRACHOMA

Trachoma is a disease caused by a virus so large in size that it shares some characteristics with bacteria in so far as it can be seen with the ordinary microscope after staining and it can be affected by antibiotics. The disease is endemic in many parts of the world, particularly the Middle East, Far East and South America, where a large part of the population has the infection at some time. The effects can be mild or severe. The disease may also occur in epidemic form. It can be carried to temperate countries where it may be passed on, thus occasional cases are found in Britain. The acute stage, which is a very red eye with discharge, large follicles in the conjunctiva lining the eyelids to give an appearance almost like sago-grains. The upper part of the cornea may also be affected and later the lining of the lids (palpebral conjunctiva) becomes scarred, leading to an entropion, and further damage is caused by the eyelashes rubbing. Secondary infection may be a further cause of serious corneal damage so that in a world-wide context, this is the cause of blindness for thousands of people.

## NEW GROWTHS

At birth, small dermoids may be found at the junction of the conjunctiva and cornea, and dermolipomas may be found in the posterior parts of the conjunctiva. Other benign growths are small melanomas (naevi). Malignancy is rare, though there is a type of malignant melanoma *in situ* and there may be a spread of basal cell carcinoma from the lids. An epithelioma may occur at the junction with the cornea.

## DISEASES OF THE CORNEA

### CORNEAL ULCERS

Corneal ulcer is a loss of the covering epithelium. Such loss may be caused by injury, where it is called an abrasion. Such an abrasion usually heals rapidly and the eye is normal again

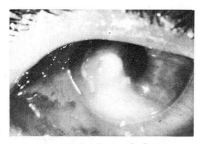

FIG. 51.3    Corneal ulcer.

within 24 to 48 hours. However, infection delays the healing and may cause advancing invasion of the substance of the cornea and then it is called a corneal ulcer.

An ulcer of this type can be due to infection with the ordinary pus-forming organisms, such as *Staphylococcus* and *Pneumococcus*, but some varieties of the Gram-negative organisms may also enter the substance of the cornea if the covering epithelium is damaged. The bacteria will rarely penetrate the intact cornea, though occasionally do so in a severe purulent conjunctivitis. Virus infections will, however, penetrate the cornea even when it is intact. Fungi are always secondary invaders after preliminary damage has been done by viruses, bacteria or injury. Drying of the cornea due to inability to close the lids because of prominence of the eye or failure of the eyelid closure (facial palsy) will lead to ulceration. Loss of the nerve supply also carries great risk of ulceration (neurotrophic keratitis).

*Symptoms and signs*

The eye is red and painful with watering and photophobia. The vision is impaired. The ulcerated area may show as a grey patch on the cornea, but in milder cases it is more easily shown by staining with fluorescein. Treatment is by antibiotics locally either by surface application or by subconjunctival injection, and sometimes systemic treatment also is required if there is a danger of the infection spreading into the interior of the eye. Severe corneal ulceration may lead to iritis and this also requires its own treatment. Virus infections may require treatment with chemical cauterisation, though now some antiviral agents are available. Treatment is also aimed at preventing secondary infection by other invaders. Fungus may be a secondary invader, and then if it will not respond to antifungal agents, local excision or even corneal grafting may be indicated. Corneal ulcer may heal by scarring which, if it is in the central part of the cornea, can seriously affect the vision. failure to heal may lead to perforation of the cornea, and loss of contents of the eye. On other occasions, infection spreads to the interior of the eye with serious damage and even loss of the eye.

### INTERSTITIAL KERATITIS

This is deep inflammation in the cornea with an intact epithelium, i.e. there is no ulceration. There is more than one cause for this, but the term is most commonly used to describe the inflammation of the cornea occurring in congenital syphilis. Treatment consists of general antisyphilitic remedies plus local atropine and corticosteroids.

Deep inflammation also occurs as a complication of virus infections of the epithelium.

## KERATOPLASTY

Keratoplasty means corneal grafting. In this operation, part of the diseased cornea is replaced by healthy corneal tissue either from the eye of a dead person or from an eye that has been removed for some pathological condition yet has an intact cornea. The grafting may take the form of the replacement of a small area of the cornea in its entire thickness (a penetrating graft) or the replacement of a circumscribed area of the cornea in part of its thickness only (lamellar graft). By this means, an opaque cornea interfering with vision is replaced by clear tissue.

## DISEASES OF THE IRIS

### IRITIS

The uveal tract comprises the iris, ciliary body, and the choroid. Inflammation of the various parts is called iritis, cyclitis and choroiditis respectively, and in the usual course of events one tissue is involved with the others, so that an iritis has some degree of cyclitis with it, and a choroiditis is likely to be accompanied by some degree of cyclitis as well. Uveitis may be due to many causes. The cause may be transmitted from outside, for instance as an indirect infection carried in by a perforating injury (exogenous). The disease may develop because of organisms or allergy spread via the blood stream (endogenous uveitis). Iritis may also develop as a reaction to other local eye disease, for instance corneal ulcer or scleritis (secondary). Infective organisms in the form of bacteria or viruses, fungi and protozoa may be involved. However, sometimes the iritis is a state of reaction in an allergic manner.

In iritis, the blood vessels of the conjunctiva around the cornea are inflamed. The iris is swollen and inflamed and the pupil is small leading to adhesions between the posterior surface of the iris and the lens behind. Inflammatory cells appear in the anterior chamber, and if these are profuse an exudate may be seen with the naked eye. Iritis is accompanied by a varying amount of pain and impairment of vision. Severe pain usually indicates some complication, for instance secondary glaucoma. In choroiditis, inflammatory cells enter the vitreous humor, producing cloudy vision.

*Treatment*

Ideally, this is directed at the systemic cause in the first instance, but it is also important to give local treatment to the eye in the form of atropine drops to dilate the pupil and keep it dilated, plus local corticosteroids in most instances. Systemic corticosteroids may be necessary.

## MELANOMA

This is a malignant tumour that arises in the uveal tract, usually the choroid. Dissemination occurs widely throughout the body, but the commonest site of secondary deposits is the liver.

## DISEASES OF THE RETINA

### DETACHMENT OF THE RETINA

The retina becomes separated in part from the choroid, which carries a great deal of its blood supply. The condition may arise as a result of trauma, but usually there is a predisposing weakness in the retina, which leads to holes in the retina and spontaneous detachment. It may be secondary to other disease in the eye when it is displaced by tumour or exudate. Sometimes there are general systemic causes. Partial loss of the field of vision or distorted vision are prominent symptoms and complete blindness of the affected eye may ensue. Myopic eyes are more liable to retinal detachment than normal eyes.

*Treatment*

If there are no underlying systemic or intraocular conditions to treat and the detachment is due to a tear in the retina, then surgery is undertaken to replace the retina to the choroid. Scarring is caused by diathermy, by cryothermy or by light coagulation. In most cases a shortening or infolding operation may be necessary on the outer scleral part of the eye—scleral resection or plication. Plastic materials are now being used to cause indentation. Both eyes are usually bandaged for a period afterwards so as to prevent movements of the eyes and strict bed rest is essential. Afterwards the patient is warned to avoid bending and stooping, or any severe exertion that might cause a recurrence of the detachment.

### RETINOBLASTOMA

Retinoblastoma is also called a glioma retinae, although there is no relation to the gliomas of the brain. It is a malignant growth of the retina that occurs in young children, usually in the first few years of life. The condition may necessitate the excision of the eye, but irradiation from cobalt plaques and chemotherapy, plus sometimes light coagulation, may enable the eye to be preserved with safety. The condition may be bilateral.

## RETROLENTAL FIBROPLASIA

Retrolental fibroplasia is a condition that sometimes occurs in premature babies treated with oxygen at a concentration exceeding 30 per cent. It affects both eyes and is characterised by the formation of fibrous tissue behind the lens and detachment of the retina is often present.

## RETINOPATHY

A number of conditions previously described as retinitis are not inflammations and are now classed 'retinopathy'.

**Hypertensive.** The most severe changes appear in malignant hypertension. Using the ophthalmoscope, oedema of the optic disc (optic nerve head) appears as a swollen disc with blurred margins, loss of the normal central pit (physiological cup) and the vessels may be obscured on the disc by exudates. The retina near the disc shows flame-shaped haemorrhages and exudates of cotton wool appearance. The oedema affects the retina also and in severe forms the central retina is affected causing a drop in visual acuity and later hard exudates in a star distribution may appear at the macula (centre of the retina).

**Arteriosclerotic.** The vessels show thicker walls than normal and alter the veins where the retinal artery crosses a vein. Lesser degrees of hypertensive changes may be shown and the veins may be obstructed leading to multiple retinal haemorrhages and oedema in the area of retina served by the vein. Arterial obstruction or failure which may also be due to embolus or to failure of the blood supply to the ophthalmic artery.

**Diabetic.** The individual features visible with the ophthalmoscope can be found in other conditions, but the overall pattern is typical enough to suspect the diagnosis. Tiny round (dot), or slightly larger (blot) haemorrhages can be seen in the retina. Some of these are microaneurysms of the capillaries, not haemorrhages. Hard-edged white or yellow exudates appear, particularly in the macular area. In general, the younger patients show a tendency to the formation of new blood vessels on the retina and optic disc producing vitreous haemorrhage and retinal detachment. Diabetic retinopathy is the largest cause of blindness in young adults in .Europe and North America.

## AFFECTIONS OF THE LACRIMAL APPARATUS

The lacrimal gland secretes tear fluid which is shed as a fine film over the conjunctiva and cornea. The fluid drains by way of the lacrimal punctae into the canaliculi to the lacrimal sac and duct into the inferior meatus of the nose. If there is block-age in any of these structures, then the tears are unable to drain away and pour on to the face, resulting in epiphora. The stagnation of tears may become secondarily infected, causing a lacrimal abscess, or a mucocele may result, and the infection may cause a unilateral conjunctivitis. Treatment con-sists of treating the secondary infection. If this is unsuccessful, then a new drainage channel may be made into the nose (dacrycocystorhinostomy) or in some cases removal of the in-fected duct altogether (dacrycocystectomy). In small children, probing the ear duct may be sufficient.

## GLAUCOMA

Glaucoma is a term that indicates an increase of pressure with-in the eye above the normal limits. Where the rise of tension is associated with some known pathological event, such as a dislocated lens or an intraocular tumour, then the condition is known as secondary glaucoma, but when no cause can be found, the condition is called primary glaucoma.

### PRIMARY GLAUCOMA

(1) Acute closed angle glaucoma or (2) an insidious quiet-type chronic glaucoma called open angle glaucoma. The in-creased pressure in the eye can, if unrelieved, lead to blindness.

**Acute glaucoma.** Occurring most often in elderly subjects, the onset is sudden, accompanied by severe pain and redness of the eye. Rainbow halos around white lights may be an early warning symptom. The cornea is 'steamy' due to alteration within the cornea, and the pupil may be fixed and dilated. The intraocular pressure is markedly raised. Miotic drops should be used. Usually pilocarpine is given intensively. The intraocular secretion of fluid should be reduced by the syste-mic use of drugs such as Diamox. If the tension still remains high, then some form of drainage operation has to be done urgently on the eye, as the vision can fail rapidly and perman-ently. If the pressure comes down with medical treatment, then an iridectomy is performed which prevents recurrence of the acute attacks.

**Chronic glaucoma.** The onset of this condition is gradual, with the result that the extent of permanent damage to vision may be very great before the condition is noticed. The eye may appear superficially normal, but curtailment of the field of vision may be very marked and blindness may result.

*Treatment*
Treatment consists of the use of miotic drops and the

patient must be kept under observation. If the raised tension in the eye is not controlled, then surgery is advised.

## STRABISMUS

Strabismus, or squint, is due to many causes. It may be paralytic, due to damage to the nerves supplying the extrinsic muscles of the eyeball, or it may be due to maldevelopment of one group of muscles or their faulty insertion. It may follow an uncorrected refractive error or be a manifestation of some cause of defective vision in an eye such as a corneal scar or a congenital cataract. A concomitant squint is one in which the degree of convergence or divergence of the eyes is the same in all positions of gaze. In a paralytic or incomitant squint, the degree of deviation varies with the direction of gaze. Squints are common in children and if uncorrected may lead to grave deterioration of vision in the squinting eye (amblyopia).

*Treatment*

Refractive errors must be corrected with suitable spectacles, and this often corrects a part or all of the squint. In some cases operation is necessary to alter the muscles that move the eye. Orthoptic treatment is of value in improving the vision of the squinting eye and in the reinforcement of binocular vision.

## NYSTAGMUS

Nystagmus is the name given to oscillatory movements of the eyes. These movements may be in any direction, but most often occur laterally. The condition may be due to many causes. It may be congenital, be a manifestation of some defect of vision such as congenital cataract or defect in the retina, part of a nervous disease such as disseminated sclerosis or cerebellar tumour, or follow some disease of the inner ear when the semicircular canals are implicated. It can also arise as an occupational condition in miners.

## CATARACT

The normal lens is a soft, clear structure. With age it becomes harder but remains clear. The development of opacity is the condition known as cataract.

A cataract may occur as a congenital condition, and infection of the mother with rubella in the early stages of pregnancy is one such cause. It may be secondary to some underlying disease of the eye such as iridocyclitis, glaucoma, retinal detachment or injury, and may occur as a manifestation of some general disease such as diabetes. Most commonly, cataract arises as a senile condition.

As the cataract extends, light is unable to penetrate into the eye and vision becomes increasingly worse.

*Treatment*

Removal of the lens is usually necessary in advanced cases. This results in inability to focus, so that strong fixed lenses must be supplied in spectacles after operation.

CARE OF THE PATIENT FOR CATARACT SURGERY

The general condition is improved as much as possible, paying attention particularly to diabetes mellitus. Conjunctival swabs are no longer routinely carried out, but the eyes must be carefully examined to exclude possible infection and it is usual to give broad-spectrum antibiotic drops for at least 48 hours preoperatively. The operation is carried out under local or general anaesthesia.

POSTOPERATIVE CARE

This has been simplified by the increased suturing of the cataract wound so that it is now possible to mobilise the patient more or less immediately and only the operated eye is covered. It is useful to have the eye covered with a pad, a shield, and with a bandage at night in order to reduce the risk that the patient may knock his eye during sleep. The eye is dressed daily and a local antibiotic drop instilled. Other treatments are given according to the decision of the surgeon.

## Complications

1. Postoperative mania is not uncommon in elderly patients. It may subside with sedatives, but may require the uncovering of the eye.

2. Prolapse of the iris may occur, and the importance of avoiding straining is very great in the prophylaxis. Further

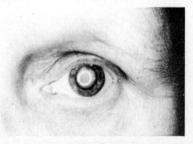

FIG. 51.4   Cataract.

operation is necessary if it occurs, and consists of the excision of the prolapsed portion and resuturing.

3. Intraocular infection is damaging and can lead to the loss of the eye.

4. Chest complications may arise as in any operation performed on a patient of advancing years who, of necessity, has been confined to bed.

5. Haemorrhage into the eye may result from sudden movement, clumsy application of eye drops, or squeezing of the eye after instillation.

## ORBITAL CELLULITIS

The whole orbit may be involved in a severe infection which may require drainage and systemic treatment.

## INJURIES AND FOREIGN BODIES

Injuries occur commonly as a result of lodgment of small foreign bodies like dust particles on the cornea.

*Treatment*

Early removal of the foreign body is very important, since corneal ulceration may develop. All cases are associated with some degree of conjunctivitis. A few drops of 1 per cent amethocaine are instilled and the foreign body is removed with a sharp sterile needle. Antibiotic drops are instilled and the eye is covered with a pad and bandage for twelve hours.

**Penetrating injuries.** The most serious injuries are due to penetrating wounds, and a foreign body may remain in the eye.

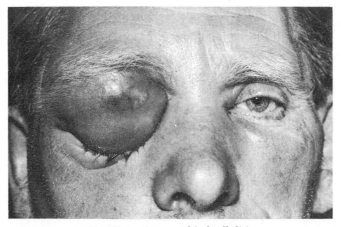

FIG. 51.5   Severe orbital cellulitis.

*Treatment*

This is on the general lines of that laid down for wounds (p. 193). Excision of the damaged tissue, removal of the foreign body and suture, together with appropriate measures to prevent infection, are carried out. Applied to the eye, this consists of:

1. Removal of the foreign body. This may require the use of the giant magnet if the foreign body is magnetic, after it has been localised by X-ray of the eye and orbit.
2. Suture of the wound with fine sutures is necessary after excision of prolapsed intraocular structures.
3. The instillation of atropine and covering of the eye.
4. The administration of antibiotics locally and systemically.

If the eyeball is damaged so seriously that conservative measures are likely to be of no avail, excision of the eyeball is necessary as there is the risk of sympathetic ophthalmia in the other eye.

*Sympathetic ophthalmia* is a severe bilateral panuveitis following perforating injury of one eye. This panuveitis can be so severe as to lose the sight from both eyes, therefore in severe injury it is often advisable to remove the injured eye prior to the eleventh day after injury, which will prevent the development of sympathetic ophthalmia.

CARE OF A CASE OF EXCISION OF THE EYE

Immediately postoperatively, a firm pad and bandage are required to reduce swelling and bruising. Subsequently, the socket will require the instillation of drops or ointment of a suitable antibiotic until healing has occurred. A plastic shell is worn for three to four weeks to prevent shrinkage and to shape the socket until an artificial eye is worn.

In most cases, a better cosmetic result is obtained by replacing the excised eye with an implant which forms a movable base for an anteriorly placed prosthesis.

# CHAPTER 52

# Gynaecology

Gynaecology is the study of diseases peculiar to women.

## STRUCTURE AND FUNCTIONS OF THE FEMALE GENITAL ORGANS

The female genital tract consists of:

1. **The external genital organs or vulva.** The vulva comprises the mons veneris, the labia majora, the labia minora, the clitoris, the vestibule with the external urethral orifice, the vaginal orifice, and the perineum.

The mons veneris is a cushion of fat occupying the midline and lying in front of the pubic bone.

The labia majora are two folds of skin enclosing fatty tissue, extending anteriorly from the mons veneris to the perineum posteriorly.

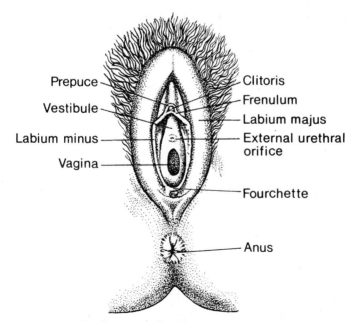

Prepuce — Clitoris
Vestibule — Frenulum
— Labium majus
Labium minus — External urethral orifice
Vagina — Fourchette
— Anus

FIG. 52.1   Female external genital organs.

603

The labia minora are two thin folds of skin lying internal to the labia majora.

The hymen, which is a septum of mucous membrane perforated eccentrically, partially closes the vaginal orifice. Occasionally it is imperforate, and may give rise to the condition of haematocolpos.

Within the substance of the posterior part of the labia majora lie the mucus-secreting glands of Bartholin, the ducts of which open on the inner side of the labia minora. The urethral orifice lies between the clitoris anteriorly and the vaginal orifice posteriorly.

The perineum is the area between the vagina and the anus.

2. **The internal genitalia.** The internal genitalia comprise the vagina, the uterus, the Fallopian tubes, and the ovaries.

The *vagina* is a muscular canal extending from the hymen below to the cervix of the uterus above. The upper end of the vagina is divided into anterior, posterior, and lateral fornices by the projecting cervix. Anteriorly is situated the urethra and bladder and posteriorly is the rectum and the recto-vaginal septum.

The *uterus* is a pear-shaped, hollow, muscular organ about 7·5 cm long, lying in the middle of the pelvic cavity supported by ligaments. It is covered by peritoneum, except laterally, where the anterior and posterior peritoneal layers pass towards the lateral pelvic wall as the broad ligaments. The Fallopian tubes and the blood and lymphatic vessels of the uterus are enclosed in these lateral folds of peritoneum.

The uterus consists of the body and the cervix. The part of the body above the insertion of the Fallopian tubes is known as the fundus.

The cavity of the uterus is lined with mucous membrane called the endometrium, the superficial layer of which is shed during menstruation.

The cervix is the lower portion of the uterus and is 2·5 cm in length. The part which projects into the vagina is conical in shape in nulliparous women, but during childbirth it is lacerated laterally, thus forming anterior and posterior lips. The cervical canal which is continuous above with the cavity of the uterus is lined with mucous membrane.

The cervix is the second commonest site of carcinoma in women, and it is not without significance that such a growth is rare in nulliparous women (women who have not borne children).

The *Fallopian tubes* are a pair of thin muscular canals, 12·5 cm in length, extending outwards and backwards from each side of the fundus of the uterus. The outer ends, which are fimbriated (fringelike structures), project into the peritoneal cavity and help to direct the shed ovum into the lumen of the tube which is lined by a specialised ciliated epithelium. The cup-like tube end lies underneath the ovary during ovulation.

It will be noted that there is a continuous canal between the vulva and peritoneal cavity.

The *ovaries* are a pair of dull white almond-shaped structures, lying in the pelvis, attached by a mesentery to the posterior layer of the broad ligaments and also by a ligament to the fundus of the uterus. They contain numerous ova or egg cells.

During the reproductive period one ovum matures each month and is extruded into the peritoneal cavity. It then enters the Fallopian tube and so reaches the uterus.

The ovaries secrete two hormones:

*Oestrogen,* which is responsible for the growth of the genital tract and breasts, the maturation of ova, and the growth of the endometrium in the first half of the menstrual cycle.

*Progesterone,* which prepares still further the endometrium for the implantation of the ovum should it be fertilised. It is also responsible for the maintenance of early pregnancy.

The secretion of the ovarian hormones is controlled by the hormones of the anterior pituitary gland, viz. follicle-stimulating hormone (FSH) and luteinising hormone (LH).

### PUBERTY

The sex characteristics of an individual slowly develop from early life, but at puberty the changes become more marked. The anterior pituitary hormones increasingly activate the ovaries, which stimulate the genital organs and the general body configuration to assume their adult form.

From puberty to the menopause menstruation normally occurs every 28 days, and the menstrual flow lasts for about four days.

### OVULATION

During most menstrual cycles one ovum activated by oestrogen grows to maturity. It approaches the surface of the ovary as it matures and is surrounded for the most part by fluid, the *liquor folliculi,* which is the source of the oestrogenic hormones. The extrusion of an ovum from an ovary into the peritoneal cavity occurs about 14 days prior to the next menstrual period. The mature ovum, *liquor folliculi,* and the wall of cells surrounding the fluid are known collectively as the *Graafian follicle.*

After extrusion of the mature ovum the ovarian cavity remaining becomes obliterated by a growth of special cells which assume a yellow pigment. This is called the corpus luteum (or yellow body) and is responsible for the secretion of progesterone.

The ovum passes into the Fallopian tube, which is the site of fertilisation, and reaches the uterus about seven days after ovulation. If it is fertilised it implants itself in the endometrium, which, due to the action of oestrogen and progesterone, has been prepared for its reception, and menstruation is suspended. Should fertilisation not occur, the ovum dies and menstruation follows normally.

## MENOPAUSE

The menopause (climacteric or change of life) occurs when the ovaries cease to function, at about the age of 50 years. Menstruation and ovulation gradually cease and atrophy of the genital organs slowly takes place. Symptoms such as hot flushes, headaches, and depression, which may occur at this time, are due to overactivity of the anterior pituitary gland and can be relieved by giving oestrogenic hormone in diminishing doses.

## DISORDERS OF MENSTRUATION

### AMENORRHOEA

Amenorrhoea is the absence of menstrual bleeding, and may be real or apparent. Real amenorrhoea is divided into:

1. **Physiological.** Before puberty, during pregnancy and lactation and after the menopause.

2. **Pathological.** (a) *General.* Any acute infection may cause amenorrhoea. Many chronic diseases such as pulmonary tuberculosis, thyrotoxicosis or myxoedema may be factors. Another important factor is a tumour of the adrenal or pituitary gland.

(b) *Local defects:*
   (i) Congenital (e.g. absence of the uterus).
   (ii) Severe tuberculosis of the genital tract.
   (iii) Masculinising tumour of the ovary—arrhenoblastoma, a very rare condition.
   (iv) Therapeutic. Operative removal of the uterus and/ or the ovaries, or destruction of the endometrium by radium or deep X-ray treatment.

3. **Psychological.** Amenorrhoea may arise from shock, sudden weight loss or changes in the environment.

Amenorrhoea is also sometimes described as primary or secondary. In primary amenorrhoea the periods have never started. Secondary amenorrhoea includes all other forms of amenorrhoea except the physiological types.

*Treatment*

Treatment consists in finding and dealing with the cause of the amenorrhoea. In some cases this may include hormonal therapy.

**Apparent amenorrhoea.** This means that although the patient has commenced menstruation there is no external evidence.

*Causes*

1. Imperforate hymen.
2. Atresia of the vagina.

There is no escape for the menstrual fluid, and the following conditions may occur:

Haematocolpos–blood collects in the vagina
Haematometra—blood collects in the uterus
Haematosalpinx—blood collects in the Fallopian tubes.

### EXCESSIVE AND IRREGULAR UTERINE BLEEDING

1. **Menorrhagia.** This is a condition of either excessive or prolonged blood loss at the time of menstruation.
2. **Epimenorrhagia.** The periods occur at excessively frequent intervals, e.g. every 14 days, are too heavy.

Both types of bleeding may be caused by:

Overactivity of the ovaries
Upset of the oestrin-progesterone balance
Inflammatory conditions such as endometritis
Uterine growths such as fibroids and polyps
Uterine displacement, e.g. retroversion
Life in hot climates
Diseases such as cardiac and renal lesions, anaemia, pulmonary tuberculosis and diabetes mellitus.

*Treatment*

Treatment depends on the cause and includes curettage of the endometrium, myomectomy, or hormonal therapy. In severe and intractable cases the induction of an artificial menopause by radium, X-rays, or even hysterectomy may be advised.

3. **Metrorrhagia or metrostaxis.** Bleeding occurs between the menstrual periods. The cause is always a local one and may be a neoplasm or polyp.

4. **Post-menopausal bleeding.** An important symptom of which carcinoma is the most important cause. Polyps, ovarian tumours, senile vaginitis, and recent oestrogenic hormone therapy may also cause the condition. Oestrogen withdrawal causes bleeding when used for inhibiting lactation or in the contraceptive pill.

*Treatment*

Treatment is that of the cause, and in every case the nurse should urge the patient to seek medical advice at once as delay may render the condition inoperable.

## DYSMENORRHOEA (MENSTRUAL PAIN)

About 50 per cent of women complain of some pain with the periods, but only a very small percentage are incapacitated.

Clinically the types of dysmenorrhoea which may be differentiated are:

Primary (spasmodic or true dysmenorrhoea)
Secondary (acquired or congestive dysmenorrhoea).

1. **Spasmodic dysmenorrhoea.** This usually occurs in healthy girls at about 17 or 18 years of age, several years after the onset of menstruation. The pain occurs in violent spasms accompanied by sweating, vomiting and fainting. The pain which comes on at the beginning of the period lasts from 12 to 24 hours, is responsible for much misery and many cases of drug addiction can be traced back to this cause. The nurse with easy access to drugs should be extremely careful to seek medical advice and not to treat herself—unless she does this, it may be the beginning of drug addiction.

*Treatment*

MEDICAL

The most effective treatment is suppression of ovulation by means of oestrogens or progestogens.

Analgesics and warmth may help but antispasmodics are ineffective.

SURGICAL

Dilatation and curettage may be tried not always with success and involve the risk of an incompetent cervix in subsequent pregnancy.

Presacral neurectomy is a major operation but the results are good.

2. **Congestive dysmenorrhoea.** The pain is less acute than in the spasmodic type and is due to the congestion of blood in the pelvic organs. Congestion is more marked and pain more severe where there are inflammatory conditions, a growth in the generative organs, malposition of the uterus or habitual constipation. The patient complains of headache, backache, pain in the thighs and the symptoms are usually relieved when the menstrual period begins.

*Treatment*

The patient should be encouraged to continue her normal routine. Any underlying cause should, of course, be treated.

# COMPLICATIONS OF PREGNANCY

## ABORTION OR MISCARRIAGE

DEFINITION. The interruption of pregnancy before the 28th week, i.e. before the fetus is legally viable (capable of living a separate existence), is known as an abortion or miscarriage.

The causes of abortion are many, but abnormality of the embryo, certain maternal diseases, abnormalities of the uterus and hormonal disturbances are the most common. In 60 per cent no cause is found.

The majority of abortions occur between the eighth and twelfth weeks of pregnancy.

## Types of abortion

1. *Threatened.* Vaginal bleeding occurs, but the cervical canal remains closed and there are no painful uterine contractions. Pregnancy continues in about 50 per cent of cases if effective treatment is given with no increased risk of fetal abnormality.

2. *Inevitable.* There is severe bleeding with painful uterine contractions. The cervix dilates and the fetus and placenta are expelled (complete abortion). Sometimes part of the products of conception are retained (incomplete abortion), and this is diagnosed by the presence of continued bleeding.

3. *Missed abortion.* The fetus dies, but the uterus, instead of expelling it immediately, retains it for a varying length of time.

After a period of weeks or months the cervix dilates and the fetus is expelled. In some cases the products of conception are either partially or completely retained and necessitate removal.

*Treatment*

1. *Threatened.* The patient is put on immediate bed rest until the heavy bleeding ceases when she is allowed up for toilet purposes. Observations of temperature, pulse and blood pressure are taken as necessary and the vaginal loss is checked. A specimen of early morning urine is taken for an immunological pregnancy test. Blood samples are taken for cross-matching and for checking the haemoglobin level. Sedatives may be given if the patient is anxious and mild analgesics may also be required. A high protein, high residue diet should be given and vitamin and/or iron supplements may be necessary (e.g. Pregaday). Progesterone is sometimes given but it is of doubtful value.

2. *Inevitable abortion.* In the majority of cases both the fetus and placenta are expelled naturally.

Operative interference is undertaken when bleeding is severe or continuous, or if on inspection of the products passed the abortion is thought not to be complete. The operation consists of removal of the retained products *per vaginam* together with ergometrine 0·5 mg given by intramuscular or intravenous injection. Blood transfusion may be necessary.

3. *Missed abortion.* The uterus should be encouraged to empty itself by the administration of an oxytocin drip. Following such treatment the uterus contracts, the cervix dilates, and the products of conception are expelled.

Occasionally, however, dilatation of the cervix and removal of the products may be necessary. In such cases postoperative haemorrhage may occur. Habitual abortions (three consecutive abortions) at mid-term may be due to an incompetent patulous cervix. The Shirodkar's operation may be performed in the early weeks of pregnancy. A non-absorbable purse string suture is inserted around the cervix at the level of the internal os; this must be removed if labour starts.

## Complications of abortion

1. Infection, which may take the form of endometritis, salpingitis, peritonitis, and septicaemia. It is usually controlled by chemotherapy.

2. Haemorrhage.

3. Pelvic thrombophlebitis.

4. Injury to the cervix and perforation of the uterus may occur during operative interference, but is much more common as a result of a criminal abortion.

5. Secondary infertility.

### TUBAL PREGNANCY (ECTOPIC GESTATION)

Occasionally the fertilised ovum, instead of becoming implanted in the uterus, may embed itself in the wall of the Fallopian tube. This is known as a tubal pregnancy. It may also be referred to as an ectopic gestation because it is a pregnancy outside the uterine cavity. Owing to the unsuitability of the Fallopian tubes for the implantation and growth of the developing ovum, either rupture of the tube occurs (tubal rupture) or the developing ovum is extruded into the peritoneal cavity through the fimbriated end of the tube (tubal abortion). Both processes are associated with abdominal pain, haemorrhage, and acute circulatory failure but these symptoms are more severe in cases of tubal rupture.

*Signs and symptoms.* There is usually a definite history of amenorrhoea or an overdue period although in 20 per cent of cases this may not be present. When tubal rupture or tubal abortion occurs the patient complains of sudden lower abdominal pain, which may be sufficiently severe to cause fainting. The pain may also be felt in the epigastrium or be referred to the shoulder. The associated internal haemorrhage leads to collapse, pallor, a weak rapid pulse and a falling of blood pressure. On examination the patient is shocked, the lower abdomen is tender with some fullness and muscle guarding. Vaginal examination, which should only be carried out in hospital, shows extreme tenderness in the fornices and marked tenderness on movement of the cervix from side to side.

*Treatment*

Intravenous therapy is commenced and blood samples are taken for haemoglobin estimations and cross-matching in case blood transfusion is necessary. A quarter-hourly pulse and blood pressure are recorded. The patient is prepared for theatre for diagnostic laparoscopy and once findings are confirmed laparotomy is essential to remove the affected tube.

### DISPLACEMENT OF THE UTERUS

The normal position of the uterus is described as being anteverted and anteflexed. Displacement may be of slight or severe degree.

**Downward displacement or prolapse.** This arises most commonly after the menopause in women who have borne children, but it may occur in nulliparous women.

Prolapse of the anterior vaginal wall together with the base of the bladder is known as a cystocele.

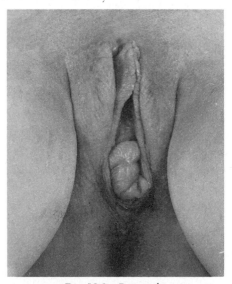

FIG. 52.2   Rectocele.

Prolapse of the lower part of the posterior vaginal wall, with bulging of the rectum into the vagina, is known as a rectocele. Bulging of the upper portion is known as an enterocele.

When the uterus protrudes outside the vulva the condition is known as procidentia.

Elongation of the cervix frequently accompanies a case of long-standing prolapse.

*Clinical features*

1. The patient complains of a lump in the vagina which is larger at the end of the day.

2. Disturbances of micturition, frequency and incontinence of urine on straining and coughing, i.e. stress incontinence. Rarely there is retention of urine.

3. Backache, aggravated by exertion and relieved by rest, but this is usually due to other causes.

4. A bearing-down sensation.

5. Vaginal discharge or bleeding if ulceration due to congestion occurs.

6. Bulging of the anterior and posterior vaginal walls with or without descent of the uterus will be found on asking the patient to strain down.

*Treatment*

The choice of treatment is determined by the degree of prolapse and the general condition and age of the patient. Postnatal care is specially important in its prevention.

1. REST AND GENERAL MEASURES such as tonics (vitamins and iron) to improve the general health, and exercises to improve the tone of the abdominal and pelvic floor muscles may cure mild cases of prolapse.

2. MECHANICAL PESSARIES. A pessary will never cure a prolapse, but, like its counterpart, the truss for a hernia, it may relieve symptoms. The ring pessary acts by keeping the vaginal walls taut and prevents them from becoming evaginated. In severe cases of prolapse, especially where the perineum is deficient, a pessary may not be retained.

There is a danger of ulceration of the vagina or fistula into neighbouring organs with the use of mechanical pessaries unless their use is carefully supervised. The risk of carcinoma of

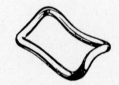

FIG. 52.3    Jessop pessary.

the vagina following prolonged use is a very real one and if at all possible operation is the treatment of choice.

Disposable pessaries are generally used and should be replaced every six to eight weeks. Rubber or vulcanite pessaries, if used, should be cleaned and reinserted every six to eight weeks. Douching is not necessary unless there is an excessive discharge, for which the patient should use normal saline or a simple antiseptic.

*Sterilisation of pessaries.* The rubber ring pessaries are sterilised by boiling. The vulcanite pessaries are sterilised by placing in an antiseptic solution, e.g. biniodide of mercury (1:10,000) or 0·5 per cent Savlon for half an hour.

3. OPERATIVE TREATMENT. Curative operative treatment consists of an anterior colporrhaphy and colpoperineorrhaphy, with or without amputation of the cervix (the former being known as Fothergill's or the Manchester operation); in some cases a vaginal hysterectomy is necessary and the prolapse is cured at the same time. Other operative treatment includes the Le Fort operation, in which the anterior and posterior vaginal walls are sutured together after a certain amount of redundant tissue has been removed. In elderly patients the vaginal epithelium is so atrophic that whatever is done may cause more injury.

In many cases vaginitis or ulceration of the cervix must be treated first by rest and local treatment, e.g. magnesium sulphate and glycerine vaginal packs, until infection has been controlled. In cases of vaginitis a high vaginal swab is taken for bacteriological investigations and the appropriate chemotherapy given.

In long-standing cases it is essential that a full urinary investigation, including pyelography, be carried out, as the presence of a hydroureter or hydronephrosis may be a contra-indication to operation.

**Retroflexion and retroversion.** Backward displacement is usually a combination of retroflexion and retroversion. The condition is fairly common and may be symptomless. Present-

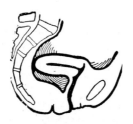

FIG. 52.4    Retroversion of uterus.

ing symptoms include leucorrhoea, backache, and dyspareunia due to prolapsed ovaries or to tenderness of the congested uterus.

*Treatment*

The condition is symptomless in 25 per cent of cases. If symptoms are present, then treatment is dependent on whether the retroverted uterus is fixed or mobile. If mobile, the uterus is first replaced digitally and then a Hodge pessary is inserted to maintain the uterus in its correct position. In other cases the mobile retroverted uterus may be replaced by operation and held permanently in its new position by one of the uterine suspension operations.

In cases of fixed retroversion with symptoms an operation for treatment of the underlying condition is essential; for example, pelvic inflammation or endometriosis.

*Acute inversion of the uterus* is associated with labour, occurring either immediately after delivery of the child or the placenta. Severe circulatory failure results. The uterus must be replaced immediately.

*Chronic inversion of the uterus* is usually caused by a pedunculated fibroid polyp situated in the fundus pulling part of the uterine wall with the tumour when it is being extruded.

*Treatment*

In the older patient (over 40 years) who doesn't want any further children a vaginal hysterectomy may be performed. Otherwise replacement is by surgery following the treatment of any existing infection or occasionally gradual reposition with an Aveling's repositor may be achieved.

## DISEASES OF THE VULVA

The principal diseases of the vulva are inflammatory conditions which may result in cyst formation, urethral caruncle and neoplasms.

*Vulvovaginitis* is usually caused by gonococcal infections though it can be caused by other organisms. It almost invariably occurs in young girls and the symptoms are swelling and inflammation. It may reach epidemic proportions in nursery schools by infection from towels. Treatment is usually chemotheraphy. In addition to the common form of vulvovaginitis, all the specific infections may affect the vulva.

*Pruritus vulvae* is only a symptom, and sometimes no definite cause can be found. The obvious general causes such as diabetes must be excluded. Local causes include leukoplakia which may be precancerous.

If a vaginal discharge is present, bacteriological examination is indicated and the cause treated.

*Kraurosis vulvae* is a condition of atrophy of the vulva including the skin and subcutaneous tissues and is sometimes associated with stenosis of the vaginal orifice.

## TUMOURS OF THE VULVA

### 1. Simple

(a) *Cysts*, e.g. Bartholin's cysts and sebaceous cysts.

(b) *Solid*, e.g. urethral caruncle, which is a small bright red, usually tender, swelling the size of a small bean arising from the posterior lip of the external urethral meatus. It is a granulomatous condition due to *Trichomonas*. It causes frequency, painful micturition, and dyspareunia.

*Treatment*

It is treated with metronidazole (Flagyl) which must also be given to the sexual partner.

Other solid tumours are: fibromas, lipomas, and papillomas.

A true papilloma is rare, but wart-like growths due to excessive vaginal discharge, either venereal or non-venereal, occur.

### 2. Malignant

(a) Squamous cell carcinoma (epithelioma) of the vulva usually arises in women past the menopause. Leukoplakia sometimes precedes it. It occurs in either the labia, the clitoris, the urethra, or Bartholin's glands.

Treatment is a wide excision of the growth and removal of the inguinal lymphatic glands on both sides. Radium and deep X-ray therapy are used for advanced cases.

(b) Sarcoma occurs, but is rare.

(c) Melanoma occurs, but is also rare.

## DISEASES OF THE VAGINA

Injuries and prolapse of the vagina may occur as a result of childbirth. Prolapse is considered with prolapse of the uterus of which it is usually an integral part (p. 611).

**Inflammatory conditions.** Senile vaginitis is seen in women after the menopause and is due to a low-grade infection, often caused by mixed organisms. It is primarily due to the lowered resistance of the atrophic epithelium.

*Treatment*

Small doses of oestrogen hormone and mild local applications are all that is necessary. If pyometra is present as the cause this must be treated.

**Trichomoniasis.** This is caused by *Trichomonas*, a protozoal organism. The vagina becomes inflamed and a greenish-yellow frothy, irritating discharge is present. The condition may affect women of any age, and even young children.

*Treatment*

Metronidazole (Flagyl) is given orally (200 mg t.d.s.) for seven days. No local treatment is necessary.

The male partner, although symptomless, may be given the same treatment to prevent recurrence.

### VAGINAL DISCHARGES (LEUCORRHOEA)

Normally the vaginal transudation is not evident at the orifice. It is increased pre-menstrually and post-menstrually, and always during pregnancy. The reaction of this secretion is highly acid, due to the formation of lactic acid, which inhibits the growth of pathogenic organisms.

The cervical mucosa also secretes mucus which, if excessive, passes downwards into the vagina to become an opaque coagulum before escaping as a vaginal discharge.

**Abnormal vaginal discharge.** It may be an excess of the normal secretions, i.e. leucorrhoea, or it may be purulent or bloodstained.

*Purulent.* This may be due to infection by the *Gonococcus*, *Trichomonas* or *Candida albicans* (thrush). Disease of the cervix or uterus, senile vaginitis, pessaries, or other foreign bodies are other causes.

*Bloodstained and offensive.* Carcinoma of the body of the uterus, carcinoma of the cervix, and sloughing fibroids are the commonest causes. The cervical mucosa secretes mucus which may be thick and sticky or watery and sticky, depending on the stage of the menstrual cycle.

A careful history should be obtained and a thorough examination of the genital tract, including bacteriological examination of the discharge, should be carried out.

*Treatment*

The treatment of a vaginal discharge depends on the cause. For those vaginal discharges due to infection by the *Gonococcus*, *Trichomonas* or *Candida albicans* there are specific measures as already described.

### TUMOURS OF THE VAGINA

1. **Simple.** For example, fibromas and cysts.
2. **Malignant.** Usually a secondary growth from carcinoma of the cervix.

Sarcoma is rare.

# DISEASES OF THE UTERUS

## INFECTIONS OF THE UTERUS

Infections of the uterus may affect the body, the cervix, or both.

1. **The cervix.** Acute infection may occur, the acute attacks being commonly due to gonococcal infection. The treatment is that of the cause.

2. **Erosion of the cervix** (adenomatosis). Consists of an overgrowth of the mucous membranes and glandular elements of the cervix. The mucous membrane grows outwards beyond the external os, replacing the stratified squamous epithelium in that area. This gives a red appearance around the external os. In addition the glands inside the cervix overgrow and often become cystic. These cysts can sometimes be seen as pearly round areas beneath the surface of the vaginal cervix. They are called Nabothian follicles.

The condition is very common during pregnancy and in multiparous patients as well as patients on oral contraceptives. It is also seen occasionally in a patient who has never been pregnant and has an intact hymen. It is then said to be congenital. The cause is doubtful. It was once thought to be inflammatory in origin, but it is now believed to be due to excess hormones. Treatment is diathermy or cautery to the affected area. In more severe lesions the infected tissue may be excised or the cervix amputated.

3. **The body of the uterus.** Acute endometritis is usually puerperal in origin.

Chronic endometritis may be senile or tuberculous.

The senile variety of endometritis is found after the menopause, and is a cause of slight post-menopausal bleeding. It is due to a low-grade infection consequent on menopausal atrophy, and is treated by establishing free drainage of the uterus and the administration of oestrogens.

The tuberculous variety, found in young patients, is diagnosed on biopsy of the endometrium.

## TUMOURS OF THE UTERUS

Both simple and malignant tumours affect the cervix and the body of the uterus, but they show a great difference in their incidence between the two sites. A carcinoma is the commonest new growth in the cervix, whilst an innocent growth, a fibromyoma (fibroid), is the commonest new growth in the uterine body.

Carcinoma of the cervix uteri is the second commonest malignant growth in women.

### Simple tumours

*Polyps* of the uterine and cervical mucous membrane occur. They are usually simple, but occasionally become malignant.

CLINICAL FEATURES are irregular haemorrhage and leucorrhoea. A cervical polyp may be seen protruding from the cervical canal.

Endometrial polyps may be removed with a curette during a diagnostic exploration of the uterine cavity.

TREATMENT. Simple excision is adequate, but the tumour must be examined microscopically to exclude malignant changes.

### FIBROMYOMAS

Fibroids or fibromyomas commence in the muscular wall of the uterus. They are firm in consistency, frequently multiple, and vary in size from a pin head (seedling fibroid) to a mass weighing several kilograms.

As they increase in size they grow either towards the peritoneal cavity (subperitoneal) or towards the cavity of the uterus (submucous). Both types may develop pedicles, and the submucous type form the so-called fibroid polyps.

#### Clinical features

Fibroids may be symptomless, but the common symptoms complained of are menorrhagia, and pressure symptoms due to their weight or impingement on the bladder or the rectum. Infertility may be the first complaint, due to failure of the fertilised ovum to implant in the wall of the uterus. Degeneration or torsion of the pedicle of a subperitoneal fibroid will give rise to symptoms of an acute abdomen. A submucous fibroid may give rise to a foul vaginal discharge owing to the occurrence of sloughing and menorrhagia because it is covered with endometrium.

#### Treatment

Myomectomy is performed if possible if the patient is in the child-bearing period, but if the fibroids are multiple hysterectomy is necessary.

## MALIGNANT NEOPLASMS

### CARCINOMA OF THE CERVIX

This occurs about eight times more frequently in women who have borne children, because laceration and chronic inflammation of the cervix are the chief predisposing factors. While carcinoma of the cervix may occur at any age, the majority of growths arise in women between 40 and 50 years of age. With

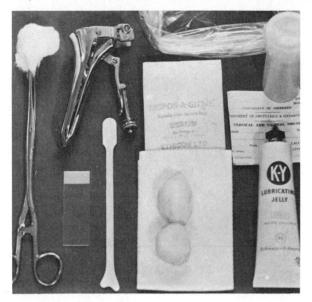

FIG. 52.5    Requirements for Papanicolaou cervical smear.

| | |
|---|---|
| 1 Sponge holder | Container for slide with alcohol |
| 1 Vaginal speculum | ether |
| 1 Ayre's spatula | 3 Wool balls |
| 1 Glass slide | 1 Disposable glove |
| 1 Laboratory form | Bag for discard |
| | Tube of lubricant. |

mass screening, diagnosis of malignancy in younger women is increasing.

*Clinical features*

1. A watery discharge which soon becomes bloodstained and offensive.

2. Irregular vaginal bleeding.

3. In the later stages pain occurs, and indicates that the lesion has spread beyond the cervix.

4. As the disease advances urinary disturbances such as frequency and incontinence of urine occur, due to invasion of the bladder.

5. Cachexia in the late stages of the disease.

6. Renal failure is a terminal condition due to involvement of the ureters.

On examination the cervix is found in the later stages to be friable, indurated, and bleeds easily when touched.

*Treatment*

The results of treatment are good in cases which are treated

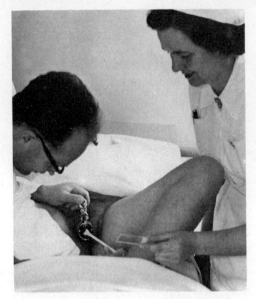

FIG. 52.6   Method of taking cervical smear.

early (over 50 per cent of all patients given radical treatment may now expect to survive for five years) and with mass screening using exfoliative cytology in the form of cervical smears many early cases are discovered. If a smear is positive from a cervix which looks normal, a cone biopsy is performed.

SURGICAL

For carcinoma limited to the cervix amputation of the cervix or a cone biopsy may be sufficient. In more extensive invasion Wertheim's hysterectomy may be performed. Besides removing the uterus, tubes, and ovaries, a wide excision of the surrounding pelvic tissue, including the removal of the pelvic lymph glands, is carried out.

Surgery is undertaken in early cases in young patients and for operable cases where radium is contraindicated or where the growth is radio-resistant.

RADIUM AND DEEP X-RAY THERAPY

Before commencing treatment with radium part of a large fungating growth is sometimes cut away. Occasionally radium is applied preliminary to operative treatment.

Local sepsis is eradicated before radium is applied. In all cases except very early growths a combination of deep X-ray and radium therapy is the usual method of treatment.

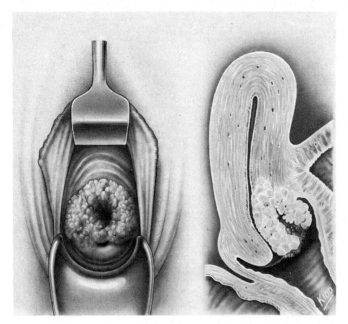

FIG. 52.7   Carcinoma of the cervix. A large carcinoma as seen through a vaginal speculum. Note that the bladder is already invaded by the growth.

### CARCINOMA OF THE BODY OF THE UTERUS

This condition usually occurs in women past the menopause, and occurs as frequently in nulliparae as in women who have borne children. It is the most important cause of post-menopausal bleeding.

*Symptoms*

In order of development symptoms are:

1. Vaginal bleeding.
2. Pain. This is earlier in onset than in the case of carcinoma of the cervix.
3. A foul vaginal discharge.

*Signs*

The uterus may be enlarged, and in advanced cases becomes fixed. Some early cases are discovered only after microscopical examination of endometrial curettings or of the vaginal discharge.

*Treatment*

Total hysterectomy, with removal of both tubes and ovaries, or combined with radium and deep X-ray therapy, gives good results in those cases where the growth is confined to the uterus.

Some measure of success with radiotherapy is obtained in inoperable cases. Cytotoxic drugs may also be used.

## RELIEF OF PAIN IN UTERINE CARCINOMA

Severe pain accompanies the late stages of the disease, and various procedures, such as section of certain of the spinal cord nerves, are of value in the relief of pain. The injection of absolute alcohol into the spinal canal is sometimes performed. Presacral neurectomy is occasionally advised.

## CHORION-EPITHELIOMA

Chorion-epithelioma is a rare uterine tumour consisting of chorionic elements. It follows an abortion of a hydatidiform mole or full-term pregnancy in which a piece of placenta has been left behind.

### Clinical features

Uterine haemorrhage persists after parturition or an abortion. Metastases quickly occur in the lungs. Immunological tests for pregnancy are positive in dilution 1 : 500.

### Treatment

Chemotherapy with methotrexate may give a complete cure in some cases. Hysterectomy is also frequently required, either as the sole measure or in combination with methotrexate therapy.

## ENDOMETRIOSIS

This is a condition in which endometrial-like growths occur in the myometrium, the ovaries, and other pelvic organs and ligaments. It is not malignant.

### Clinical features

These growths behave as endometrium, i.e. they menstruate. Patients complain of sterility, irregular menstruation, backache, lower abdominal pain, pain on defaecation, and dysmenorrhoea. The diagnosis from pelvic infection is often difficult.

### Treatment

A definite diagnosis can be made only by laparoscopy or laparotomy. Conservative surgery is undertaken in young women and it may be controlled with progestogen therapy. Pregnancy usually cures the condition. In older patients hysterectomy with oöphorectomy may be carried out.

The ovaries are inactivated by radiotherapy.

## SALPINGITIS

This condition may be acute or chronic.

**Acute salpingitis.** While most commonly due to gonococcal infection, it may also occur as a result of:

1. Infection at childbirth, miscarriage and especially criminal abortion.
2. Spread from an abdominal focus, e.g. the appendix.
3. Tuberculosis (a relatively rare occurrence).

The attack may be the first or an exacerbation of an old infection.

### Clinical features

The patient complains of sudden, severe, lower abdominal pain. Tenderness and rigidity of the lower abdomen may be present. Fever is usually well marked, the temperature rising in severe cases to 39° to 40° C (103° or 104° F). Menstrual irregularities are not uncommon, and a purulent vaginal discharge is occasionally present. On examination the lower abdomen is found to be acutely tender on either side; on pelvic examination movement of the cervix to either side produces pain, and bimanual palpation through the fornices is excruciatingly painful. Examination of the blood shows a raised white blood cell count and an increased erythrocyte sedimentation rate.

Frequency of micturition and scalding due to an associated urinary infection may also be symptoms.

### Treatment

This is conservative. The patient is confined to bed and treated on the usual lines for an acute febrile condition. The pulse and temperature are carefully charted and a careful note made of any complaint of increasing pain or spreading tenderness which may indicate spreading peritonitis.

Analgesics are required until the pain settles. Sedatives may be necessary. Chemotherapy is usually curative. Once the pain subsides and the white blood count and erythrocyte sedimentation rate improves the patient is allowed up for toilet purposes. Short-wave diathermy is frequently used in the convalescent period to promote resolution.

### Complications

1. Tubo-ovarian abscess (which may require drainage).
2. Hydrosalpinx.
3. Pelvic abscess.
4. Narrowing of the tube due to adhesions.
5. Ectopic gestation later (as a result of scar tissue).
6. Sterility.

**Chronic salpingitis.** With treatment the acute condition localises and resolves, or passes into the chronic stage. It may manifest itself as a pyosalpinx, chronic interstitial salpingitis, or
a hydrosalpinx. The ovary is often affected simultaneously
(tubo-ovarian disease).

*Clinical features*

The patient is often pale, due to the presence of latent sepsis. A history of previous infection may be obtained. The main
symptoms are lower abdominal pain, dragging backache,
general ill-health, menstrual irregularities, and leucorrhoea.

*Treatment*

In the majority of cases symptoms can be relieved by palliative measures such as rest, short-wave diathermy, analgesics
and chemotherapy. The severe cases require operative treatment, which in young women should be as conservative as
possible. Radical treatment such as total hysterectomy or bilateral salpingo-oöphorectomy may be carried out in older
women.

### TUBERCULOSIS

Tuberculosis usually arises by infection from the blood
stream, from a primary focus in the lungs, bronchial or mesenteric glands. Less commonly, direct spread from the pelvic
peritoneum occurs.

Tuberculosis of the genital tract usually commences as a bilateral salpingitis. A tuberculous pyosalpinx may form and
the pelvic peritoneum may be infected, forming dense adhesions between the pelvic organs and the intestines. Ascites may
develop. Tuberculosis of the endometrium usually co-exists.

*Clinical features*

The signs and symptoms of general tuberculosis may be
present—cough, loss of weight, night sweats. Locally, lower
abdominal pain may be present together with amenorrhoea
or menorrhagia.

A definite diagnosis is made on biopsy of the endometrium, at laparotomy, or on microscopical examination of the
diseased Fallopian tubes. In women complaining of infertility, tuberculosis of the pelvic organs should always be excluded and dilatation and curettage performed.

There may be evidence of tuberculosis in the lungs.

*Treatment*

Streptomycin, INAH, and PAS are given. In cases which do
not react favourably surgical treatment may be required, but

may be impossible because of adhesions. X-ray therapy may be of value.

## DISEASES OF THE OVARIES

### INFLAMMATION

The ovaries may be involved in any pelvic inflammatory process. Tubal infection often involves the ovary, causing a tubo-ovarian abscess.

### OVARIAN CYSTS

Cysts of the ovaries are common. They vary considerably in pathology from simple cysts to highly malignant neoplasms.

*Clinical features*

Ovarian cysts occur at all ages. Symptoms are few, unless the cyst reaches a size sufficient to be noticeable and to give rise to pressure symptoms such as oedema of the legs and dyspnoea. An ovarian cyst may obstruct labour.

Complications include:

1. Torsion.
2. Haemorrhage.
3. Rupture and infection.
4. Malignant changes may develop in a simple cyst.

*Treatment*

Excision is the usual treatment. In the presence of complications urgent operation is necessary. The preparation and after-care are similar to those for any abdominal operation. In cases of malignant changes cytotoxic drugs are sometimes given after surgery.

### INFERTILITY (SUBFERTILITY)

Many patients consult gynaecologists because, after two years, their marriages are not fertile.

Infertility may be due to faults in either or both partners. In the female, hormonal dysfunction may cause irregular menstruation or amenorrhoea, or abnormalities or disease of the pelvic organs may be the cause. In the male, disease or abnormalities of the testes and ducts may be present, resulting in defects in the spermatozoa.

*Treatment*

An examination is made to exclude any general disease. The male partner should be investigated first. In the female, endometrial biopsy, tubal insufflation, and hysterosalpingography may be undertaken; also laparoscopy to view pelvic organs and to take a biopsy of the ovaries. Operative treatment may consist of dilatation of the cervix, replacement of a misplaced uterus, and plastic operations on diseased tubes. In the male, semen analysis and plastic operation on the testicular ducts may be carried out.

In both partners improvement of the general health, reassurance and the relief of anxiety, the addition of vitamins, especially vitamin E in the diet, and hormonal therapy may be successful. Human gonadotrophins may be given and have resulted in a high incidence of multiple pregnancy. The reason for this is unknown.

## PREPARATION AND AFTERCARE OF PATIENTS

Prior to any operative procedure the patient must be suitably prepared.

*Preoperative care for vaginal and abdominal operations*
1. General observations should be made on admission, e.g. temperature, pulse and blood pressure.
2. A routine specimen of urine is tested for any abnormalities, especially for glucose.
3. When there is a foul discharge, a swab should be taken for bacteriological investigation and the appropriate chemotherapy given.
4. In most cases the abdomen and vulval areas should be shaved, taking particular care of the cleft of the buttocks.
5. A bath or a bed-bath is necessary the evening before operation and the morning of surgery.
6. Bowel preparation is important, e.g. enemas or suppositories (in some cases) are necessary.
7. The patient should be seen by the physiotherapist before surgery.
8. The doctor checks the patient's haemoglobin estimation and blood is cross-matched.
9. Night sedatives are given to ensure that the patient has a good sleep before surgery.
10. The patient is fasted for six hours before going to the theatre. In some major cases the surgeon prefers to perform catheterisation in the theatre after anaesthesia has been induced.

*Postoperative care for minor surgery*
1. Immediate care is as for any postoperative theatre case.
2. The patient is allowed up to the toilet and to the bidet four hours after surgery if her condition is satisfactory.
3. Careful observation of vaginal loss is necessary.

4. Normally all minor cases are discharged from hospital on the day after surgery. They attend the gynaecological clinic six weeks later for a check-up.

*Postoperative care for major surgery*

1. Immediate postoperative care is as for minor cases.

2. Observations of pulse, temperature, blood pressure, the wound condition and vaginal loss are made and recorded.

3. Analgesics are given as prescribed by the doctor.

4. Intravenous therapy may be ordered.

5. Fluid intake and output is observed and recorded carefully. In cases of urine retention the patient is catheterised and the catheter may be left on free drainage for up to five days. When it is removed the output is observed very closely and catheterisation for residual urine may be required.

6. Vulval toilet should be carried out initially and then the patient is taken to the bidet.

7. The patient is seen by the physiotherapist as soon as possible after surgery.

8. Early mobilisation is important for all cases, e.g. up the day after surgery and allowed to have a bath on the second to third day.

9. On the third day after surgery a haemoglobin estimation is carried out by the doctor. An enema is given and a routine mid-stream specimen of urine is taken and sent for bacteriological investigation.

10. On the seventh to tenth day abdominal clips or sutures are removed. With pelvic floor repairs catgut sutures are generally inserted.

11. Patients are usually discharged from hospital on the tenth to fourteenth day. They are advised to avoid any heavy lifting and to take as much rest as possible. They are asked to attend a gynaecological follow-up clinic six weeks after discharge.

The physiotherapist can aid the patient's recovery by exercises both in bed and when she is ambulant.

## RADIUM IN GYNAECOLOGICAL CASES

The use of radium in the treatment of carcinoma of the body of the uterus and cervix has already been mentioned.

The nurse must be familiar with the radium rules, which provide that all dressings and excreta, etc., from the patient must be preserved until the radium has been removed from the patient's body, checked and found to be correct. The patient is kept on bed rest until the radium is removed. All excreta are inspected before disposal.

Radium for intrauterine use is contained in a platinum case which is inserted into a rubber tube to which silk-nylon sutures are attached. The sutures are strapped to the groin.

For radium treatment the patient is prepared as for a general anaesthetic. She is given an aperient followed by an enema. The vulva is shaved, a douche of sterile water is given and the bladder must be emptied before the patient goes to the theatre. When the radium has been inserted the vagina is plugged with gauze and the patient is usually catheterised. The gauze and radium are removed in 24 hours and a douche of sterile water is given. Between the applications of radium the patient should be observed for symptoms of reaction such as vomiting, pyrexia, lassitude and weakness.

*Reduction of radium hazards in the ward*

Howes and Osborne have drawn attention to the practical measures which may be taken to reduce the hazards to the nurse. They include:

1. Reduction of the time the nurse must spend close to the patient—for example by using anaesthetics with a short recovery time, avoiding transport of the patient to the X-ray department and careful positioning in the wards.

2. The use of mobile lead screens which give adequate protection to the nurse even while close to the patient during such procedures as bed-making.

Downies are now being used in some units to cut down on the bed-making time.

### COMPLICATIONS OF RADIUM THERAPY

The constitutional disturbances have already been mentioned (p. 221). These especially apply to its use in the uterus, as a comparatively large dose is given on several occasions, e.g. the first two doses at weekly intervals and the third dose two weeks after the second.

**Local complications**

1. *Early*. Adhesive vaginitis, cystitis, pyelonephritis, or a proctitis giving rise to diarrhoea and tenesmus may occur. Other complications are pelvic cellulitis, pelvic abscess, peritonitis, septicaemia, or pyometra.

2. *Late*. Atresia of the vagina, atrophy of the cervix and pelvic tissues, constriction of the rectum, and a recto-vaginal fistula. Late complications in the urinary tract include a vesico-vaginal fistula, ureteric obstruction, hydronephrosis, and uraemia. Premature menopausal symptoms are also a late manifestation.

CHAPTER 53

# Iatrogenic Disorders

There were always conditions which arose directly or indirectly from treatment. Admission to hospital has always exposed the patient to the risk of infection and the simplest and apparently most innocuous treatment may produce artificial conditions. Something is restricted, prohibited or added in the form of diet or drugs. The whole of the patient's metabolic processes may be altered. As physiological processes are better understood there is a constant stimulus to design new operations or to invent new drugs and machines which take over temporarily or permanently certain bodily functions.

Radioactive material is used in an ever-increasing variety of forms to investigate function and to treat disease. It is not surprising that many side effects occur and some are so important as to constitute a group of diseases induced by or directly attributable to therapy. Others are minor but none the less troublesome. All, however, are iatrogenic conditions.

In some instances mishaps occur which could easily have been avoided. In other cases a condition arises which could not have been foreseen. Here are considered together conditions arising from treatment whether preventable or otherwise.

They may be:

1. Physical injuries from surgical apparatus or a surgical environment.
2. Chemical injuries.
3. Drug toxicity and idiosyncrasy.
4. Direct operative complications.
5. The effects of surgical ablation.

## PHYSICAL INJURIES

These are numerous and fairly obvious. They include burns.

**Burns.** These may occur from:

1. *Chemicals* used on the wrong tissue or in too concen-

trated a strength. There is no substitute for personal check of the label on the container.

2. *Hot-water bottles.* These burns can be avoided by not using hot-water bottles. They are unnecessary.

3. *Surgical diathermy* incorrectly used. A high-frequency current generates heat passing through the body but does not cause an electric shock. This has already been considered in detail (p. 96).

**Explosions.** See page 96.
**Scalds.**
**Loss of foreign bodies.** See page 93.

**Pressure and traction.** These injuries may arise from:

1. *Tourniquets.* Their use is rarely required for control of haemorrhage and if used to provide a bloodless operation field they must be removed by the person who applied them.

2. *Plaster casts and splints.* If too tight, plaster casts and splints act as tourniquets with the most devastating effects.

3. *Pressure sores.* These may occur from the roughened edges of a plaster. Even more important are bed sores in which the body weight is one factor. Others are loss of sensation, incontinence, excessive sweating, oedema and an impaired circulation.

4. *Nerve paresis.* This is particularly liable to occur if the brachial plexus is stretched or the radial nerve suffers pressure from lying on the edge of the table. The lateral popliteal nerve may be damaged by severe pressure or may be stretched from traction over the neck of the fibula. Drug injection into the radial or sciatic nerves may also cause paresis.

**Confinement to bed.** This may cause no special trouble, but it may initiate a chain reaction giving rise to conditions such as:

1. *Thrombosis and embolism.* The incidence of these is diminishing but not abolished by early postoperative ambulation and the measures mentioned on page 129.

2. *Diminished blood volume.* This occurs from confinement to bed and, in general, patients should be up and about before operation or, if this is impossible, the blood volume should be restored preoperatively. If it is not, drugs used for the induction of anaesthesia which cause vasodilation may bring on early circulatory collapse. A small amount of bleeding will cause a similar effect.

3. *Retention of urine.* This is commonly due to some degree of prostatic obstruction, particularly in elderly men.

4. *Bed sores and deformities*, such as drop foot.

5. *Faecal impaction.*

**The surgical environment.** The best surgical environment is
that in which the access of infective organisms to wounds is
prevented. This ideal is rarely achieved completely.


## DRUGS AND THERAPEUTIC SUBSTANCES

A few general principles are important. They are:

### 1. *Identification*

This is fundamental. If a drug is to be injected the solution
must be drawn into the syringe after the label has been read.
The same care is essential with fluid for infusion. Mixtures
dangerous for infusion should be coloured, for example, sodium citrate for use in the bladder.

Blood is particularly important. The most essential precaution is that the correct cross-matched bottle for the patient is
the one being handled. Then it should be checked that:

(a)  It is the correct group.
(b)  The Rh typing is correct.
(c)  That it is not out of date.

Most important of all a careful watch should be kept that
the first 50-100 ml are causing no reaction.

### 2. *Drug therapy in progress when surgery is necessary*

This should always be reviewed in the light of possible
consequences. Particularly important are:

(a) ANTICOAGULANT THERAPY. This must always be temporarily reversed by the intravenous administration of protamine sulphate for heparin, or of vitamin K in the case of
warfarin.

(b) CORTICOSTEROID THERAPY. This delays healing, but if the
dosage is reduced too rapidly the original condition for
which the patient is being treated may flare up in a fulminating form. Therefore before surgery corticosteroid therapy
must be increased so that the response to injury (p. 243) can
occur. Afterwards it is reduced gradually.

**Drug reactions.** There are many complications of steroid
therapy which may be of surgical importance. The commonest are:

(i)  Reactivation of quiescent pulmonary tuberculosis.
(ii)  Bleeding from a peptic ulcer.
(iii)  Development of fulminating infections, such as appendicitis, which progress silently.
(iv)  The rapid development of cardiac failure.

Other complications include thrombosis, osteoporosis, psychosis, myopathies and skin reactions such as acne and hirsutism.

(c) THE CORRECT DRUG BY THE WRONG ROUTE. This may cause great harm. Thiopentone, so effective intravenously, causes arterial thrombosis with gangrene of the hand if given into the brachial artery.

(d) THE CORRECT RATE. This must be determined for any substance given intravenously.

**Complications of drug therapy:**

*Sensitivity* in some individuals is almost inevitable; there is almost no drug to which an individual may not be sensitive. This may vary from a severe anaphylactic reaction to a mild skin rash.

*Resistant organisms may develop.*

*Normally suppressed organisms may proliferate.*

*Anaemia* and damage to the blood-forming tissues may occur. Chloramphenicol, the sulphonamides and most of the cytotoxic drugs used in malignant disease, as well as radiotherapy, are particularly notable.

*Crystallisation in the kidney* may occur from some sulphonamides associated with an inadequate fluid intake, particularly with an acid urine.

*Damage to the nucleus* of the VIIIth cranial nerve is almost always due to streptomycin.

*Vitamin B deficiency* is most liable to occur from alteration of the intestinal flora by the tetracycline group of antibiotics.

*Jaundice* may occur from blood plasma (infective) or drugs. Notable are:

Halothane—used in anaesthesia.
Methyldopa—used for hypertension.
Chlorpromazine—an anxiolytic drug.
Phenylbutazone—an anti-inflammatory agent.
Ampicillin
Tetracycline }—antibiotics.

*Intestinal ulceration* with stricture formation may result from enteric-coated diuretic capsules containing potassium chloride.

*Gastric erosions* are common from the irritation of aspirin as well as phenylbutazone.

*Coma and respiratory failure* may be quite alarming following small doses of morphia in a sensitive patient.

*Abdominal pain* may be severe from excessive dosage of vitamin D, while constipation may result from ganglion-blocking drugs used in the treatment of hypertension.

*Retrolental fibroplasia* may result from the administration of oxygen in excess of 35 per cent, to the newborn.

*Gangrene* may result from severe spasm produced by ergot.

*Glaucoma* is aggravated by atropine.

*Citrate intoxication* after massive blood transfusion. In addition to causing reduction of serum calcium stored blood contains excess of potassium ions.

## DIRECT AND INDIRECT OPERATIVE COMPLICATIONS

These are similar to the general processes outlined in this work.

1. Direct damage from trauma.
2. Obstruction postoperatively.
3. Fluid leakage from the (i) blood vessels, (ii) the suture line in visceral anastomosis.
4. Metabolic changes from surgical intervention. Re-operation may be indicated for (a) fluid leakage (including haemorrhage) and (b) obstruction.
5. Infections.

### OPERATIVE ABLATION

The effects which arise from operative ablation depend on the extent of the ablation, to what extent the functional reserves of the body are adequate and to what degree, if any, disability can be overcome or minimised by artificial means. Many of the physiological consequences which arise take time to manifest themselves. The longer the results of many ablations are studied, the more wide-reaching their effects are discovered to be.

### MISCELLANEOUS IATROGENIC LESIONS

The obvious sequelae of amputation of the limbs or the breast need no special stress except the importance of ensuring that such mutilation is undertaken only for compelling indications.

Even where the functional reserve is adequate, as in the kidneys, the ovaries or the testes, a conservative attitude to removal is essential, since time may bring similar or more severe disease to the contralateral organ.

Ductless gland ablation can be largely overcome by administration of the appropriate hormone if its removal causes a deficiency. More difficult and more complicated are the effects of extirpation of large amounts of gastrointestinal tract.

### Physiological and anatomical shortening of the digestive tract

**The stomach.** The greatest effects in proportion to the amount removed are seen after gastrectomy, partly due to anatomical and physiological exclusion of the duodenum. The main effects are:

1. Limited intake of food.
2. Anaemia.
3. Vitamin deficiency.
4. Intestinal hurry.
5. Defective absorption.
6. Enterocolitis (possibly from achlorhydria).
7. Other syndromes:
   (a) Face flushing.
   (b) Hypoglycaemia.
   (c) Bilious vomiting.
8. Osteoporosis.

**The small intestine.** Resection of large lengths of the small intestine results in loss of weight and some frequency of stools.

Intestinal hurry occurs in all conditions of physiological shortening of which gastrectomy is one of the most important examples.

**The large intestine.** This has a considerable functional reserve and more than half can be removed without any great effect.

**The gall-bladder.** Cholecystectomy results in dilute bile dribbling into the duodenum as it is formed. Most patients after cholecystectomy have no great disability although there may be a certain amount of windy discomfort and a bowel action which is freer than usual.

After removal of the gall-bladder the patient should be able to eat a reasonable amount of fat but not excessive quantities. In the immediate postoperative phase fat should be liberally supplied to encourage biliary drainage and to avoid further colic from inspissated mucus or a tiny fragment of gravel which may form the nidus of a further stone.

**The pancreas.** Pancreatectomy, which is usually undertaken for neoplasm, causes:

1. Diabetes, control of which presents no great difficulty.
2. Steatorrhoea, diminished by giving pancreatic enzymes.
3. Diminished calcium absorption.
4. Fat and protein absorption is also disturbed.

Most operative procedures produce after-effects which are usually of a minor nature. The more seriously ill the patient beforehand the more ready he is to accept these discomforts, but where preoperative symptoms, and especially pain, have been slight the less tolerant the patient is likely to be later of postoperative symptoms. It is rightly said that the bad results of operations for peptic ulceration are more frequently the results of bad selection of patients than of bad surgery.

# CHAPTER 54

# Some Biographical Notes

HIPPOCRATES (460–370 BC) is considered to be the father of modern medicine for he severed medicine from witchcraft and superstition and transformed it into a science based on observation. He travelled widely throughout Greece setting up teaching centres and left model clinical records for posterity (his descriptions of epilepsy and puerperal septicaemia could be found in any modern textbook). His work was assisted by his emphasis on good nursing and a balanced diet. The Hippocratic oath is a tribute to the high ethical standards he brought to the profession.

GALEN (AD 130–200). Prior to 1500, Galen was second only to Hippocrates in medicine, and his theories, both correct and erroneous, were accepted without question. After serving the Roman Emperor Marcus Aurelius as personal physician, he retired to write and to study. He was the first experimental physiologist and discovered that the arteries contained blood and that contraction of muscle occurred independently of the nerve supply. Among his other important discoveries were his explanations of respiration and inflammation. His work on anatomy was less successful for he based all his findings on the dissection of animals. As a physician he placed great reliance on drugs, notably opium, sugar and alcohol. While some of his teaching misled, his collection of 80 books preserved much that was finest in ancient medicine throughout the Dark Ages.

AMBROISE PARÉ (1510–90). By his own skill and personality, Paré raised the status of surgery from a despised mechanical art to that of a major profession, using the new discoveries in anatomy to advance surgery. By the discovery that gunshot wounds were not poisonous and required soothing applications rather than boiling oil and by his advocacy of artificial limbs for wounded soldiers, he brought much relief to the surgery of the battlefield. To prevent bleeding after amputation, he replaced the indiscriminate use of a red hot cautery with a simple ligature. Among his other work was the invention of artery forceps, detailed discussion of the treatment of fractures and dislocations and the suggestion that syphilis was the cause of aneurysm. He established himself in a position of great authority as surgeon to four French kings, and riled the established physicians of the time by scorning such remedies as powdered mummy and a unicorn's head.

ANDREAS VESALIUS (1514–64). By freeing anatomy from many of Galen's errors, Vesalius laid the foundation on which many subsequent advances in medicine and surgery could take place. At the age of 23 he was Professor of Anatomy at Padua University and his great work, the *Fabrica*, published in 1543, corrected Galen on many points, completely destroying Galen's osteology and muscle anatomy. For instance, he found the lower jaw consisted of a single bone, that loss of the spleen was compatible with life, and he destroyed such fallacies as the double bile duct and the five-lobed liver. His work on the spinal cord showed the means by which the brain acts on the various muscles of the limbs and trunk. By 1555 he had laid the basis of Harvey's discovery of the circulation by denying the existence of interventricular pores and by noting the existence of valves in the vein without appreciating their significance. His later years were spent as physician to the Emperor Charles V.

ST VINCENT DE PAUL (1576–1660) was the founder of the Sisters of Charity. Destined for the Church he was sold into slavery on his capture by pirates. After his release he returned to Paris to fight against poverty, ignorance and infection. Initially 120 well-to-do ladies would visit the poor in teams of four but no nursing was undertaken until St Vincent widened the membership of the Order to include peasant women, known as Sisters of Charity, who were taught simple nursing procedures. The ladies and Sisters of Charity were then amalgamated and the first Nursing Order had been formed, performing heroically on the battlefields of seventeenth-century France. After St Vincent's death the Order waned because it failed to follow the advances in surgery and medicine, but at the time of the Crimean War the Sisters of Charity inspired Florence Nightingale to provide a similar standard of nursing of British soldiers in the Crimea.

WILLIAM HARVEY (1578–1657). It was as Lumelian lecturer that William Harvey delivered the following statement in 1616 which revolutionised the whole of medical science: 'The movement of the blood is constantly in a circle and is brought about by the beat of the heart.' With a sound knowledge of anatomy, Harvey saw that the valves in the veins would permit the blood to pass only to the heart while those in the great arteries permitted blood to flow only away from the heart. He then calculated that the quantity and velocity of the blood was such as made it physically impossible for the blood to do other than return by a venous route. His conclusions were published in his famous book *De Motu Cordis*. His *De Generatione Animalium*, published in 1651, was the first English work on embryology, also containing the first chapters in English on obstetrics. As a staunch Royalist, Harvey compared the heart to his king, Charles I—'the centre of all strength and power'.

JOHN HUNTER (1728–93) was not only one of the foremost surgeons of all time but the most versatile of scientists. He raised surgery to a technical science firmly grounded in physiology and surgical pathology. To assist him in his work he founded a great menagerie of 13,000 specimens and it was his study of the capillary system of the deer which led to his treatment for aneurysm which is still in use today. Among his other discoveries were the arterial supply of the gravid uterus, the olfactory nerve in the nose and many features of the lymphatic system. As a surgical pathologist his descriptions of phlebitis, pyaemia and shock were revolutionary and his technical inventions, such as artificial feeding by a tube in the stomach and apparatus for forced respiration, were of the highest order. As a biologist his work led him to the principle that functional activities in the lower forms of life were simplifications of those in the higher. His love of science caused his death which was as a result of a mistaken inoculation of syphilis and gonorrhoea. A certain incoherence in writing was more than compensated for by his work as a teacher, as three famous doctors (Jenner, Abernethy and Astley Cooper) were his pupils.

EDWARD JENNER (1749–1823) was a country doctor in Berkeley, Gloucestershire, who noticed that those who had had cowpox (a mild form of pox contracted by milkmaids from cows) never became infected with smallpox. In May 1796 he conducted a crucial experiment by vaccinating an 8-year-old boy with pus from the hand of a dairymaid infected with cowpox. The boy failed to develop smallpox following inoculation eight weeks later. Cowpox was technically known as vaccinia so it was inevitable that Jenner's process became known as vaccination. Not only was one of the most terrible diseases banished from this country but a principle had been established which eventually led to the immunisation of man against many infectious diseases.

JAMES BLUNDELL (1790–1877) was the pioneer in the field of blood transfusion. He discovered the value of transfusion by injection of the blood of a dog into the circulation of another dog but discovered that a dog would die if injected with the blood of a sheep. This established the incompatibility of the blood of different species and prevented the practice of injecting animal blood into human beings. By further experiment he showed that a smaller quantity of blood than the amount lost would resuscitate an animal. The first transfusion of human blood took place on 12 December 1818 on a patient who was fatally ill. His first successful recovery was for a postpartum haemorrhage for which the patient received 8 oz of blood, recorded in the *Lancet* of 1829. Blundell showed, contrary to existing belief, that the blood was not injured by its passage through instruments and that a few air bubbles in the circulation were quite harmless. The problem of coagulation proved difficult and later led to his invention of a special apparatus enabling the blood to be transferred from donor to recipient with minimal physical interference.

THEODOR FLIEDNER (1800–64) was a Lutheran clergyman responsible for the experiment which began nursing reform. In 1826 he founded an association to help discharged prisoners and relieve the sick poor of his parish. This association led in 1836 to the development of a new hospital which was founded at Kaiserswerth, where Fliedner trained women called deaconesses to help him in his work. It was the first nursing experiment to exist independently of a religious order. The deaconesses were examined in medicine and pharmacy but, unlike the nursing training of Florence Nightingale, this was more on the lines of a comprehensive social service including training in cooking, laundering and gardening. Kaiserswerth was the first school of nursing and left a lasting impression with its spirit of dedicated service. At the time of Fliedner's death 1600 deaconesses were nursing as far apart as Turkey and the U.S.A.

WILLIAM THOMAS MORTON (1819–68) was a dental partner of Horace Wells (1815–48), whose career was ruined when he gave an unsuccessful public demonstration using nitrous oxide to anaesthetise a patient. A Boston chemist recommended to Morton the use of sulphuric ether and the first successful public demonstration was given at the Massachusetts General Hospital on 16 October 1846 when an operation for a vascular tumour was successfully performed. Morton ruined his reputation by attempting to patent the drug and made no further contribution to the subject.

In Edinburgh, the Professor of Midwifery, JAMES SIMPSON (1811–70), found ether unsatisfactory in midwifery and used a new drug, chloroform. His first experiment was upon himself and, on recovering consciousness, rightly remarked, 'This is far stronger than ether.' The drug was first administered on a child for an operation for osteomyelitis on 15 November 1847. More powerful and pleasant than ether, chloroform became the standard anaesthetic drug in Britain for the next 50 years and the new medical science of anaesthetics was born with far-reaching effects for the development of surgery.

FLORENCE NIGHTINGALE (1820–1910) was the first outstanding figure in the history of nursing. Before she went to the Crimea nursing did not exist as a profession of high ethical and technical standards. She was able to overcome the social barriers which prevented women entering nursing. In 1854 she was able to go to the Crimea where, amid the filth of the hospitals in Scutari, she courageously fought her own battle for cleanliness and care of the patients. She never ceased to fight for sanitary conditions in the army medical service, being influential in later Royal Commissions. Her *Notes on Nursing* and *Notes on Hospitals* emphasise the principles of personal and communal hygiene as well as administrative efficiency.

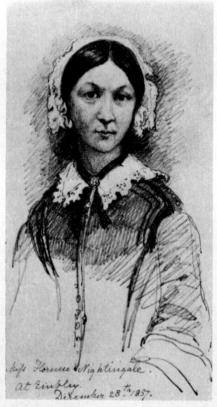

Florence Nightingale, aged 37, by Sir George Sharf—one of the first Directors of the National Gallery.

By 1860 a grateful nation had contributed £50,000 to the Nightingale Fund which was used to establish a nursing school at St Thomas's Hospital, London. The great medical advantages of this period could only be of benefit to mankind with trained and educated nurses. Her most notable administrative reform was the removal of nurses from the supervision of the medical staff to that of the matron. She set a standard of nursing education which was a model for all subsequent English and Commonwealth schools. After choosing the probationers herself, she ensured that they would be instructed in the basic sciences by the medical staff and would receive practical instruction in the wards under the supervision of the sisters. In later years she pressed for many reforms in workhouse nursing and was responsible for the grant of a Royal Charter to the Royal British Nursing Association in 1893.

LOUIS PASTEUR (1822–95) is considered to be the founder of modern bacteriology for by extensive study of milk and beer he proved that organisms naturally present in the air are alive and can produce putrefaction, but on heating lose their power and are killed—a discovery fundamental to aseptic surgery. By injecting anthrax bacilli, greatly reduced in strength, into a sheep, he was able to immunise it against subsequent infection by the virulent bacillus. This, and similar experiments, led him to conclude that the origin or extinction of infectious disease in the past may have simply been due to the strengthening or weakening of its virulence by external conditions, and the principle was applied with success in the case of preventive vaccination against hydrophobia. In 1885 the Pasteur

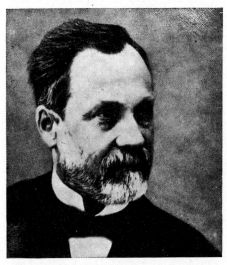

Louis Pasteur.

Institute was opened and Pasteur surrounded himself with brilliant pupils—among them:

*Emile Roux*, responsible for epoch-making work on the diphtheria antitoxin;

*Yersin*, who found a vaccination against plague, and

*Calmette*, who discovered preventive inoculation against snake bites.

Truly Pasteur was one of the pioneers of modern preventive inoculation.

LORD LISTER (1827–1912) was the greatest surgical figure of modern times. As Professor of Surgery in Glasgow, he studied the work of Pasteur from which he deduced that infection in wounds was analogous to putrefaction in wine, and selected carbolic acid as a means of destroying the organisms in the wound. Thus Lister discovered the principle involving the prevention and cure of sepsis in wounds. He insisted that everything touching the wounds should be treated with antiseptic and sought constantly to improve his dressings, eventually deciding on a gauze containing the oxides of mercury and zinc. The effects of the new principle were shown by a dramatic drop in the mortality rate of amputations and compound fractures. Abdominal, cranial and chest surgery date from the invention of the antiseptic system which had made possible the surgery of the hollow cavities of the body. Lister's antiseptic principle was later developed into an aseptic system by Halsted and Spencer Wells.

Among Lister's other achievements were the invention of the sinus forceps, probe pointed scissors and the catgut liga-

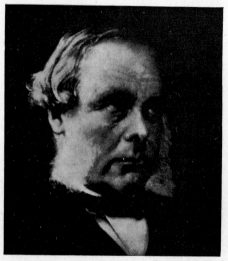

Joseph Lister

ture. He further showed that an uninfected clot if undisturbed can be organised into living tissue, and a piece of dead bone may be absorbed in an aseptic wound.

He was President of the Royal Society 1895–1900 and became the first medical peer in 1897.

HUGH OWEN THOMAS (1834–91) spent his whole professional life in the poorer areas of nineteenth-century Liverpool, but no one did more to advance the treatment of bones and joints. In his day excision and amputation were the remedies for the chronic diseases of the joints but, instead, Thomas applied the principle of complete rest for the treatment of tuberculous joints and this prevented many amputations. To ensure that the diseased part was not compressed or the circulation of the blood impaired, Thomas invented his famous fracture splint, now known as the Thomas splint (Fig. 47.7). His other inventions included a wrench for the reduction of fractures and an osteoclast to break deformed bones before resetting them. The effect of the Thomas splint was not seen until World War I when it was responsible for the reduction of the mortality rate of fracture of the femur from 80 per cent in 1916 to 7 per cent in 1918—only now was Thomas seen as a great pioneer. His work was continued by his nephew, Sir Robert Jones, who developed the modern methods of tendon transplantation and bone grafting.

ROBERT KOCH (1843–1910). When he delivered his paper on the anthrax bacillus in 1876, Robert Koch had produced the greatest discovery in bacteriology for he had proved that an infectious disease can often be caused by a specific microorganism. He also showed how to fix and stain bacteria. In 1882 he announced the discovery of the tubercle bacillus which made possible all subsequent work on the cure for tuberculosis. On his visits to India and Egypt as the head of the German cholera Commission of 1883 he discovered the cause of cholera—the *Vibrio cholerae*—and its transmission by water and food. His work on rinderpest, tropical malaria and bubonic plague was extremely valuable and for his services to medicine he was awarded the Nobel Prize in 1905.

WILHELM CONRAD ROENTGEN (1845–1923) was Professor of Physics at Würzburg who, while working with a Crooke's tube, discovered that shadows were forming on a photographic plate. After careful experiment he found that, by making his tube light-proof, a greenish fluorescent light would be thrown on a platino-barium screen 9 feet away. These rays passed through substances ordinarily opaque, such as the soft parts of the body, revealing the bones. He read his paper to the Würzburg Society and when Professor Kolliker submitted his own hand to be photographed all doubts were allayed,

Kolliker suggesting the new rays, which had been called X-rays, be known as Roentgen rays.

Among the many honours he was to receive for this discovery were the Rumford Gold Medal of the Royal Society and the Nobel Prize.

SIR ALEXANDER FLEMING (1881–1955) was responsible for the greatest contribution to the science of medical treatment

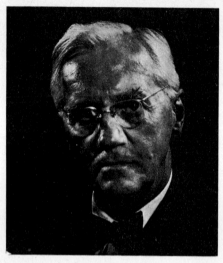

Alexander Fleming

made in the first half of the twentieth century—the development of antibiotics. In 1928, on examining one of his culture plants in his laboratory at London University, he found that the growth of the mould was the same as on other culture plates but the microbes near the mould, instead of forming into a yellow opaque mould, had dissolved. He then placed various microbes near the mould with different effects—for instance the diphtheria microbe was among those destroyed whilst the typhoid and influenza microbes were not so affected. Thus an antibiotic had been discovered—something alive in the mould was killing other living microbes. Fleming called this substance penicillin and it has been responsible for inhibiting the growth of the causative organisms of many common infectious diseases. During the Second World War it was used to great effect in the treatment of war wounds and gas gangrene.

Fleming was knighted in 1944 and received the Nobel Prize in 1945.

# Table of Approximate Normal Values

**Haematology**
Haemoglobin—14·6 g/100 ml or 100 per cent
Red cells—5 million/mm³
White cells—
    Adults—4 to 10,000/mm³
    Infants—10,000 to 25,000/mm³
Differentiated white cell count—
    Polymorphs 40 to 75 per cent
    Lymphocytes 20 to 50 per cent
    Monocytes 1 to 6 per cent
    Eosinophils 1 to 6 per cent
    Basophils 1 per cent
Platelets—150,000 to 350,000/mm³
Bleeding time—1 to 5 minutes
Coagulation time (capillary) 2 to 8 minutes
Erythrocyte sedimentation rate (E.S.R.).
    Men 0 to 10 mm/hour
    Women 0 to 20 mm/hour

**Blood chemistry**
*S.I. Units are given in brackets*
*Electrolytes—*
    Serum sodium ($Na^+$) 136 to 144 mEq/litre (136–144 mmol/litre)
    Serum potassium ($K^+$) 3·5 to 4·5 mEq/litre (3·5–4·5 mmol/litre)
    Serum chloride ($Cl'$) 100 mEq/litre (100 mmol/litre)

*Acid/Base balance—*
    Plasma alkali reserve (or carbondioxide combining power)—
        50 to 75 ml $CO_2$/100 ml plasma, often referred to as 50 to
        75 volumes per cent
        *or* 20 to 30 mEq/litre (20-30 mmol/l)
    Arterial $pCO_2$—35 to 45 mm Hg
        *or* 1 to 1·35 mEq/litre
    Standard bicarbonate 21 to 25 mEq/litre
    Base excess of blood—2·3 to +2·3 mEq/litre (± 2 mmol/l)
    $pH$—7·35 to 7·42.
*Blood urea*—20 to 40 mg/100 ml (2·50–6·5 mmol/litre)
*Blood glucose*—80 to 120 mg/100 ml (4·44–6·67 mmol/litre)
*Serum calcium*—9 to 11 mg/100 ml (2·25–2·62 mmol/litre)
*Serum phosphate*—2·5 to 4·5 mg/100 ml (0·81–1·4 mmol/litre)
*Serum cholesterol*—150 to 250 mg/100 ml (3·35–6·46 mmol/litre)
*Plasma uric acid*—2 to 4 mg/100 ml (0·12–0·40 mmol/litre)
*Serum amylase*—75 to 150 Somogyi units/100 ml
*Serum acid phosphatase*—1 to 3 K.A. units/100 ml
*Serum alkaline phosphatase*—5 to 11 K.A. units/100 ml
*Serum proteins—*
    Total—6 to 8 g/100 ml (60–80 g/litre)
    Albumin—3·6 to 5 g/100 ml (36–50 g/litre)
    Globulin—2 to 3 g/100 ml (20–30 g/litre)
*Liver function tests—*
    Serum bilirubin—0·1 to 0·5 mg/100 ml (1·7–15·4 $\mu$mol/litre)
    Thymol turbidity—0·4 units
*Serum transaminases—*
    Glutamate oxalacetate transaminase—(SGOT)—10 to 35
        units/ml
    Glutamate pyruvate transaminase (SGPT)—0 to 35 units/ml
    Serum protein bound iodine (PBI) 4 to 8 $\mu$g/110 ml

**Cerebrospinal fluid**
Protein—20 to 40 mg/100 ml (200–400 mmol/litre)
Chloride—700 to 740 mg/100 ml (119–126 mmol/litre)
Glucose—40 to 80 mg/100 ml (2·2–4·4 mmol/litre)
White cells—0 to 5/mm³

# Index

## A

Abdominal conditions, complications of, 343
Abdominal pain, extra-abdominal causes of, 334
Abnormal discharges, 11
Abortion, 609 *et seq.*
  complications, 610
Abscess, alveolar, 270
  cerebral, 517
  cold, 74
  dental, 270
  of appendix, 339
  of breast, 289
  of liver, 386
  of lung, 309
  pelvic, 345
  perianal, 424
  perinephric, 459
  periurethral, 486
  psoas, 528
  residual, 345
  subcutaneous, 204
  subperiosteal, 558
  subphrenic, 346
  thyroid, 284
Accelerated reaction, 44
Actinomycosis, 273
Acute, abdomen, 333 *et seq.*
  appendicitis, 337 *et seq.*
  cholecystitis, 392
  circulatory failure, 135 *et seq.*
  dilatation of stomach, 374
  epididymo-orchitis, 487
  ethmoiditis, 584
  gangrene, 231
  glaucoma, 598
  infections of chest, 304
  intestinal obstruction, 350 *et seq.*
  lymphadenitis, 248
  mastitis, 288
  maxillary sinusitis, 584
  osteomyelitis, 557
  otitis media, 574
  pancreatitis, 397
  parotitis (non-suppurative), 267
  peritonitis, 334 *et seq.*
  renal failure, 450
  retention of urine, 466
  salpingitis, 623
  sialadenitis, 267
Adeno-carcinoma, 213
Adrenal glands, diseases of, 286
Adrenalectomy, 298
Agranulocytosis, 41
Amenorrhoea, 606
Amnesia, 510
Amputations, 234 *et seq.*

Amputations (*cont.*)
  complications of, 235
  stump, care of, 235
Amyloid disease, 559
Anaesthesia, 21
  care of patient under, 20
  induction of, 22
Anaesthetics, explosions and burns, 96
Analgesia, 21
Anaphylaxis, 44
Anatomical narrows, 241
Aneurysms, 225
  cirsoid, 227
Angiocardiography, 324
Angiogram, cerebral, 507
Ankylosis, 567
Anthrax, 72
Antibacterial agents, 52
Antibiotics, 52
Anticoagulants, 130
Anuria, 444
Anus, and rectum, operations on, 431
  diseases of, 423 *et seq.*
Aortic valve disease, 321
Aortography, 449
Appendix mass, 339
Approximate normal values, table of, 645
Arteriogram, 225
Arteriosclerosis, 225
Arthritis, acute infective, 567
  rheumatoid, 571
  tuberculous, of hip, 568
  of knee, 569
Artificial respiration, 164
Artificial ventilation, 165
Arvin, 131
Ascites, 356
Asepsis and theatre technique, 86 *et seq.*
Asiatic cholangio hepatitis, 504
Aspiration,
  gastric, 378
  pleural cavity, 306
Astigmatism, 586
Atresia, intestinal, 498
  oesophageal, 497
  posterior choanal, 496
  rectal, 499
Atrial septal defect, 319
Auscultation, 9
Autograft, 252

## B

Bacteria, 48
Bacteraemia, 68
Barium enema, 414

Barium meal, 364
Bed sores, 198 *et seq.*
Bee and wasp stings, 203
Bell's palsy, 534
Bilharzia, 504
Biographical notes, 637 *et seq.*
Biopsy, 215
  rectal, 431
Birth injuries, 535
Bladder, care of, before operation, 24
  diseases of, 466 *et seq.*
  diverticulum, 476
  irrigation of, 474
Blepharitis, 590
Blood
  and blood products, clinical use of, 124
  and the rhesus factor, 119
  cross matching, 117
  grouping, 117
Blood transfusion, 116 *et seq.*
  collection of blood for, 119
  complications of, 123
  precautions during, 123
  procedure after, 123
Blood urea, estimation of, 446
Boils, 204
  Delhi, 502
Bone, diseases of, 557 *et seq.*
Brain, diseases of, 517 *et seq.*
Breast, congenital abnormalities of, 288
  diseases of, 287 *et seq.*
  male diseases of, 302
Bronchiectasis, 309 *et seq.*
Bronchogram, 310
Burns and scalds, 181 *et seq.*
  chemical, 189
  special complications, 188
Burnt areas, care of, 184
Bursae, 208
Burst abdomen, 347

C

Caecostomy, 417
Caecum, diseases of, 408 *et seq.*
Calculi, *see* Stones
Cancer, predisposing factors, 210
Carbuncles, 204
Carcinoma
  of bladder, 476
  of breast, 292 *et seq.*
  of bronchus, 312
  of cervix, 618
  of colon, 412
  of ear, 574
  of gall-bladder, 397
  of jaw, 273
  of kidney, 460
  of liver, 387
  of lung, 312
  of male breast, 302
  of oesophagus, 330
  of pancreas, 400
  of penis, 485

Carcinoma (*contd.*)
  of peritoneum, 355
  of prostate gland, 483
  of rectum, 434
  of stomach, 373
  of testicle, 490
  of thyroid, 284
  of tongue, 264
  of uterus, body of, 621
  of vulva, 615
Cardiac arrest, 142
  resuscitation trolley, 144
Cardiac catheterisation, 323
Cardiac disease, acquired, 320
Cardiac pacemaker, 325
Cardiospasm, 328
Cartilage, torn semilunar, 564
Caruncle, urethral, 615
Cataract, 599 *et seq.*
Catheter, correct method of passing, 471
  indwelling, 471
Catheterisation, 468 *et seq.*
  ureteric, 448
Cellulitis, 67
  orbital, 601
Central nervous system, diseases of, 505 *et seq.*
Cerebral compression, 509
Cervical rib, 535
Cervical smear, 620
Cervix, erosion of, 617
Chancre, 76
  of lip, 77
Changes in personality and behaviour, 13
Charcot's joints, 569
Chemotherapeutic agents, 52
Cholangiogram, 393
Cholangiography, percutaneous trans-hepatic, 394
Cholecystectomy, 395
Cholecystogram, 393
Cholecystostomy, 395
Chondromas, 559
Chorion-epithelioma, 622
Choroiditis, 595
Chronic, cholecystitis, 392
  epididymo-orchitis, 448
  glaucoma, 598
  lymphadenitis, 248
  osteomyelitis, 559
  otitis media, 575
  pancreatitis, 399
  peritonitis, 355
  pyothorax, 309
  renal failure, 451
  salpingitis, 624
  sialadenitis, 267
  sinusitis, 584
Circo-electric bed, 201
Circulatory collapse, prevention of, 141
Circulatory failure, prevention and treatment, 29
Circumcision, 484
Cleft lip, and palate, 259 *et seq.*

Clinical examination, 8
Clutton's joints, 569
Coarctation of aorta, 319
Colic, biliary, 395
 intestinal, 405
 renal, 442
 ureteric, 458
Colon, diseases of, 408 et seq.
 diverticular disease of, 411 et seq.
 inflammatory conditions of, 408
 investigations, 414
Colonic operations, care of patient, 415
Colostomy, 417
 closure, 421
 complications of, 420
 instructions to patient, 420
 opening of, 418
 orifice(s), 418
Coma, 12
Complications, of antibiotic therapy, 53
 result of recumbency in bed, 30
Conjunctiva, diseases of, 592
Consciousness, level of, 509
Constrictive pericarditis, 321
Contractures, 554
 Dupuytren's, 208
 hour-glass, 372
Cornea, diseases of, 593
Corns, 209
Coronary arterial disease, 324
Corticosteroids, surgical significance of, 300
Craniotomy, 520 et seq.
 care of a case of, 520
Crohn's disease, 404
Cryosurgery, 429
Cryotherapy, 216
Cyclitis, 595
Cyst, Bartholin's, 78
 branchial, 274
 dermoid, 258
 hydatid, of liver, 387
 in mouth, 264
 meibomian, 591
 of face, 257
 of ovary, 625
 of vulva, 615
 sebaceous, 257–491
 thyroglossal, 274
Cystic hygroma, 274
Cystitis, 472
Cystocele, 611
Cystodiathermy, 476
Cystography, 447
Cystoscopy, 447
 preparation of patient, 448
Cystotomy, suprapubic, 471
Cytological examination, 369

D

Deafness, 577
Defaecation, difficulty with, 31
Dental caries, 271

Desensitisation, 44
Diagnosis, nurse's special contribution, 11
 radiological, 9
 surgical, 7 et seq.
Dialysis, 452
 peritoneal, 452
Diathermy, care of patient, 97
 surgical, 96
Dilatation, anal, 428
 of cervix uteri, 617
 of rectum, 430
 urethral, 486
Diminution or elimination of infection, 28
Disease, the nature of, 240 et seq.
Dislocations, 562
 causes of, 562
 congenital of hip, 564
 of shoulder, 563
 pathological, 562
 traumatic, 563
Diverticulum, Meckel's, 403
Dog bite, 203
Drainage, postural, 311
 tubes, 316
Drains, surgical, 106
Dressing procedure, 103
Dressing trolley, preparation of, 102
Dressings, surgical ward, 102 et seq.
Drug reactions, 631
Drugs and therapeutic substances, 631
Drug therapy, complications of, 632
Duodenum, diseases of, 359 et seq.
Dysentery, amoebic, 504
Dysmenorrhoea, 608
Dysuria, 443

E

Ear, diseases of, 572 et seq.
 inner, diseases, 577
 middle, disease, 574
 outer, 573
 wax in, 573
Ectopic, gestation, 610
Ectropion, 591
Electricity failure, 99
Electrolytes, 147 et seq.
Embolism, 131 et seq.
 air, 133
 fat, 133
 pulmonary, 131
Emotion, relation to disease, 5
Endocrine glands, 275 et seq.
Endometriosis, 622
Enemas, diagnostic, 12
Enterectomy, 407
Entero-anastomosis, 407
Enterostomy, 407
Entropion, 591
Epididymo-orchitis, 487
Epiphyses, separated, 540
Epistaxis, 581
Erb's paralysis, 535

Excision, of eyeball, 602
  of tongue, 266
Exophthalmos, 283
External female genital organs, 603
Eyeball, section of, 587
Eyelids, diseases of, 590
  ptosis of, 591
Eyes, basic nursing of eye conditions, 589
  diseases of, 586 et seq.
  examination of, 587
  following craniotomy, 522
  injuries and foreign bodies, 601

**F**

Face, 257 et seq.
  inflammatory conditions, 257
Familial polyposis, 412
Fibreoptic colonoscopy, 415
Fibro-adenosis, 291
Fibromyomata, 618
Filariasis, 503
Fissure in ano, 425
Fistula in ano, 424
  faecal, 347
  gastro-colic, 373
Fluid administration, 153 et seq.
  complications of, 158
  enteral, 153
  parenteral routes, 154
  rate of infusion, 157
Fluid, and electrolyte balance, 146 et seq.
  balance chart, 148
  replacement, Wallace's 'Rule of Nine', 183
Foreign bodies, 203
  in ear, 573
  in eye, 601
  in heart, removal of, 321
  in ileum, 405
  in oesophagus, 326
Fothergill's operation, 613
Fractures, 539 et seq.
  anatomical varieties of, 539
  birth, 552
  causes of, 540
  Colles's, 550
  complications of, 541
  compound, 540
  immobilisation of, 544
  of carpal bones, 550
  of clavicle, 547
  of femur, 551 et seq.
  of foot, 556
  of humerus, 548
  of jaw, 272
  of mandible, 272
  of metacarpals and phalanges, 550
  of metatarsals and phalanges, 556
  of olecranon process, 549
  of os calcis, 556
  of patella, 555
  of pelvis, 550

Fractures (contd.)
  of radius, shaft of, 549
  of ribs, 303
  of scapula, 548
  of skull, base of, 512
  of spine, 522
  of tibia, 556
  of ulna, shaft of, 549
  of vault of skull, 512
  pathological, 540
  pond shaped, 513
  Pott's, of ankle, 556
  reduction of, 543
  restoration of functional activity, 546
  supracondylar, 549
  symptoms and signs of, 541
Function, restoration of, 33

**G**

Gall-bladder, diseases of, 390 et seq.
  investigations of, 392
Ganglion, 207
Gangrene, 230 et seq.
  common clinical types, 231
  gas, 72
Gastrectomy, partial, 374 et seq.
  post-, syndrome, 382
  postoperative treatment, 376
  preoperative treatment, 376
  total, 375
Gastric secretory function tests, 365
Gastro-jejunostomy, 374
Gastroscopy, 368
Gastrostomy, 331 et seq.
Genital organs, male, 466
Glaucoma, 598
  primary, 598
Glossitis, 263
Gloves, surgical, putting on, 93
Goitre, 275
Gonorrhoea, 78 et seq.
Grafts, corneal, 595
  Thiersch, 186
Gram's stain, 49
Gynaecology, 603 et seq.

**H**

Haematemesis, 370
Haematocele, 490
Haematocrit reading, 183
Haematoma, 125
Haematuria, 442 et seq.
Haemodialysis, 452
Haemorrhage, 108 et seq.
  arrest of, 114
  common causes of, in gastrointestinal tract, 370
  danger of, in jaundiced patients, 385
  extraperitoneal, 355
  following extraction of teeth, 271
  following rectal and anal operations, 433

Haemorrhage (*cont.*)
 from special sites, 125
 from varicose veins, 239
 gastrointestinal, 370
 in scalp wounds, 512
 in tonsillectomy, 579
 into eye, 601
 intraperitoneal, 355
 natural arrest of, 111
 post-gastric operation, 380
 post-prostatectomy, 479
 symptoms and signs, 113
 treatment of, 114
 types of, 108
 uterine, 616
Haemorrhagic diseases, 126
Haemorrhoids, 427 *et seq.*
Haemothorax, 304
Hallux rigidus, 566
 valgus, 566
Hammer toe, 565
Head injuries, 508 *et seq.*
 advice to patients leaving hospital, 517
 assessment of, 509
 complications, 516
 local treatment, 515
 of newborn, 513
Heart, congenital disease of, 318
 cyanotic disease of, 318
 surgery of, 318 *et seq.*
Heart-lung machines, 323
Heller's operation, 329
Hemicolectomy, 415
Hepatitis, viral, 385
Hernia, 437 *et seq.*
 causes of, 438
 diaphragmatic, 500
 hiatus, 329
 incisional, 348
 strangulated, 352
 treatment, 439
 types, 437
Hernioplasty, 450
Herniorrhaphy, 450
Herniotomy, 450
Heterograft, 253
Hip, congenital dislocation of, 564
Hirschsprung's disease, 500
Hodgkin's disease, 248
Homograft (allograft), 253
 reaction, 253
Hordeolum, 590
Hydrocele, 488
Hydrocephalus, 519
Hyperbaric oxygen chamber, 229
 therapy, 177
Hypermetropia, 586
Hypophysectomy, 299
Hypothermia, 22
Hypoxia, causes of, 174
Hysterectomy, total, 621

Identification, of patient, 14 *et seq.*
 of specimens, 15
Ileostomy, 409
Immune response, types of, 41
Immunisation programme, 43
 prophylactic and therapeutic, 43
Immunity, clinical application, 43
Incontinence of urine, 443
 types, 443
Infection and immunity, 40 *et seq.*
 localised, of the skin, 204
 of kidney, 455
 prevention and control, 45
 pulp space, 206
 specific surgical, 70 *et seq.*
 spread in tissues, 67
 susceptibility to, 42
Infertility, 625
Inflammation, 63 *et seq.*
 failure of reaction of, 65
 symptoms and signs, 66
 treatment and nursing care, 69
Ingrowing toe-nails, 209
Injuries, abdominal, 402
 multiple, 191
 physical, 629
Injury, metabolic response to, 149
Inoperable malignant disease, treatment of, 223
Inspection(s), 8
 endoscopic, 11
Intensive care, after heart or lung surgery, 322
 general view, 176
Intensive care units, 179 *et seq.*
Intermittent cardiac pumping or com-
  pression, 143
Internal female genitalia, 604
Interstitial keratitis, 594
Intestine, small, diseases of, 402 *et seq.*
 inflammatory conditions, 403
 injury to, 402
 operations on, 407
Intramuscular injection, site for, 56
Intussusception, 405
Investigations, gastric, 364
 neurological, 505
 renal, 445
 special, 506
Iris, diseases of, 595
Iritis, 595
Irrigation, continuous, dangers of, 11

J

Jaundice, 384 *et seq.*
 classification of, 384
Jejunostomy, 154
Joints, diseases of, 562 *et seq.*
 injuries to, 564
 syphilitic disease of, 569

I

Iatrogenic disorders, 630 *et seq.*

K

Keloids, 196–197

Keratoplasty, 595
Kidney, congenital abnormalities, 453
    diseases of, 441 *et seq.*
    injuries to, 454
    operations, 460
        care of patients, 460
    surgical diseases of, 454
    transplants, 254
Koenig-Rutzen bag, 410
Kraurosis vulvae, 615

**L**

Lacrimal apparatus, affections of, 597
Laringectomy, 581
Le Fort operation, 613
Leprosy, 502
Leucopenia, 41
Limbs, care of, during anaesthesia, 24
Liver, disease of, 384 *et seq.*
    function tests, 387 *et seq.*
    injury to, 384
    puncture biopsy, 387
Lobectomy, 313 *et seq.*
Ludwig's angina, 274
Lumbar puncture, 507
Lungs, and thorax, diseases of, 303
Lymphangitis, 67
Lymphatic glands, 248
Lymphatic system, 248 *et seq.*

**M**

Malaria, 504
Malignant new growths, 213
    palliative treatment, 216
    radical treatment, 216
    spread of, 214
    symptoms and signs of, 214
Manometer, for measuring pressure of
    spinal fluid, 507
Mastectomy, radical, nursing care, 295
Mechanical ventilators, types of, 165 *et
    seq.*
Meconium ileus, 499
    peritonitis, 499
Melaena, 370
Melanoma, 596
Mendelsohn's syndrome, 25
Meningioma, 518
Meningocele, 526
Meniscectomy, 565
Menopause, 606
Menorrhagia, 607
Menstruation, disorders of, 606
Metrorrhagia, 607
Microbiology, 48
Micturition, difficulty in, 443
    frequency of, 443
    postoperative, 30
Mouth, 257 *et seq.*
    care of, after operations, 26
Mouth-to-mouth respiration, 164

Mucoviscidosis, 499
Muscle, diseases of, 206
    relaxants, 22
Myelomeningocele, 527
Myopia, 586
Myositis ossificans, 549
Myringotomy, 575
Myxoedema, 276

**N**

Naevi, 211
Narcotic and non narcotic analgesics,
    37
Nasal obstruction, causes of, 583
Nasal septum, deflected, 583
Nasogastric intubation, modifications
    of, 379
Nasotracheal intubation, 168
Neck, swellings in, 274
Neo-natal surgery, 492 *et seq.*
Neonates, pre and postoperative care,
    493
Nerves, lesions of individual, 534 *et seq.*
Neuralgia, 533
Neuritis, femoral, 537
Neurofibromatosis, multiple, 533
Neurological examination, 505
New growths, 210
    of bladder, 476
    of colon and caecum, 412
    of eyes, 593
    of face and lips, 259
    of glands, 249
    of kidney, 460
    of lung, 312
    of rectum, 434
    of stomach, 373
    of testicle, 490
    of thyroid gland, 284
    of tongue, 264
    simple, 212
    types, 212
Nitrofurans, 62
Nose, diseases of, 581 *et seq.*
Nutrition, maintenance of, 159 *et seq.*
    in ulcerative colitis, 409
Nystagmus, 599

**O**

Observation, general, 13
Obstruction, common bile duct, 390
    intestinal, 404
    large bowel, 352
    of the newborn, 498
    peripheral arterial, 227
    prostatic, 477
    pyloric, 359
    respiratory, 168
    small bowel, 351
Ochsner-Sherren regime, 339
Odontomes, 270
Oedema, pitting, 32

Oesophagus, diseases of, 326 *et seq.*
  removal of, 330
  simple stricture of, 328
Oligaemia, 135
Omphalocele, 499
Operative ablation, 633
Operative complications, direct and in-
  direct, 633
Ophthalmia neonatorum, 592
Organ and tissue transplantation, 252
  *et seq.*
  nursing management of, 255
Organisms, access of, 42
  artificial growth of, 48
  common pyogenic, 50
  effect of temperature on, 48
  proteus, group of, 51
Osteitis deformans, 560
Osteitis fibrosa cystica, 561
Osteoarthritis, 570 *et seq.*
Osteoma, 559
Otosclerosis, 576
Ovaries, diseases of the, 625
Ovulation, 605
Oxygen masks, 178
Oxygen therapy, 174 *et seq.*
  special precautions, 176


P

Paediatric drip set, 495
Pain, 35
  chronic, persistent or recurrent, 38
  clinical management of, 36
  drugs for relief of, 37
  gate control theory of, 35
Palpation, 8
Pancreas, diseases of, 397 *et seq.*
Paracentesis, 356
  pack for, 357
Paralysed limbs, care of, 525
Paralytic ileus, 344
Parathyroid glands, diseases of, 285
Parkinson's disease, 520
Paronychia, 206
Patent ductus arteriosus, 311
Penicillin, 54 *et seq.*
Penis and urethra, 484
Percussion, 8
Periarthritis, 566
Peripheral arteries, diseases of, 225 *et
  seq.*
Peripheral nerves, 531 *et seq.*
  resuture of, 538
  types of injury, 531
Peripheral neuritis, 532
Peritonitis of the newborn, 499
Phlebitis, 238
Phlebography, 129
Phlyctenular conjunctivitis, 592
Pilonidal sinus, 426
Pituitary gland, diseases of, 285
Plague, 502
Plaster of Paris, application of, 545
Pneumonectomy, 313

Pneumothorax, 303
Polydipsia, 13
Polypi, nasal, 583
Portal hypertension, 387
Post-menopausal bleeding, 607
Postoperative period, special points, 4
Pregnancy, complications of, 609
Premedication, 20
Preoperative breathing exercises, 313
Pre- and postoperative care, 18 *et seq.*
Preparation and after-care of gynaeco-
  logical patients, 626
Pressure areas, 199
Proctitis, 430
Prolapse
  of haemorrhoids, 428
  of rectum, 429
  of uterus, 611
Prostate gland, diseases of, 477 *et seq.*
Prostatectomy, 478 *et seq.*
  care of drainage tubes, 481
  complications of, 482
  methods of, 478
Pruritus ani, 426
Pruritus vulvae, 614
Pseudomonas aeruginosa, 51
Puberty, 605
Pulmonary embolus, 131
Pulmonary tuberculosis, surgical treat-
  ment of, 311
Pulmonary valve stenosis, 319
Pupillary changes, 510
Pyaemia, 69
Pyloric stenosis, 372
  congenital, 361
Pyloroplasty, 376
Pyothorax, 304
Pyrexia, postoperative, 33


Q

Queckenstedt's test, 529
Quinsy, 577


R

Radiation reaction, 221
  in sterilisation, 81
Radioactive isotopes, 220–283
Radiography, cine, 9
Radiological examination of women
  of reproductive age, 10
Radiotherapy, 218 *et seq.*
Radium application, 219 *et seq.*
  care of patient, 221
  complications of, 628
  gynaecological uses of, 627
  needles in mouth, nursing care, 266
  protection of nursing staff, 222
Ramstedt's operation, 362
Raynaud's disease, 234
Reception of patient, 3
Rectum, resection of, 435
Refractive errors, 586

Renal control, 149
Renal failure, 449
Residual urine, 446
Respiration, 162
Respiratory complications, 31
Respiratory failure, 162 et seq.
Resuscitative therapy control of, 180
Retina, detachment of, 596
  diseases of, 596
Retinoblastoma, 596
Retinopathy, 597
Retroflexion of uterus, 613
Retrognathia, 496
Retrograde pyelography, 448
Retrolental fibroplasia, 176–597
Retroperitoneal fibrosis, 465
Retroversion of uterus, 613
Ripple bed, 201
Rupture, of muscle or tendon, 206
  of spleen, 250
  of urethra, 486
  of urinary bladder, 472

S

Salivary glands, 267 et seq.
Scar, complications of, 202
Sciatica, 536
Scrotum, 491
Senile vaginitis, 615
Septic fingers, 205
Septicaemia, 68
Sequestrum, 558
Serum, reactions, 44
  sickness, 44
Shirodkar's operation, 610
Shortening of digestive tract, physio-
    logical and anatomical, 634
Sinusitis, 583
Skin, diseases of, 198 et seq.
  localised infection of, 204
Skin extension, application of, 553
Skin grafting, 186 et seq.
Skull and scalp, injuries to, 511
Spermatic cord, diseases of, 490
Spina bifida, 526
Spinal cord, injuries of, 523 et seq.
    symptoms and signs, 523
    treatment of, 524
    transection of, 523
Spine and spinal cord, diseases of, 526
    acquired, 527
    congenital, 526
Spitz-Holter valve, 519
Spleen, diseases of, 249
Splenectomy, 250
Splints, care of the patient in, 544
Sprains, 562
Sterilisation, 80 et seq.
  checks, 83
  methods of, 81
  of electrical apparatus, 85
  of equipment, 83
  of syringes, 85
Stitches, removal of, 105

Stomach, diseases of, 359 et seq.
  operations on, 374
Stones, in bladder, 475
  in gall-bladder, 390
  in kidney, 457
    types of, 457
  in prostate gland, 484
  in ureter, 458
  in Wharton's duct, 268
Strabismus, 599
Stricture, of rectum, 430
  of urethra, male, 486
Subluxation, 562
Sulphonamide group of drugs, 60
  toxic reactions, 61
Surgery, aims of, 3
  day, 33
  spare part, 256
  the nurse and the patient, 1
Surgical diagnosis and the nurse, 7
Surgical lesions of skin and subcu-
    taneous tissue, 203
Synovitis, syphilitic, 569
  frontal, 584
  traumatic, 564
Syphilis, 76 et seq.
  congenital, 76

T

Talipes deformities, 500
  equino-varus, 500
Teeth and jaws, 269 et seq.
Tendons, cut, 206
  diseases of, 206
Testicle, diseases of, 487
  undescended, 487
Tetanus, 70 et seq.
Tetracyclines, 59
Theatre, dress, 87
  nurse, duties of, 90
  technique, 87
  ward nurse and, 88
Therapeutic fluids, tablets and other
    agents, 16
Thomas' splint, application of, 554
  care of patient in, 555
Thoracoplasty, 312
Thorax, injuries to, 303
Throat, diseases of, 577 et seq.
Thromboangiitis obliterans, 234
Thrombosis, 125 et seq.
  mesenteric, 406
  postoperative, 31
Thyroid gland, diseases of, 275
  inflammation of, 284
  simple enlargements of, 276
Thyroidectomy, complications of, 282
Thyrotoxicosis, 278 et seq.
Tongue, 263 et seq.
Tonsillectomy, 578
Tonsillitis, 577
Tourniquet, application of, 114
Tracheostomy, 166 et seq.
  care of patient with, 172

Tracheostomy (*cont.*)
  rules for management of, 172
Trachoma, 593
Transfusion, intra-arterial, 122
Trauma, 190 *et seq.*
Treatment, principles of, 19
Trichiniasis, 503
Tropical diseases, surgical aspects of, 502
Tuberculosis, of female genital tract, 624
  of kidney, 459
  of spine, 528
  of tendon sheaths, 207
  surgical, 74
Tuberculous arthritis, 568 *et seq.*
Tumours, cerebral, 518
  gastrin secreting, 401
  islet cell, 400
  of adrenal glands, 286
  of blood vessels, 227
  of bone, 559
  of breast, simple, 292
  of ear, 574
  of eyelids, 592
  of jaw, 273
  of kidney, 460
  of larynx and pharynx, 580
  of nerves, 533
  of parotid glands, 269
  of skin, 205
  of spine and spinal cord, 529
  of uterus, 617
  of vagina, 616
  of vulva, 615
  Wilms', 460


U

Ulceration, 202
Ulcer, aphthous, 264
  corneal, 593
  Curling's, 189
  definition of, 202
  dental, 264
  duodenal, 363
  gastric, 363
  parts of, 202
  peptic, 363 *et seq.*
  perforated, 348
  rodent, 259
  specific infective perforation of, 403
  stomal, 382
  syphilitic, 264
  tongue, 265
  tuberculous, 264
  types of, 202
  varicose, 239
Ulcerative proctocolitis, 408
Ultrasonic devices, 11
Ureter, diseases of, 441
  transplantation of, 463
Urethritis, non-specific, 79
Urinary disease, symptoms and signs, 441
Urinary diversion, 463

Urinary tract, papillomatous disease of, 476
Uterine bleeding, excessive and irregular, 607
Uterus, displacement of, 611
  infections of, 617


V

Vagina, diseases of, 615 *et seq.*
Vaginal discharge, 616
Vagotomy, 375
Valvotomy, mitral, 320
Varices, oesophageal, 329
Varicocele, 491
Varicose veins, 237 *et seq.*
  complications of, 238
  treatment of, 238
Vascular obliterative diseases, 227 *et seq.*
Vasectomy, 488
Vasomotor (syn allergic) rhinitis, 582
Venereal diseases, 75 *et seq.*
Ventricular septal defect, 319
Vertigo, 573
Viruses, 51
Volkmann's ischaemic contracture, 542
Vomiting, postoperative, 25
Vulva, diseases of, 614
Vulvo-vaginitis in children, 614


W

White blood corpuscles, 40
Wounds, accidental, 191
  care of, 193
  complications of, 196
  healing of, 195
  of eyelids, 591
  of face, 257
  of neck, 274
  of scalp, 512
  open, 194
  penetrating, of chest, 304
  protective dressings of, 104
  types of, 191


X

Xenograft, 253
X-irradiation, 219
X-ray burns, 189


Y

Yaws, 502
Yttrium, 220


Z

Zollinger-Ellison syndrome, 366